Cognitive-Behavioral Therapy

Theory into Practice

Adam M. Volungis

ROWMAN & LITTLEFIELD
Lanham • Boulder • New York • London

Executive Editor: NA
Associate Editor: Katie O'Brien
Production Editor: Darren Williams
Interior Designer: Rhonda Baker
Cover Designer: Sarah Marizan
Cover Art: Getty/VICTOR DE SCHWANBERG/SCIENCE PHOTO LIBRARY

Credits and acknowledgments of sources for material or information used with permission appear on the appropriate page within the text or in the credit section on page XXX.

Published by Rowman & Littlefield
An imprint of The Rowman & Littlefield Publishing Group, Inc.
4501 Forbes Boulevard, Suite 200, Lanham, Maryland 20706
www.rowman.com

Unit A, Whitacre Mews, 26-34 Stannary Street, London SE11 4AB

British Library Cataloguing in Publication Information Available

Library of Congress Cataloging-in-Publication Data

Names: Volungis, Adam M., author.
Title: Cognitive-behavioral therapy : theory into practice / Adam M. Volungis.
Description: Lanham : Rowman & Littlefield, [2019] | Includes bibliographical references and index.
Identifiers: LCCN 2018007121 (print) | LCCN 2018009164 (ebook) | ISBN 9781442274112 (electronic) | ISBN 9781442274099 (cloth : alk. paper) | ISBN 9781442274105 (pbk. : alk. paper)
Subjects: | MESH: Cognitive Therapy—methods | Evidence-Based Practice | Professional-Patient Relations | Models, Psychological
Classification: LCC RC489.C63 (ebook) | LCC RC489.C63 (print) | NLM WM 425.5.C6 | DDC 616.89/1425—dc23
LC record available at https://lccn.loc.gov/2018007121

Printed in the United States of America

To Yeonjoo:
My wife and best friend

To Kai:
My son and angel from heaven

Contents

List of Figures   vii

List of Tables   ix

List of Sample Forms   xiii

List of Activities   xv

List of Video Vignettes   xvii

Preface   xix

Acknowledgments   xxiii

1   The CBT Model   1

2   Establishing a CBT Therapeutic Alliance: Collaborative Empiricism   11

3   CBT Assessment, Case Formulation, and Treatment Planning   31

4   CBT Session Structure: Purposeful and Flexible   71

5   Psychoeducation: Teaching, Supporting, and Motivating   105

6   Behavioral Activation: Monitoring, Scheduling, Moving,
and Getting Things Done   121

7   Automatic Thoughts: Eliciting, Identifying, Evaluating,
and Modifying Maladaptive Thought Patterns   157

8   Core Beliefs: Identifying and Modifying the Source of Maladaptive
Thought Patterns   209

9   Behavioral Exposure: Relaxing, Testing Thoughts, and Confronting
    Fears and Anxieties   259

10   Homework: Therapy Between Sessions   299

11   CBT and Technology   311

12   Common CBT Myths   321

13   Being a Competent CBT Therapist   329

Index   335

About the Author   351

List of Figures

1.1   Reciprocal Cognitive-Behavioral Model   4

1.2   Reciprocal Cognitive-Behavioral Model—Maladaptive
      Functioning Individual   5

1.3   Reciprocal Cognitive-Behavioral Model—Adaptive
      Functioning Individual   5

2.1   Therapist–Client Activity Level Across Three Phases of Therapy   20

6.1   Behavioral Inactivity and Distress   123

6.2   Graded Task Assignment Worksheet   149

7.1   Guided Discovery: Using Emotions to Elicit Automatic Thoughts   166

7.2   Emotion Intensity and Negative Automatic Thought Believability Scale   174

7.3   Attributional Style Worksheet   186

7.4   Responsibility Attribution Pie   187

8.1   Core Belief Development   213

8.2   Downward-Arrow Technique   221

8.3   Core Belief Flowchart   226

8.4   Negative Core Belief Continuum Worksheet   241

9.1   Cognitive and Behavioral Avoidance Reinforcing Anxiety   261

List of Tables

2.1 Questions to Consider While Expressing Empathy   14

2.2 Presenting Symptoms and Challenges to the Therapeutic Relationship   22

2.3 Using the Collaborative Relationship for Conceptualization and Treatment   26

2.4 Common Challenges in Establishing a Therapeutic Alliance   27

3.1 Common Intake Information Gathered   33

3.2 Specific CBT Assessment Information   36

3.3 Basic Intake Questions to Assess Thoughts, Emotions, Physiological Arousal, and Behaviors   41

3.4 Treatment Goals: Poor Versus Better   64

3.5 Treatment Interventions: Poor Versus Better   65

3.6 Common Challenges for CBT Assessment, Case Formulation, and Treatment Planning   68

4.1 Therapy Session Stages   73

4.2 Common Challenges for CBT Session Structure   102

5.1 Early Phase Psychoeducation Worksheet   108

5.2 Common Challenges for CBT Psychoeducation   119

6.1	Psychoeducation for Activity Monitoring and Scheduling	125
6.2	Weekly Activity Monitoring Log	126
6.3	Daily Activity Monitoring Log Evaluation Questions	132
6.4	Daily Activity Schedule	134
6.5	Daily Activity Schedule Evaluation Questions	143
6.6	Common Challenges for Behavioral Activation	154
7.1	Key Elements of Automatic Thoughts	159
7.2	Validity and Utility of Negative Automatic Thoughts	160
7.3	Negative Emotions and Negative Automatic Thoughts Worksheet	170
7.4	Negative Emotions and Associated Events Worksheet	171
7.5	Negative Automatic Thoughts Tracker	172
7.6	Socratic Techniques and Common Questions for Automatic Thoughts	180
7.7	Examining the Evidence Worksheet—Automatic Thoughts	181
7.8	Decatastrophizing Worksheet	183
7.9	Possible Alternatives Worksheet	184
7.10	Cognitive Distortions and Examples	194
7.11	Negative Automatic Thought Record	196
7.12	Cognitive Rehearsal Steps Worksheet	204
7.13	Common Challenges for Automatic Thoughts	207
8.1	Three Categories of Core Beliefs	210
8.2	Key Elements of Core Beliefs	211
8.3	Core Belief Flowchart Domain Questions Worksheet	227
8.4	Core Beliefs Tracker	234
8.5	Socratic Techniques and Common Questions for Core Beliefs	237
8.6	Examining the Evidence Worksheet—Core Beliefs	238
8.7	Advantages and Disadvantages Worksheet	239

8.8	Old Core Beliefs Versus New Core Beliefs	246
8.9	Common Challenges for Core Beliefs	256
9.1	Examples of Safety Behaviors	264
9.2	Anxious Patterns Record	265
9.3	Progressive Muscle Relaxation Template	271
9.4	Hierarchy of Feared Situations Goals: Poor Versus Better	283
9.5	Hierarchy of Feared Situations for Graded Exposure	285
9.6	Common Challenges for Behavioral Exposure	296
10.1	Common Challenges for Homework	308
11.1	Smartphone Applications with CBT Utility	315

List of Sample Forms

3.1   CBT Case Formulation and Treatment Plan Template   60

4.1   Therapy Session Worksheet   75

4.2   Client Therapy Notes Worksheet   83

8.1   Behavioral Experiment Worksheet   251

9.1   Exposure Tracking Form   288

List of Activities

1.1	Examples of Adaptive and Maladaptive Functioning	4
1.2	Develop Examples of Adaptive and Maladaptive Functioning	6
2.1	Empathy (Observer Perspective) Scenario 1	14
2.2	Empathy (Individual Perspective) Scenario 2	15
2.3	Environmental Stressors (Internalization) Scenario 1	24
2.4	Environmental Stressors (Externalization) Scenario 2	24
3.1	CBT Assessment—Presenting Problems	48
3.2	CBT Assessment—Measures	57
3.3	CBT Case Formulation and Treatment Plan	67
4.1	Early Session Stage	89
4.2	Late Session Stage	101
5.1	Psychoeducation	116
6.1	Behavioral Activation—Weekly Activity Monitoring Log	131
6.2	Behavioral Activation—Review Completed Activity Monitoring Log	142
6.3	Behavioral Activation—Daily Activity Schedule	142
6.4	Behavioral Activation—Review Complete Daily Activity Schedule	147
6.5	Behavioral Activation—Introducing and Reviewing Weekly Activity Monitoring Log and Daily Activity Schedule	147

6.6   Behavioral Activation—Graded Task Assignment   154

7.1   Automatic Thoughts—Eliciting, Identifying, and Evaluating   178

7.2   Automatic Thoughts—Modifying   192

7.3   Automatic Thoughts—Modifying 2   192

7.4   Automatic Thoughts—Negative Automatic Thought Record—"Before"   202

7.5   Automatic Thoughts—Negative Automatic Thought Record—"After"   203

8.1   Core Beliefs—Identifying—Downward-Arrow Technique   224

8.2   Core Beliefs—Identifying—Core Belief Flowchart—Part A   233

8.3   Core Beliefs—Modifying—Evidence and Advantages and Disadvantages   244

8.4   Core Beliefs—Modifying 2—Core Belief Flowchart—Part B   248

8.5   Core Beliefs—Modifying 3—Behavioral Experiment   255

9.1   Behavioral Techniques—Assessment of Anxious Patterns   269

9.2   Behavioral Technique—Relaxation—Progressive Muscle Relaxation   272

9.3   Behavioral Techniques—Relaxation—Diaphragm Breathing   276

9.4   Behavioral Techniques—Modifying Anxious Thoughts   281

9.5   Behavioral Techniques—Imaginal and In Vivo Exposure   295

10.1   Responding to Clients Not Completing Homework   307

11.1   Practice Using CBT   319

12.1   Refuting CBT Myths   327

13.1   Practice for CBT Competence   334

List of Video Vignettes

Note: PDA = panic disorder and agoraphobia; MDD = major depressive disorder

3.1   PDA-1: CBT Assessment—Presenting Problems   42

3.2   MDD-1: CBT Assessment—Presenting Problems   45

3.3   PDA-2: CBT Assessment—Motivation to Change   50

3.4   MDD-2: CBT Assessment—Motivation to Change   51

3.5   PDA-3: CBT Assessment—Measures   54

3.6   MDD-3: CBT Assessment—Measures   55

4.1   MDD-6: Early Session Stage—Early Phase Therapy   85

4.2   MDD-13: Early Session Stage—Middle Phase Therapy   86

4.3   MDD-18: Early Session Stage—Late Phase Therapy   88

4.4   PDA-5: Late Session Stage—Early Phase Therapy   93

4.5   PDA-8: Late Session Stage—Middle Phase Therapy   97

4.6   PDA-10: Late Session Stage—Late Phase Therapy   99

5.1   MDD-4: Psychoeducation—Therapy Expectations and Cognitive Model   110

5.2   PDA-4: Psychoeducation—Diagnosis   114

6.1   MDD-5: Behavioral Activation—Psychoeducation and Introducing Weekly Activity Monitoring Log   128

6.2 MDD-6: Behavioral Activation—Reviewing Completed Activity Monitoring Log 137

6.3 MDD-7: Behavioral Activation—Introducing Daily Activity Schedule 139

6.4 MDD-8: Behavioral Activation—Reviewing Completed Daily Activity Schedule 144

6.5 MDD-8: Behavioral Activation—Graded Task Assignment 150

7.1 MDD-9: Automatic Thoughts—Psychoeducation 161

7.2 MDD-10: Automatic Thoughts —Eliciting and Identifying 166

7.3 MDD-10: Automatic Thoughts—Evaluating 176

7.4 MDD-11: Automatic Thoughts—Modifying 188

7.5 MDD-12: Automatic Thoughts—Negative Automatic Thought Record 200

8.1 MDD-14: Core Beliefs—Psychoeducation 215

8.2 MDD-15: Core Beliefs—Identifying—Downward-Arrow Technique 222

8.3 MDD-16: Core Beliefs—Identifying 2—Core Belief Flowchart—Part A 230

8.4 MDD-17: Core Beliefs—Modifying—Evidence and Advantages and Disadvantages 241

8.5 MDD-17: Core Beliefs—Modifying—Core Belief Flowchart—Part B 246

8.6 MDD-18: Core Belief—Modifying 3—Behavioral Experiment 253

9.1 PD-6: Behavioral Techniques—Assessment of Anxious Patterns 266

9.2 PD-7: Behavioral Techniques—Relaxation—Diaphragm Breathing 274

9.3 PD-9: Behavioral Techniques—Modifying Anxious Thoughts 279

9.4 PD-11: Behavioral Techniques—In Vivo Exposure 290

Preface

I have been a cognitive-behavioral therapist for more than 15 years, working with a diverse age range of clients (i.e., children, adolescents, and adults) suffering from significant distress (e.g., depression, trauma, phobias, and disruptive/aggressive behaviors) using a variety of modalities (i.e., individual, couple, family, and group), in multiple settings (i.e., outpatient, residential, and psychiatric). Although a good portion of my graduate training was cognitive-behavioral, I found I was craving a stronger emphasis on the applied nature of specific cognitive-behavioral therapy (CBT) skills by the time I started working with clients. This also seemed to be the sentiment of many of my colleagues from a variety of graduate programs. Luckily, with good supervision and training and much practice and critical self-evaluation based on client outcomes, I was able to develop my CBT skill set with high self-efficacy. Having become professor in a graduate program that specializes in CBT, I have realized that although many great books are available for developing a sound CBT theoretical foundation, few books truly address explicitly the applied nature of basic CBT skills.

Cognitive-Behavioral Therapy: Theory into Practice is unique because a very limited number of books address the application of CBT skills and techniques for mental health professionals. It is designed for graduate students in training and mental health professionals who want to learn the basic foundations of applied CBT. However, this book can also be helpful to those who are experienced with CBT but want to improve their skills. The primary purpose of this book is to translate CBT theory into actual practice with clients in a clear and practical manner. Although every mental health disorder has its own idiosyncratic treatment approach, this book provides a thorough review of the most common and pertinent CBT skills necessary for most clients encountered in practice, from establishing a sound therapeutic alliance and structuring sessions to modifying negative automatic thoughts and behavioral exposure.

Each skill is first presented with a sound evidence-based rationale followed by specific steps to follow. Most of the CBT skills covered include therapist–client therapy dialogue vignettes and many hours of supplemental videos. (Two separate clients are followed from the early phase of therapy to the late phase of therapy.) Each chapter includes multiple discussion questions to process these vignettes and related topics. Additionally, there are activities and worksheets to practice each of these CBT skills individually and with a peer. Throughout, there are also multiple tables and figures to help conceptualize and summarize key themes and skills, including common challenges.

The following highlights the key themes for each of the 13 chapters in this book:

Chapter 1 provides a brief review of the history and theory of CBT. This includes a reciprocal cognitive-behavioral model of how thoughts, emotions, and behaviors interact with the environment. The general cognitive model is also introduced as a means to conceptualizing clients' problems and presenting distress.

Chapter 2 focuses establishing a therapeutic alliance and the therapist–client activity nature of CBT through collaborative empiricism. The role of Rogerian qualities and interpersonal skills in developing a CBT therapeutic relationship is addressed. Collaborative empiricism is explained through therapist–client activity level, depending on the phase of therapy (i.e., early, middle, or late), responding to client specific factors, and conceptualization and treatment. Overall, although the therapeutic alliance is not the primary means for change in CBT, it is still essential for desired treatment outcomes.

Chapter 3 addresses CBT assessment, case formulation, and treatment planning. CBT requires a purposeful process in determining the most effective treatment approach. Beyond gathering basic information with the intake interview, CBT assessment strategies include compatibility with CBT (to inform the approach to psychoeducation and interventions, not to screen out), obtaining detailed information about presenting problems, motivation and responsibility for change, and formal symptom measures. This information aids in the process of developing a CBT case formulation, a cognitive-behavioral conceptualization of the presenting problems, associated symptoms, and contributing factors. Finally, a CBT treatment plan includes developing measurable treatment goals that can be obtained by evidence-based interventions that are client specific.

Chapter 4 explains the purpose and process for providing session structure from the first session to the final session. It is important that therapy remain focused on the problems and treatment goals most relevant to each client's distress. Consistent session structure also socializes clients to therapeutic expectations and provides an opportunity to model the collaborative nature of CBT. Individual sessions are broken down into four stages (i.e., pre-session, early session, middle session, and late session) to provide a template to structure sessions that are purposeful yet flexible enough to be responsive to clients' needs. Examples of topics include (but are not limited to) reviewing assessment information, setting an agenda, reviewing homework, problem-solving strategies, summarizing, and assigning homework.

Chapter 5 addresses the important role of psychoeducation throughout CBT. Clients will need to learn new skills as they collaboratively participate in their own therapy and long after therapy is over. This chapter is divided into two parts: early phase CBT psychoeducation and CBT skill psychoeducation. Early phase CBT psychoeducation focuses on reviewing therapy expectations, the cognitive model, clients' diagnosis, case formulation, and treatment plan. CBT skill psychoeducation broadly approaches the process of teaching new skills in session and to be used between sessions, including the use of bibliotherapy and technology.

Chapter 6 discusses the key CBT components for behavioral activation, often a common intervention used during the early phase of therapy for clients with depression and/or those that have difficulty getting things done. Behavioral activation gets clients moving in the "opposite direction" to break their maladaptive behavioral patterns by completing daily tasks and activities, including experiencing a sense of accomplishment and pleasure. Two of the most common and effective formats of behavioral activation are addressed in detail: activity monitoring and scheduling and graded task assignments.

Chapter 7 addresses automatic thoughts, one of the most important concepts for CBT therapists. At the heart of long-term change for CBT is being able to change clients' maladaptive thinking patterns, otherwise known as negative automatic thoughts. Most clients experiencing psychological distress often perceive and interpret particular events as negative (even those that are neutral or positive). Successful modification of clients' negative automatic thoughts can result in reducing clients' distress by improving emotions, reducing physiological arousal, and replacing maladaptive behavior patterns with more adaptive behaviors. However, clinically, multiple steps are required to appropriately address negative automatic thoughts. After providing clients psychoeducation, appropriate negative automatic thoughts need to be elicited and identified. Thereafter, such thoughts require evaluation before they are modified. Finally, sometimes clients have valid negative automatic thoughts where utilizing coping skills and acceptance strategies are more appropriate.

Chapter 8 provides an extensive review of conceptually understanding core beliefs from an applied perspective. In order to enhance long-term change for CBT, it is sometimes necessary to go beyond clients' negative automatic thoughts by exploring their negative core beliefs. Core beliefs are all-or-nothing statements that are typically rigid, global, and overgeneralized views about the self, others, and how the world "works." Some clients have patterns of thinking that are so pervasive that it may be an extension of a negative core belief. Thus, sometimes it may be necessary to "dig deeper" to get at the true source (at least in part) of their distress. Similar to automatic thoughts, core beliefs, after they are identified, need to be evaluated and modified.

Chapter 9 discusses the key components for behavioral exposure and related techniques. Exposure techniques can be very effective for a variety of anxiety and anxiety-related disorders. Many times when clients are anxious, they have negative automatic thoughts (e.g., catastrophizing) and increased physiological arousal, resulting in eventually avoiding (cognitively and/or behaviorally) their source of distress because they perceive it as threatening. Exposure confronts the source of avoidance to stop this maladaptive behavioral pattern as clients learn that the situation is no longer threatening. In addition to reviewing behavioral exposure techniques (e.g., hierarchy of feared situations, imaginal exposure, and in vivo exposure), this chapter first focuses on assessing anxious and fearful cognitive and behavioral patterns. Relaxation techniques (progressive muscle relaxation, diaphragm breathing, and visualization) are also reviewed as possible options for some clients, depending on their type of anxious distress. Finally, options for modifying specific anxious thoughts are presented.

Chapter 10 addresses the general process of integrating homework as a key component of CBT. Homework is a necessary component for effective CBT. Clients only typically spend about 1 hour per week in therapy. They will need to practice what they learn in session between sessions. This chapter addresses the process of assigning homework and maintaining client compliance.

Chapter 11 highlights a variety of modes of technology that are commonly used by CBT therapists for multiple therapeutic techniques. Examples of technology include smartphone and tablet applications, video and audio recordings, internet videos and pictures, and virtual reality. These technologies are not meant to replace therapy. Rather, their purpose is to supplement therapy to enhance the effectiveness of CBT.

Chapter 12 reviews some of the most common CBT myths. Although CBT is a well-established effective treatment approach for most mental health problems, there remain some common myths about its nature. Knowledge of such myths helps those entering training in CBT avoid any possible self-filling prophecies and/or negatively biased influences. Such myths can also be refuted while ensuring that clients are receiving high-quality care.

Chapter 13 addresses key domains to consider, both professionally and personally, while developing your competency as a CBT therapist throughout your career. Your training does not stop after reading a few books or after graduation. Being a competent CBT therapist requires a high level of therapeutic skill that comes from continuous training and personal growth.

Overall, it is desired that after reading *Cognitive-Behavioral Therapy*, you will be able to develop (or improve) a strong foundational application of CBT skills to use with your clients presenting with a variety of mental health distress. There are many fundamental CBT skills to learn throughout one's career as a mental health professional. It is hoped that this book will allow for a smoother and easier practical application of CBT skills to build your self-efficacy. Being a competent CBT therapist requires much practice and patience; it requires a high therapeutic skill set. However, the time you put into developing your CBT skills is well worth it, as with additional training and experience you will have the skills to reduce client distress and improve quality of life by competently providing robust evidence-based practice.

Acknowledgments

Writing this book and integrating multiple hours of therapy vignettes was an exhausting but enjoyable endeavor. I am grateful for my graduate research fellows who dedicated much time and thought in assisting with the development of the therapy vignettes. Mark Joyce was a great "depressed client" and assisted with video editing. Likewise, Lindsey Fox was a great "anxious client," and assisted with video transcribing. Brenden Knight was extremely helpful with video recording and editing. Colleen Popores put much time and effort into video transcribing. Finally, Emily Morse provided much help in deciphering some of my written diagrams into attractive electronic documents and assisted with video transcribing.

I am most grateful for my loving and understanding wife, Yeonjoo Son. Her support and sacrifice was invaluable in making this book a reality.

1

The CBT Model

An extensive review of the history and theory of cognitive-behavioral therapy (CBT) is not necessary and is beyond the scope of this text (see A. T. Beck, 1964, 1976; J. S. Beck, 2011). The focus of this text is to translate the theory of CBT into practice with your clients. This will be done by learning how to conceptualize your clients' distress through a CBT lens, develop a therapeutic alliance, structure your sessions, and effectively apply a variety of key CBT concepts and skills. Thus, the following provides a brief history of Aaron T. Beck's development of cognitive therapy (now often referred to as cognitive-behavioral therapy) and concise review of the CBT model, the latter of which will be the driving force to conceptualizing and treating your clients' problems and presenting distress.

BRIEF HISTORY

Aaron T. Beck, a psychiatrist, was trained in psychoanalysis but had concerns about its effectiveness. By the late 1950s and early 1960s, he had tested the psychoanalytic approach for depression and found that it was conceptually inaccurate (i.e., not about hostility and need to suffer but instead distorted thinking) and did not do much to reduce client distress (A. T. Beck, 1967). Rather, he found that his depressed clients had very quick and brief negative self-evaluative thoughts. Additionally, he discovered such thoughts to be strongly related to their distressing emotions. He soon referred to such thinking as "negative automatic thoughts." He noticed that when he helped his clients identify, evaluate, and modify these negative automatic thoughts, their depressed mood significantly improved.

Beck also found that psychoanalysis focused too much on the past and was too long term (i.e., from many years to the rest of your life), resulting in clients thinking that they would always need a professional to help them with their life stressors and problems (A. T. Beck, 1976). This approach to therapy ultimately inhibits generalization and maintenance of change after therapy (assuming therapy ever does end!). In other words, clients were not able to develop their own independent problem-solving skills and manage future life stressors. Thus, Beck began working on developing a short-term and present-oriented form of therapy for depression that focused on modifying negative automatic thoughts and using problem-solving skills (A. T. Beck, 1964). At this point, he also developed a conceptualization of the development of depression in which client distress is due to a negative thinking pattern across three domains: self, world, and future.

During this time (1950s–1970s), behavioral therapists were employing the work of experimental behaviorists, such as Pavlov (classical conditioning) and Skinner (operant conditioning). Many behaviorists at the time viewed all human behavior as learned from the environment. More specifically, behavior was considered the result of a "simple" stimulus–response association (Watson, 1970). Additionally, behaviorism at the time was concerned primarily with observable behavior while viewing internal events, such as thinking and emotions, with minimal utility. This school of thought resulted in such behavioral interventions as systematic desensitization, reciprocal inhibition, and relaxation training, which were found to be effective in treating some anxiety disorders with minimal focus on cognitive processes (Eysenck, 1966; Wolpe, 1958, 1982; see also Jacobson, 1938). These behavioral interventions focused on modifying desired measurable behavior with reinforcement and extinguishing fearful/anxious responses with exposure.

While Beck was developing his theoretical approach and treatment for depression, other theorists were also developing treatment programs that incorporated cognitive and behavioral components. Most notably, both Meichenbaum's (1977) concept of internal dialogue and self-instructional training and Ellis and Harper's (1975) perspective of irrational thinking and rational emotive behavior therapy (a theoretical approach on its own) were instrumental in the development of CBT. Both theories acknowledged the importance of internal events (i.e., thoughts) and their influence on emotions and behaviors. Furthermore, both Meichenbaum and Ellis and Harper recognized that modification of distressing thoughts can reduce distressing emotions and behaviors. Bandura's (1976) social cognitive theory, which recognized the importance of learning through observing others, was also influential in the transition from behaviorism to CBT. Bandura also coined the term "reciprocal determinism" to explain how behavior both influences and is influenced by thoughts, emotions, and the social environment.

Beck, Rush, Shaw, and Emery's (1979) seminal book *Cognitive Therapy of Depression* provided a solid theoretical approach for treating depression with supportive empirical evidence. When this book was published, CBT research was already active at this time and showing promising results. However, Beck's recent books and studies appeared to spark a big wave of research in 1980s. At this point, research moved beyond depression to include other distressing mental health problems, especially anxiety-related disorders, with a more explicit integration of cognitive and behavioral methods. While there are certainly other theoretical approaches that are effective for specific disorders, CBT is now the most well-established theoretical approach for the most mental health problems (APA Presidential Task Force on Evidence-Based Practice, 2006 (see www.div12.org/psychological-treatments/); Butler, Chapman, Forman, & Beck, 2006; Hofmann, Asnaani, Vonk, Sawyer, & Fang, 2012). Furthermore, CBT has been shown to be more effective than other theoretical approaches for treating anxiety and depressive disorders (Tolin, 2010).

Although Aaron Beck was influenced by philosophers (e.g., Cicero, Epictetus, and Kant) and other cognitive and social-cognitive theorists (e.g., Albert Bandura, Albert Ellis, George Kelly, Donald Meichenbaum, and Richard Lazarus), he was the first person to develop a coherent evidence-based theoretical approach that now targets both thoughts and behaviors for treating a variety of psychological disorders. A driving force for the effectiveness of CBT across multiple disorders is its focus on the importance of conceptualizing clients' problems in a coherent manner, which then becomes the driving force for the treatment plan and interventions. Overall, CBT is purposeful, flexible, goal directed, and based on tangible client evidence and requires active collaboration between both the therapist and the client. Having a good understanding of the CBT model provides a solid foundation for conceptualizing and effectively reducing your clients' distress and improving overall well-being.

CBT MODEL

Presently, there are many slight variations of the CBT model depicting human adaptive and maladaptive functioning. Nevertheless, there are many more similarities than differences in these models, especially with regard to the primary role of cognitive processing and appraisal. Figure 1.1 provides a concise visual depiction of how thoughts (including mental images), emotions (including physiological arousal), and behaviors are related and interact with the environment (including social interactions). According to the CBT model, our emotions and behaviors are influenced by how we perceive situations (or, more broadly, the environment). This means that it is not the situation itself that affects how we feel. Rather, our thoughts act as a mediator between the situation and resulting emotions. The reciprocal interaction between our thoughts and emotions in turn influences our behaviors, which then interact with the environment. This interaction with the environment and its outcomes then reciprocally influence our thoughts and emotions. Thus, although our thoughts are the primary factor that initially influences our emotions and behaviors, once the process begins, all contributing elements can have a reciprocating influence on each other. For individuals who are maladaptively functioning, the reciprocal interaction of thoughts, emotions, and behaviors can negatively feed into each other. This results in an escalation of psychological distress, where each element gets worse over time. Consider Activity 1.1, which follows two individuals (maladaptive and adaptive) responding to the same situation. Thereafter, Activity 1.2 has you complete your own examples. Discussion questions follow both activities.

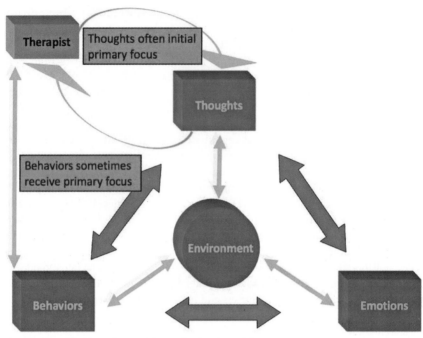

Figure 1.1.   Reciprocal Cognitive-Behavioral Model

ACTIVITY 1.1: EXAMPLES OF ADAPTIVE
AND MALADAPTIVE FUNCTIONING

While heading to class, a college student walks by her peer in the hallway and says, "Hi," while briefly making eye contact. The peer does not respond and keeps walking in the opposite direction.

College student 1 (Debbie; see Figure 1.2) walks into her classroom thinking, "Wow, she completely ignored me. She's probably annoyed and doesn't want to be associated with me." Debbie then starts to feel sad and has difficulty concentrating in class while ruminating over her thoughts and emotions. Later in the evening, Debbie realizes that she took poor notes while in class and does not feel prepared for the next quiz. This results in her feeling frustrated and anxious while thinking, "Why do I do this to myself? I'm probably going to fail this quiz." Debbie then decides to not go out to dinner with her friends and stays in her dorm room for the night.

College student 2 (Mary Jane; see Figure 1.3) walks into her classroom thinking, "Wow, she must be really busy. She usually acknowledges me when we walk by each other. I'll check in with her later today to see how she's doing." Mary Jane feels content while in class and is able to focus on the class lecture. Later in the evening, Mary Jane feels prepared for the next quiz because she took good notes and takes the time to text her friend to see how she

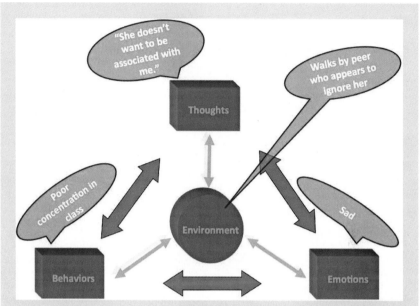

Figure 1.2.   Reciprocal Cognitive-Behavioral Model—Maladaptive Functioning Individual

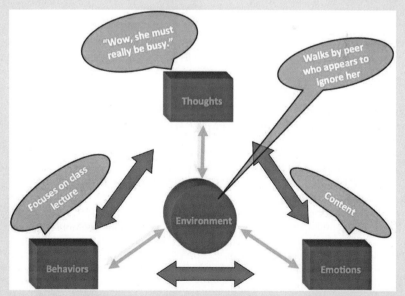

Figure 1.3.   Reciprocal Cognitive-Behavioral Model—Adaptive Functioning Individual

(*continued*)

ACTIVITY 1.1: *Continued*

is doing. Her friend states that she is very stressed out about her midterm exam and did not even see Mary Jane in the hallway. Mary Jane offers to hang out with her friend during the weekend after her exam is over. She then goes out to dinner with her friends feeling happy and thinking, "I'm glad I have friends who are supportive of each other."

Discussion Questions 1.1

- What was Debbie's negative automatic thought? Was there any evidence to support her thought based on the situation?
- What was Mary Jane's automatic thought? How was her cognitive processing different from Debbie's?
- How did the difference between Debbie's and Mary Jane's thoughts result in different emotions and behaviors? In other words, discuss the difference in the relationship between their thoughts, emotions, and behaviors based on Figures 1.2 and 1.3.
- Explain how Debbie's thoughts, emotions, and behaviors "feed into each other" in a reciprocal manner. How could Debbie's thoughts, emotions, and behaviors continue to feed into each other beyond the described scenario?
- Although you do not know much about Debbie, what are some possible alternative thoughts and behaviors (at any point in the scenario) that could potentially "break" her negative reciprocal interaction cycle?

ACTIVITY 1.2: DEVELOP EXAMPLES OF ADAPTIVE AND MALADAPTIVE FUNCTIONING

Now that you completed reviewing examples of adaptive and maladaptive (i.e., negative automatic thought) functioning using the reciprocal cognitive-behavioral model, create your own examples. Create a scenario that is not too complicated but ambiguous enough that it is open to multiple interpretations. Next, use Figure 1.1 to complete each part of the reciprocal cognitive-behavioral model for both the adaptive and the maladaptive response: first thought, second emotion, and third behavior. Do not worry if your thought is a true negative automatic thought, as you will learn about this later. Also, be sure that you can clearly differentiate between thoughts (usually a phrase or sentence) from emotions (usually a single word). Finally, pick a behavior that has the potential to have a direct impact on the environment (i.e., it will have some form of an outcome).

Discussion Questions 1.2

- Discuss how each example is (or can be) reciprocal. In other words, go beyond your initial thought, emotion, and behavior and discuss how these elements can affect each other (i.e., "feed into each other").
- Similar to Activity 1.1, for your negative automatic thought example, what are some possible alternative thoughts and behaviors (at any point in the scenario) that could potentially "break" this person's negative reciprocal interaction cycle?
- What example was more difficult for you to create: the negative automatic thought or the adaptive automatic thought? Share any thoughts on why this may be the case.

Within the context of the general cognitive model, Beck and Haigh (2014) have posited that the difference between adaptive and maladaptive functioning is largely quantitative, not qualitative. In other words, all individuals have negative biases (or thoughts) and positive biases, in many ways on a continuum ranging from maladaptive to adaptive. In maladaptive functioning individuals, their negative biases can be extreme and amplify perceived threats. Likewise, their positive biases can be reduced and minimize rewards or gains. These biases tend to get exaggerated and eventually activated after experiencing a particular stressor or series of stressors. Thus, when clients are experiencing psychological distress, their thoughts tend to be distorted (i.e., negative automatic thoughts), resulting in associated distressing emotions and maladaptive behaviors. The consequence is negative environmental outcomes that can reinforce and/or maintain negative automatic thoughts (and biases) and maladaptive behaviors, continuing the cycle of psychological distress.

The primary goal of CBT is to help clients identify, evaluate, and modify their negative automatic thoughts and corresponding behaviors. In other words, you want your clients to "think about thinking." The eventual recognition and modification of negative automatic thoughts is often the driving force for clients to "break" their negatively reciprocating relationship of thoughts, emotions, and behaviors. Additionally, part of this awareness is having a good understanding of how thoughts, emotions (including physiological arousal), and behaviors are interrelated within themselves and between the environment. For long-term change, this process can also include working on overarching, global, and rigid core beliefs (including biases) about themselves, other people, and the world. These core beliefs are developed from past significant events and influential individuals. Having more rational and adaptive thoughts results in feeling better and engaging in fewer maladaptive behaviors. There are also times (e.g., some anxiety disorders) when targeting primarily behaviors (although thoughts are often still addressed) can have a strong effect on changing thoughts and emotions. Ultimately, successful therapy is when clients are able to independently make these modifications to their thoughts and behaviors while developing effective coping and problem-solving skills. You will want your clients to be able to generalize and maintain their skills across many other facets of life beyond what was addressed in therapy over time. In other words, clients should eventually be their "own therapists" through the long-term maintenance of skills.

It is important to note here that CBT is not positive thinking (e.g., "Don't worry, be happy!"). It is helping clients think more rationally. There are times when rational thoughts are negative—this happens in life—and may require acceptance. On the other hand, emotionally distressed clients tend to have many thoughts that are negative and irrational. Such thoughts are the ones that will receive focus for modification. Although it is helpful to focus on the positive aspects of our lives, it can be detrimental to our well-being to ignore the reality of the negative aspects.

Overall, the CBT model provides a lens to help you conceptualize your clients' problems and presenting distress. This conceptualization will be the driving force for your treatments and interventions. At the same time, it is malleable to new information as you gain a more sophisticated understanding of your clients' ways of functioning. This allows you to be up to date and flexible in your treatment approach as your clients progress through therapy.

REFERENCES

APA Presidential Task Force on Evidence-Based Practice. (2006). Evidence-based practice in psychology. *American Psychologist, 61,* 271–285.

Bandura, A. (1976). *Social learning theory.* Englewood Cliffs, NJ: Prentice Hall.

Beck, A. T. (1964). Thinking and depression: II. Theory and therapy. *Archives of General Psychiatry, 10,* 561–571.

Beck, A. T. (1967). *Depression: Causes and treatment.* Philadelphia: University of Pennsylvania Press.

Beck, A. T. (1976). *Cognitive therapy and the emotional disorders.* New York: International University Press.

Beck, A. T., & Haigh, E. A. P. (2014). Advances in cognitive theory and therapy: The generic cognitive model. *Annual Review of Clinical Psychology, 10,* 1–24.

Beck, A. T., Rush, A. J., Shaw, B. E., & Emery, G. (1979). *Cognitive therapy of depression.* New York: Guilford Press.

Beck, J. S. (2011). *Cognitive behavior therapy: Basics and beyond* (2nd ed.). New York: Guilford Press.

Butler, A. C., Chapman, J. E., Forman, E. M., & Beck, A. T. (2006). The empirical status of cognitive-behavioral therapy: A review of meta-analyses. *Clinical Psychology Review, 26,* 17–31.

Ellis, A., & Harper, R. A. (1975). *A guide to rational living* (3rd ed.). North Hollywood, CA: Wilshire Book Company.

Eysenck, H. J. (1966). *The effects of psychotherapy.* New York: International Science Press.

Hofmann, S. G., Asnaani, A., Vonk, I. J. J., Sawyer, A. T., & Fang, A. (2012). The efficacy of cognitive behavioral therapy: A review of meta-analyses. *Cognitive Therapy and Research, 36,* 427–440.

Jacobson, E. (1938). *Progressive relaxation* (2nd ed.). Chicago: University of Chicago Press.

Meichenbaum, D. H. (1977). *Cognitive-behavior modification: A integrative approach.* New York: Springer

Tolin, D. F. (2010). Is cognitive-behavioral therapy more effective than other therapies? A meta-analytic review. *Clinical Psychology Review, 30,* 710–720.

Watson, J. B. (1970). *Behaviorism.* New York: Norton.

Wolpe, J. (1958). *Psychotherapy by reciprocal inhibition.* Stanford, CA: Stanford University Press.

Wolpe, J. (1982). *The practice of behavior therapy* (3rd ed.). New York: Pergamon Press.

2

Establishing a CBT Therapeutic Alliance

Collaborative Empiricism

Probably one of the most well-known characteristics of CBT is that it is not a passive treatment. The cliché image of a client sitting on a couch pouring out any thoughts or emotions that comes to mind to a therapist who tells the client what to do is the antithesis of CBT. An explicit expectation of CBT is that both the therapist and the client are active participants throughout the therapeutic process. In other words, it is a collaborative process. For the collaborative nature of CBT to produce effective outcomes, there needs to be a strong therapist–client therapeutic alliance; it is more than just a relationship. A common definition of "alliance" is a relationship in which people agree to work together toward mutual goals. The assessment and intervention techniques used to obtain these goals are based on empirically supported research while also using information provided by clients. Hence, collaborative empiricism is an action-oriented therapeutic alliance driven by research that integrates, tests, and modifies clients' thoughts and behaviors.

The therapeutic alliance is not considered the primary process for change in CBT, but it is still essential for obtaining desired treatment outcomes for improvement in mental health and overall quality of life (Beck, Rush, Shaw, & Emery, 1979; Leahy, 2008; Wright & Davis, 1994). Research consistently shows that across theoretical approaches, there is a strong relationship between the therapist–client relationship and treatment outcomes (Ardito & Rabellino, 2011; Arnow et al., 2013; Raue, Goldfried, & Barkham, 1997). Interestingly, this relationship means that the quality of the therapeutic alliance can have either a negative or a positive impact on client well-being. More specifically, just as much a strong positive therapeutic alliance can improve clients' well-being, a strong negative therapeutic alliance can make clients worse. In fact, with regard to the latter, clients will most likely terminate prematurely and seek therapy elsewhere or, even worse, decide that therapy is not a viable option and no longer pursue the necessary help to work on their mental health distress. These outcomes have been observed in studies specifically examining the CBT therapeutic alliance (Evans-Jones, Peters, & Barker, 2009; Kazdin, Marciano, & Whitley, 2005; Keijsers, Schaap, & Hoogduin, 2000). Furthermore, it is especially important to establish a quality relationship early in the therapeutic process. Studies examining CBT outcomes over time have noted that relationship measures early in treatment predicted symptom improvement (Arnow et al., 2013; Klein et al., 2003).

Developing a strong therapist–client therapeutic alliance is not as easy as some may believe. The skills necessary for therapeutic alliance are ever evolving throughout your career as a therapist. Although many people who choose to enter the field of therapy may already "naturally" have many of these skills based on their non-therapeutic relationships (e.g., friends and family), the dynamics of a therapeutic relationship are often very different. In other words, adjustments need to be made when working with clients who are struggling with a variety of mental health issues. Such skill development requires significant training and practice, introspection, and supervision. The following two sections of this chapter address the necessary skills to develop effective therapeutic alliances with clients. First, nonspecific factors are used in most therapeutic approaches and include key skills that come naturally to most therapists. Second, CBT-specific factors contribute to the therapeutic alliance and are necessary for collaborative empiricism.

NONSPECIFIC FACTORS

Treatment elements that impact therapeutic outcomes across theories are typically referred to as nonspecific factors (or common factors). There are also treatment elements that are idiosyncratic to a particular theory, known as specific factors. This section first addresses two of the most common and well-known nonspecific factors: Rogerian qualities and interpersonal skills. Although the focus of this chapter is on establishing a CBT therapeutic alliance, these nonspecific factors are still important for effectively practicing CBT. In fact, without these skills, a discussion of CBT-specific factors is moot.

Rogerian Qualities

Carl Rogers's (1959, 1995) humanistic approach to therapy was a welcome change to many, as it was a reaction to the deterministic and negativistic view of human nature by both psychodynamic and behavioral theories at the time. Rogers's approach to therapy was not directive, but he placed great emphasis on valuing clients by treating them with dignity and respect. Thus, his view of therapeutic growth centered mainly on the therapist–client relationship. Even today, the sine qua non of Rogerian qualities are considered to be largely empathy, unconditional positive regard, and genuineness. Empathy consists of understanding the thoughts and feelings of the client. It is not pity. Empathy allows the therapist to take an objective perspective of the client's presenting problems and distress. Unconditional positive regard consists of client acceptance in a nonjudgmental attitude, also known as warmth. In other words, there are no strings attached in order to be valued as a client. Finally, genuineness consists of communicating (verbally and nonverbally) and presenting oneself in a natural, honest, and sincere manner. Rogers argued that there would be minimal to no client growth without these therapeutic qualities. Although these basic therapeutic relationship skills are humanistic, there are sophisticated ways therapists can integrate these skills within a CBT framework and purpose.

Empathy and CBT

Empathy is often defined with the metaphor of "standing in someone else's shoes" or "seeing through someone else's eyes." These are valid statements; however, providing such congruent empathy takes both skill and practice. When making empathetic comments, it is important to make sure that your verbal and nonverbal expression matches how the client feels and is appropriately timed. With regard to matching the client, assumptions should not be made about how the client is feeling. In other words, the more information you can glean from your client, implicitly or explicitly, the more confident you can be in what you say and how you express empathy. An inaccurate display of empathy can potentially harm the therapeutic relationship, especially in the early stages. Even though what you may be feeling for the client is sincere, what and how it is expressed is just as important.

Related to matching is therapist timing in expressing empathy. A common mistake therapists make is coming on too strong with empathy too soon. Although your intentions may be well placed, this approach can come off an insincere and off-putting (e.g., "She is being fake. There is no way she can know how I feel right now."). On the other hand, missing an opportunity to display appropriate empathy (i.e., weak or no response) may come off as cold and disconnected from the client (e.g., "Does she even care about what happened to me?"). A final comment about expressing empathy and timing is a word of caution when validating clients' thoughts and feelings. From a CBT perspective, being overeager to express empathy can potentially reinforce maladaptive thoughts (i.e., invalid thoughts). For example, if clients are repeatedly making self-deprecating comments (e.g., "I can't do anything right. Nobody cares about me.") and you respond with empathetic validation verbally (e.g., "It makes sense that you think that way.") or nonverbally (e.g., repeatedly nodding head in agreement), some clients might think that you agree with their negative self views. Even if some clients are not put off by such empathy, they might think that change is hopeless (e.g., "Wow, even my therapist thinks I'm a loser."). Whenever you are unsure about your approach to expressing empathy, focus on validating clients' emotions instead of their thoughts. Even if they have invalid thoughts, their emotions are still very real to them. Table 2.1 provides a list of questions to consider while expressing empathy.

Table 2.1.   Questions to Consider While Expressing Empathy

1. Is the client congruent in what she is saying and her nonverbal behaviors?
2. Do I understand the context of the information shared?
3. How will my display of empathy most likely be perceived by the client?
4. What is my purpose in expressing empathy in this way?
5. Will the timing in expressing my empathy be appropriate (e.g., too soon, not enough information)?
6. Will my expression of empathy be consistent with other similar situations?
7. How can I convey empathy that validates his emotions while also providing insight into cognitive and/or behavioral patterns that may require change?
8. Is it possible to provide empathy that praises and validates adaptive thoughts and behaviors?

The utility of accurate empathy in CBT goes beyond objectively understanding a client's thoughts and emotions. For example, through a CBT lens, empathy can also help you identify maladaptive behavior patterns, negative automatic thoughts and core beliefs, and dysfunctional relational problems with greater clarity. The more you can take a client's perspective, the more you can understand where the client is "coming from," even if a particular behavior pattern or way of thinking may appear illogical on the surface. Consider Activity 2.1, broken down into two parts with discussion questions. The first part provides a description of a case from the perspective of the observers. The second part provides a description of the case from the perspective of the individual.

ACTIVITY 2.1: EMPATHY (OBSERVER PERSPECTIVE) SCENARIO 1

Jill and Richard have requested family therapy due to increasing verbal arguments over the past couple of months. The have also noticed that their children, Mike (12 years old) and Stacey (6 years old), have been distressed. Jill arrives for therapy with the children. However, you are told that Richard will be arriving a few minutes late due to work. You begin your intake by gathering some information on recent familial interactions. The following includes some highlights shared by Jill and the children.

Over the past month Richard has been coming home about 2 hours later than usual and after a quick "hello" to his family retreats to his study. When Jill checks in on him, he is often short with her and becomes increasingly irritable at her attempts to talk about his day. This often results in Jill's retreating to the bedroom, where she eventually falls asleep before Richard comes to bed. Mike waits for an opportunity to talk to his father when he occasionally steps out of the office. Mike has recently been eagerly waiting for some help on a school project. When Mike asks Richard for help, he tells him that tonight is not a good night but tomorrow might be better. Stacey looks forward to Richard reading a bedtime story with her before she goes to sleep, but this has not happened for many nights.

Each family member is concerned about Richard's change in behavior and is becoming increasingly distressed because they do not know the reason for his recent behaviors. This has resulted in all family members formulating their own reasons for Richard's behavior. Jill has reported concerns that maybe Richard is having an affair due to his lack of affection and spending more time on the computer at night. Mike is sad because he thinks his father does not think he is smart enough to help him on his project. Stacey has been recently making comments wondering if her father still loves her. You soon realize that the intake session is over, and Richard never showed up.

Discussion Questions 2.1

- What are your initial thoughts and feelings about Jill and the children?
- What are your initial thoughts and feelings about Richard?
- What information would you like to obtain from Richard?
- What options do you have to try to ensure that Richard attends the next family session?

ACTIVITY 2.2: EMPATHY (INDIVIDUAL PERSPECTIVE) SCENARIO 2

You decide to call Richard between sessions to check in and see if he is willing and able to attend therapy. Richard is apologetic for missing the session and states that he is actually very much interested in therapy. With minimal prompting, Richard starts to cry and explain why he has been acting "strangely" lately. Richard states that he has been "very stressed" about money because the mortgage rate on their house has dramatically increased, resulting in higher monthly mortgage payments. He also shares that he has heard rumors at work that there might be layoffs at his job by the end of the year. He does not know if he will be one of the layoffs and does not think he has the job skills to find another job with a comparable wage. He has been working late as much as possible to get additional overtime pay. When he comes home, he is very tired and just wants to be alone. When he has the energy, he goes online to look for possible part-time jobs and refinancing options for their mortgage. When asked why he did not share at least some of this information with his wife and children, he states that this is actually his second marriage and that he "went through the same thing" in his first marriage. He explains that during his first marriage, he also experienced financial difficulties and whenever he tried to talk about it with his ex-wife, she would get "hysterical" and become verbally abusive. Richard attributes the failure of his first marriage to these financial difficulties and putting too much stress on his ex-wife. Richard is afraid that what happened in his first marriage is about to happen "all over again." He states that he is willing to share these concerns with Jill at the next family session.

(continued)

ACTIVITY 2.2: *Continued*

Discussion Questions 2.2

- After talking to Richard, have your thoughts and feelings about Richard changed?
- What information changed your perspective of Richard?
- In what ways could you verbally express empathy to Richard over the phone that would be sincere and not off-putting?
- At the next family session, is it possible to demonstrate empathy to both Jill and Richard, without empathy being expressed to one being perceived as insulting to the other? If so, how?

Unconditional Positive Regard and CBT

Simply stated, unconditional positive regard consists of showing warmth, acceptance, and respect for clients without conditions or "strings attached." Clients will potentially share much personal information with you, some of which may be embarrassing and/or never shared with anyone else. Thus, the more clients perceive that they are not being judged by you, the more likely they are going to open up and share relevant personal information. This is especially important for CBT therapists because understanding client history, intense emotions, maladaptive (or embarrassing) thoughts, and disruptive behaviors is vital information that informs and directs the treatment process.

Genuineness and CBT

Although presenting such genuineness qualities as honesty and sincerity may seem easy for a therapist on the surface, this can be challenging when balancing your own personal thoughts/feelings and providing constructive feedback and therapeutic direction. It is important for CBT therapists to genuinely balance being hopeful and optimistic for change while also being grounded in your clients' strengths and weaknesses. Additionally, clients may share certain behaviors and thoughts that elicit strong emotional responses in you. If you are not self-aware of your own reaction, internally and/or externally, this can potentially be off-putting to clients. Self-awareness is a must for CBT therapists due to the nature of eliciting and challenging client maladaptive thoughts and behaviors. Effective CBT requires detailed discussions of sometimes distressing and off-putting content. If CBT therapists lack awareness in how they respond to such content, a key component of CBT effectiveness is lost.

In sum, these nonspecific Rogerian factors still have much utility across all modern therapeutic approaches. However, for many mental health issues, research shows that these factors are necessary but not sufficient for clients experiencing high levels of distress (APA Presidential Task Force on Evidence-Based Practice, 2006). Stated differently, these skills are needed for effective therapy, but alone they will typically not provide long-term help for many clients. With that said, these skills are still important for CBT therapists. Many of the skills in the forthcoming chapters require these nonspecific factors for enhanced therapeutic effectiveness.

Interpersonal Skills

Although seemingly obvious, interpersonal skills are important for any competent therapist. Simply put, if clients do not feel comfortable with you, they will most likely terminate prematurely. As noted above, the nonspecific Rogerian skills are naturally important for relationship development. Strong (1968) has also noted a few interpersonal influence process factors that are important to integrate into the therapeutic alliance: expertness, attractiveness, and trustworthiness. These variables are also often referred to "opinion-change" variables because they are not only important to interpersonal relationship development but also play a role in facilitating client therapeutic change over time. These interpersonal factors naturally fit well into the CBT model due to their very nature to promote change through the therapeutic alliance. In other words, these factors can greatly enhance the purposeful nature of collaborative empiricism in CBT. In fact, Evans-Jones et al. (2009) found that expertness, attractiveness, and trustworthiness were associated with a better CBT therapeutic relationship and client engagement.

Expertness

Expertness refers to explicit and implicit evidence that demonstrates a certain level of specialized training, knowledge, and expertise. Explicit examples include your diplomas and license on display in your office, membership in professional organizations, and books. More implicit and more important is evidence of expertness displayed by your behavior. Simply conducting yourself as confident in theory and practice (e.g., psychoeducation, case formulation, treatment goals, and interventions) can enhance client perception of expertise. Providing clear roles, expectations, and session structure demonstrates that you know what you are doing. Most clients feel comfortable when there is a sense of structure and purposeful treatment. These elements, especially clarifying therapist–client roles and organized session structure, are at the heart of CBT (see Chapter 4). The more clients perceive their therapists to be competent, the more clients will be engaged and willing to challenge their own maladaptive thoughts and behaviors.

Trustworthiness

Trustworthiness initially comes from your established reputation and possibly the organization you are associated with. Once face-to-face, you can initially display genuineness to establish trustworthiness. Thereafter, displaying interest in client welfare, along with optimism and instilling hope, is valued. Respecting client confidentiality and following policies and procedures also naturally produce relational trust. Additionally, following through on your word and therapeutic factors (e.g., agenda setting and homework) shows that you are a reliable therapist. Trust takes time to be established in any relationship, but a strong start provides a solid foundation to build on in anticipation of future therapeutic challenges. Achieving trust is important for CBT, as disclosure of particularly distressing and embarrassing thoughts and behaviors is vital for initiating the process of decreasing client distress. Similarly, as therapy progresses, clients will need to have much trust in you, as they will be asked to engage in new ways of thinking and behaving, which can be psychologically threatening.

Attractiveness

Attractiveness is not so much the physical attributes of the therapist as a level of likability and compatibility that comes from how you conduct yourself during client interactions. Providing unconditional positive regard and warmth are significant contributing factors to therapist attractiveness. These attributes are perceived by the client as being liked, which is then typically reciprocated back to the therapist. Similarity between the therapist and client also contributes to attractiveness. In this context, similarity often comes from your empathy by showing that you understand the client's experiences. This process can include your self-disclosure of similar experiences or common interests. Although it is not necessary for CBT therapists to disclose personal information, self-disclosure of the process of therapy (i.e., discussing your thoughts and feelings about information shared by the client or the current status of the therapeutic relationship) is a good avenue for providing and receiving feedback about therapeutic progress. Also helpful for CBT therapists is having the skill to "match" to the client with verbal and nonverbal mannerisms. Demonstrating some level of similarity in how clients verbally and nonverbally communicate can improve the therapeutic relationship. This means that you should be malleable in how you present yourself, communicate CBT-specific information (e.g., psychoeducation), and approach CBT-specific skills and interventions. Having a "canned" approach where the style and content are the same across clients tends to make you less attractive.

Overall, these three interpersonal influence processes are a nice supplement to the previously mentioned Rogerian skills; in fact, there is much overlap. CBT therapists who consider relational factors while developing a therapeutic alliance will notice that quality therapist–client relationships better facilitate client disclosure of relevant mental health content and motivation to change. A common myth about CBT is that therapeutic relationships are of little value (see Chapter 15). This is far from true. As discussed here, there are many common therapeutic relationship factors that are important for CBT. The following are key CBT-specific factors that are necessary for establishing collaborative empiricism.

COLLABORATIVE EMPIRICISM: CBT-SPECIFIC FACTORS

As briefly stated earlier, CBT espouses collaborative empiricism, an action-oriented therapeutic alliance driven by research that integrates, tests, and modifies clients' thoughts and behaviors. This working alliance is a CBT-specific factor that emphasizes the shared therapist–client responsibly in client change, including setting goals and working on interventions. Although the previously mentioned nonspecific factors are important, collaborative empiricism is the key therapeutic alliance factor that fosters the overall empirical effectiveness of CBT (Cohen, Edmunds, Brodman, Benjamin, & Kendall, 2013; Dattilio & Hanna, 2012; Kazantzis, Beck, Dattilio, Dobson, & Rapee, 2013). The primary focus of collaborative empiricism is to identify maladaptive cognitions and behaviors and then "test" for their empirical validity and/or utility. This process ultimately results in more adaptive cognitions and behaviors, a reduction in the frequency and severity of symptoms, and an improvement in overall quality of life. This section is broken down into three sequential sections that highlight the key specific factors of collaborative empiricism: therapist–client activity level, client-specific factors, and conceptualization and treatment.

Therapist–Client Activity Level

CBT requires you to be highly active throughout every session. Much effort goes into structuring and guiding treatment session by session to ensure that each client receives the most efficient and effective therapeutic experience. Additionally, it is important that clients are also actively engaged throughout therapy. Unlike other theoretical orientations that have been historically one-directional (e.g., psychodynamic—therapist very directive; humanistic—therapist very nondirective), clients are not passive recipients of "knowledge" or "insight" where they are expected to absorb information from their therapists. For some clients, the expectation that they are to be active in their own treatment may be surprising. Thus, it is vital that therapists immediately convey this expectation to their clients while emphasizing that client change and symptom improvement will come from a therapist–client "team effort" known as an alliance. In other words, expectations need to be set early by your words and actions. The therapist–client activity level will fluctuate depending on the phase of therapy. Of course, there will be variability depending on client symptoms and needs and from session to session. The following sections describe Figure 2.1, which provides a general visual depiction of therapist–client activity level across three phases of therapy. (For CBT video vignettes that integrate the three phases of therapy and session structure, see Chapter 4.)

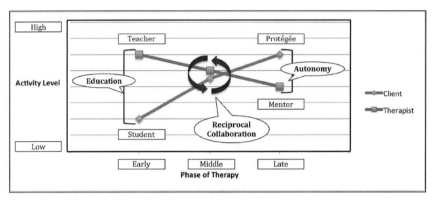

Figure 2.1. Therapist-Client Activity Level Across Three Phases of Therapy

Early Phase of Therapy

The early phase consists of a high therapist activity level and a relatively lower client activity level. In addition to the therapist and client beginning to establish their therapeutic relationship, this is when the CBT model is introduced and clients are typically more distressed, requiring more guidance. At this time, it is also important for you to instill hope and motivation for change while also developing an initial conceptualization. In many ways, the therapeutic relationship at this point resembles a teacher–student relationship that is more educative. Although the client-student is still expected to be activity engaged in therapy, it is the therapist-teacher who leads the flow and expectations of therapy. Additionally, the therapist-teacher will scaffold what is "taught" as the client-student understands key basics of CBT while also being motivated to move toward cognitive and behavioral change. (For CBT-specific psychoeducation techniques, see Chapter 5.)

Middle Phase of Therapy

During the middle phase of therapy, therapist activity may slightly decrease while client activity significantly increases to an equitable level with the therapist. At this point, you are still active with implementing treatment goals and corresponding interventions, including clients reciprocating active involvement in their own changes and improvement. Ultimately, the therapeutic relationship becomes highly collaborative. Not only are you still guiding the client during the cognitive and behavior change process, but the client is also providing direct and indirect feedback back to you, resulting in reciprocal collaboration. Thus, during this phase, the activity level of both therapist and client is truly interactive in that each action by one will affect the action (response) by the other.

Late Phase of Therapy

As the last phase of therapy approaches, therapist activity continues to slightly decrease while client activity continues to increase. This is when client cognitive and behavioral change is now a more autonomous process and begins to translate to other facets of life. Essentially, the therapeutic relationship during this phase resembles a mentor–protégé relationship that is more supportive with selective guidance. In other words, less direct action is required by the therapist-mentor as the client-protégé takes more of a lead role in flow and therapeutic focus. However, this does not mean that the therapist-mentor is not actively involved. Rather, the therapist-mentor is more judicious in providing expertise and support in order for the client-protégé to autonomously identify and respond to problems and stressors. This process is essential for client long-term change and generalization of treatment gains well after therapy ends.

Client-Specific Factors

From initial intake to termination, clients present with an extensive range of problems, psychological distress, diagnostic symptoms, life experiences, racial and cultural backgrounds, expectations, and motivation to change. Thus, although the previously mentioned discussion focused on therapist–client activity fluctuating throughout the phases of therapy, you still should be flexible and sensitive to the unique needs of each client. In addition to phase of therapy, there are three broad client-specific idiosyncratic factors to consider when building a therapeutic relationship based on collaborative empiricism: presenting symptoms, environmental stressors, and sociocultural factors.

Presenting Symptoms

When working with managed care, each client will require a formal diagnosis. Although a diagnosis does have its utility, what is more important to focus on when building a collaborative therapeutic relationship is each client's specific symptoms and associated presenting problems. Similarly, the unique personality traits of clients that may be contributing to their own distress have the potential to also influence the therapeutic relationship. Table 2.2 provides a brief list of disorders/conditions with common symptoms and associated challenges to the therapeutic relationship.

As can be observed based on the examples in Table 2.2, even a seasoned therapist will sometimes be challenged by the thoughts and behaviors of clients. Nevertheless, it is still important that a collaborative therapeutic relationship be established for the well-being of the client, even if it requires "more work" on your part. The following are a few strategies that can be helpful in responding to client symptoms and personality traits that influence the therapeutic relationship.

Be self-aware and proactive for potential problems. Part of having good therapeutic relationship skills includes good self-awareness skills. In this context, self-awareness includes both noticing how you think and feel in response to a client's comments and behaviors and noticing how you "come off" to a client. All therapists have their weaknesses and negative idiosyncrasies in response to certain personali-

Table 2.2. Presenting Symptoms and Challenges to the Therapeutic Relationship

Disorder/Condition	Challenging Symptoms/Behaviors	Challenges to the Therapeutic Relationship
Depression	Low energy, irritable, apathy, passive, pessimism, hopeless, suicidal thoughts and behaviors	Establishing rapport, expressing thoughts and emotions, engage and motivate, developing autonomy
Bipolar (mania)	Intrusive, irritable, extreme impulsivity, risky behaviors, charming, seductive, mood fluctuations, minimization, suicidal thoughts and behaviors	Boundaries, treatment adherence (including medication compliance), acknowledging problems to change
Substance use	Deceptive to self and others, manipulative, blaming others/the system, minimization, cunning, low motivation to change	Establishing trust, treatment adherence, providing empathy, acknowledging problems to change, engage and motivate
Borderline personality disorder	Chaotic and unstable relationships, seductive, impulsive, intense and erratic emotions, self-harm, demanding, suicidal thoughts and behaviors	Boundaries, treatment adherence, developing autonomy, burnout
Anger	Argumentative, insulting, stubborn, confrontational, critical/blaming others, sensitive, defensiveness	Establishing rapport, providing empathy, providing/receiving feedback, engage and motivate

ties and behaviors. Thus, effective therapist self-awareness provides opportunities to proactively avoid potential negative therapist–client interactions. More specifically, if you can recognize that a client is eliciting certain negative thoughts and behaviors in yourself, you will be more apt to make any necessary adjustments before there is any significant damage to the therapeutic relationship. Correspondingly, you also need to be able to notice potential problems that may be outside of your own interpersonal demeanor. Even if you do not have a negative response to a client, there may still be specific client behaviors/symptoms and personality traits that require you to adjust your own thoughts and behaviors accordingly. The earlier you notice and respond to such client variables, the better the chance to build an effective therapeutic alliance.

Avoid labeling clients. Labeling is when diagnostic terminology is used to identify clients (e.g., manic, alcoholic, psychotic, or borderline). Although often not intended, such labeling can come off as pejorative and condescending. Labeling puts you at risk for creating a self-fulfilling prophecy for clients where your thoughts and behaviors may actually reinforce the very symptoms that are causing the client's distress. Or, even worse, you may falsely interpret your clients' thoughts and behaviors as maladaptive when they are innocuous or even adaptive (i.e., a thought or behavior that would typically be viewed as "normal" for other clients is viewed as maladaptive for the labeled client). Furthermore, these negative client attitudes are often subtle and covert, which can make it difficult to notice and make the appropriate modifications. Eventually, labeling of clients often creates a more detached and strained therapeutic relationship. Clients typically feel less motivated for change while your efforts also decrease as you lose hope for client improvement (e.g., "This is as good as she is going to get.").

Provide vigilant empathy. As discussed earlier, therapist empathy is a key common factor for establishing a therapeutic alliance and effective treatment. However, even the most skilled therapists can struggle providing empathy with certain challenging clients. Thus, the expression "vigilant empathy" is emphasized here because empathy may not always come naturally. Rather, at times, you may have to figuratively take a step back and remind yourself of where your clients are coming from. Many clients present with symptoms and behaviors that are result of their past experiences, some of which may have been out of their control. If you are able to remind yourself of your clients' backgrounds, it will help provide perspective and understanding for why they engage in certain maladaptive thoughts and behaviors. This approach allows you to respond with alternative cognitive and emotional responses that are more conducive for empathy. In sum, if empathy is not occurring naturally for you, it is fruitful to examine why this may be the case and reevaluate if the client is being fairly perceived.

Environmental Stressors

Sometimes, clients experience life events that are completely out of their control (e.g., medical illness, death of a loved one, job loss, or traumatic accident). Other times, there are life events that clients may have at least partially contributed to (e.g., financial problems, separation or divorce, involvement with social services, or involvement with the criminal justice system). Sometimes, these "outside" environmental stressors become key factors to consider and integrate while developing a therapeutic relationship and conceptualizing client problems and treatment plans. Understanding the level of impact and control that clients perceive to have over these life events is important to consider for collaborative empiricism. If the life event is largely out of the client's control, there may be a need to shift the client's internalization of the event (e.g., feeling guilty by blaming oneself) to a more external perspective. In these cases, clients' internalizing not only is inaccurate but also is causing them undue distress. On the other hand, if the life event is largely within the client's control, there may be a need to shift the client's externalization of the event (e.g., not taking responsibility by blaming the government) to a more internal perspective.

In these cases, a client's externalizing is often a type of cognitive avoidance, which may provide short-term relief but long-term distress because no learning/changing of certain cognitive and behavior patterns is taking place. Consider Activity 2.2, broken down into two parts with discussion questions. The first part provides a description of a case from the perspective of internalization. The second part provides a description of the case from the perspective of externalization.

ACTIVITY 2.3: ENVIRONMENTAL STRESSORS (INTERNALIZATION) SCENARIO 1

John has been suffering from depression for many years. He has made some improvement in therapy but still has a tendency to overly internalize negative events that results in self-blame and sometimes guilt. He shares with you that he has been having trouble sleeping and concentrating throughout the day because he keeps ruminating about something that happened to one of his friends. John explains that about a week ago, his friend Steve asked him to come to his place to help repair the roof of his house. John declined to help because he was not feeling well that day and was looking forward to resting after having had a stressful day at work. When John spoke to Steve the following day, Steve told him that he had fell off his ladder and broke his leg. John apologized profusely to Steve. Steve told John that it was not necessary for him to apologize because it was not his fault. Nevertheless, John still thinks he is responsible for Steve's broken leg because he had declined to help him that day.

ACTIVITY 2.4: ENVIRONMENTAL STRESSORS (EXTERNALIZATION) SCENARIO 2

Billy has been mandated by court to see you for therapy related to alcohol abuse. During the intake, you ask him to share what he did to require mandated therapy. Billy initially states that he has done nothing to deserve these consequences ("It's the cop's fault."). Billy is asked to explain why he thinks the police officer is responsible for his mandated therapy. Billy shares that he was pulled over by the police officer because he was driving too fast and not keeping the car between the lines. On being pulled over, the police officer smelled alcohol on Billy's breath and requested that Billy do a sobriety test. Billy refused and verbally assaulted the police officer. Due to these behaviors, he was arrested and brought down to the local jail. At the jail, Billy took a breathalyzer test, which indicated that he was nearly twice the legal alcohol limit. Billy was ultimately charged for drunk driving, and part of his probation is to attend therapy for his alcohol abuse. During the rest of the intake, Billy acknowledges that he drinks frequently throughout the week, often resulting in multiple hangovers. However, he insists that he does not have a problem because he drinks excessively only when other people make him mad. When asked what he could have done differently the night of his arrest, Billy says, "Nothing." Billy repeatedly states that he would not be in the current position if the "cop just left me alone."

Discussion Questions 2.3

- How may John therapeutically benefit from shifting his internalizing of the event to more externalizing?
- How may Billy therapeutically benefit from shifting his externalizing of the event to more internalizing?
- What thinking pattern of these two cases do you think would be the most challenging therapeutically? Explain.
- What are possible ways to "empirically test" the beliefs of the individuals in each case?

Sociocultural Factors

Any competent and ethical therapist needs to be sensitive and considerate of their clients' sociocultural factors. If you cannot connect with your clients on a cultural level, the therapeutic relationship will be strained. Examples of cultural factors to consider include age, gender, sexual orientation, race/ethnicity, religion/spirituality, socioeconomic status, developmental disability, educational level, physical disability, and national origin. As much as any good therapist tries to be respectful when working with clients of diverse backgrounds, there is always the possibility that certain biases or stereotypes may inadvertently negatively affect the therapeutic relationship. Furthermore, just like therapists, clients may also have their own biases and stereotypes entering therapy. It is up to you to monitor the therapist–client sociocultural dynamics and respond accordingly.

Similar to being self-aware in responding to clients' comments and behaviors, you must also be aware of your own biases and stereotypes. This requires self-introspection and honesty with yourself; this is not easy. If you have greater awareness of your own biases and stereotypes, you will be better prepared to catch your thoughts and reactions before having a permanent negative effect on the therapeutic relationship. It is also best for you to be aware of therapeutic alliance dynamics and address any potential sociocultural conflicts with clients sooner than later. Such conflicts may be the result of the interaction of biases and stereotypes between yourself and your clients. Furthermore, poor self-awareness can result in difficultly with feeling and expressing empathy, not being oneself (i.e., not genuine), putting less effort into meeting clients' needs, and possibly apathy. Overall, collaborative empiricism will not be possible.

If you notice that you have a frequent pattern of biases and stereotypes with particular populations, it is highly advisable to develop a plan to make the necessary changes to be more accepting and empathetic. This can include consulting with other colleagues, supervision, additional education, increasing exposure with the population of concern, and possibly therapy to address specific negative cognitive biases. The topic of multicultural therapy is beyond the scope of this book. See Hays (2009) for a more in-depth review of multicultural therapy specific to CBT.

Conceptualization and Treatment

Although Chapter 3 addresses specific concepts in how to formally gather pertinent client information and conceptualize cases with appropriate treatment goals, the discussion here focuses on the role of collaborative empiricism in order effectively achieve these tasks. First, a good CBT case formulation requires information gained from the client through both formal and informal assessments. Keep in mind that clients are experts of themselves, as all clients have their own unique histories. Second, you are the expert in synthesizing this information into a working CBT conceptualization of the clients' precipitating and maintaining factors of their symptoms/problems and corresponding treatment plan. An honest CBT conceptualization includes not only clients' strengths but also how they may be contributing to their own distress and what they need to do to change certain life patterns that may be an integral part of their lives. This is a sensitive process and can cause potential client distress. True collaborative empiricism involves obtaining accurate information from the client, which includes client trust and willingness to monitor and "test" specific thoughts and behaviors in session and outside of session. The more clients are in agreement with their CBT case formulation, the more they will be in agreement with their treatment goals. Furthermore, clients need to have substantial trust in you when it comes to implementing interventions. A key element of CBT is identifying and modifying maladaptive thoughts and behavior patterns, which can temporarily increase cognitive and physiological distress. In order for clients to be willing to put themselves at such psychological risk, they need to trust that you know what you are

Table 2.3. Using the Collaborative Relationship for Conceptualization and Treatment

1. Remember that clients are experts of themselves and that relationship building begins with the intake/first session.
2. Be honest but respectful about clients' problems and maladaptive thoughts and behaviors in need of change.
3. When possible, recognize and implement clients' strengths into the treatment plan.
4. Continuously monitor distress and progress while providing consistent and supportive feedback.
5. It is best to keep the client informed throughout the conceptualization process in order to avoid surprises (and possible resentment) when implementing the treatment plan.
6. Be sure to take the mystery out of therapy by ensuring trust and connecting your conceptualization with treatment goals and interventions.
7. As therapy progresses, allow for greater client autonomy in the direction of therapy as progress is increasingly made with treatment goals.

doing and that the final outcome will ultimately provide improvement in quality of life. Table 2.3 provides a few suggestions on how to use the collaborative relationship for conceptualization and treatment.

COMMON CHALLENGES IN ESTABLISHING A THERAPEUTIC ALLIANCE

Table 2.4 provides some common challenges that can be experienced while trying to establish a therapeutic alliance and possible considerations for responses. It may be reassuring to keep in mind that encountering challenges in establishing a therapeutic

Table 2.4. Common Challenges in Establishing a Therapeutic Alliance

Challenge	Possible Considerations
Client having low motivation or hope for change	Increase validation, affirmative statements, and reflection of feelings; do not debate, lecture, or give unsolicited advice or solutions; normalize experiences; ask for permission to talk about particular topics and/or provide information; share possible alternative outcomes if change is made; use casual open-ended questions; summarize—link key themes
Difficulty establishing a therapeutic relationship with client	Show sincere interest in particular task/interests; reassess client's perception of your expertness, trustworthiness, and attractiveness; do you convey unconditional positive regard, genuineness, and empathy? consider possible biases or stereotypes; are environmental stressors being taken into account?
Difficulty feeling empathy for client	Recall vigilant empathy—try to remind yourself of where the client is coming from to increase understanding of particular thoughts or behaviors
Client struggling with autonomy as therapy progresses	Review effectiveness of collaboration—e.g., are you leading too much, and is the rationale for collaboration made clear? use simple behavioral experiments to "test" new thoughts and behaviors; reinforce/praise autonomous actions
Negative/interfering expectations based on client's past therapy experiences	Process past experiences and consider what worked and what can be different; set expectations for therapy early, including the CBT model; model expectations and demonstrate benefits; do not bash past therapy experiences—look at CBT as alternative to what was done in the past ("give it a shot")
Client having difficulty providing feedback	Set expectation for feedback early in therapy; provide gentle feedback to client; elicit feedback from client; praise client when feedback is provided; provide examples of how past feedback has resulted in good therapeutic outcomes

alliance does not mean that therapy will fail. In fact, research has shown that alliance levels fluctuating from high to low and then back to high after a therapeutic alliance repair is actually associated with good therapeutic outcomes (Kivlighan & Shaughnessy, 2000; Stiles et al., 2004).

REFERENCES

APA Presidential Task Force on Evidence-Based Practice. (2006). Evidence-based practice in psychology. *American Psychologist, 61,* 271–285.

Ardito, R. B., & Rabellino, D. (2011). Therapeutic alliance and outcome in psychotherapy: Historical excursus, measurements, and prospects for research. *Frontiers in Psychology, 2,* 1–11.

Arnow, B. A., Steidtmann, D., Blasey, C., Manber, R., Constantino, M. J., Klein, D. N., et al. (2013). The relationship between the therapeutic alliance and treatment outcome in two distinct psychotherapies for chronic depression. *Journal of Consulting and Clinical Psychology, 81,* 627–638.

Beck, A. T., Rush, A. J., Shaw, B. F., & Emery G. (1979). *Cognitive therapy of depression.* New York: Guilford Press.

Cohen, J. S., Edmunds, J. M., Brodman, D. M., Benjamin, C. L., & Kendall, P. C. (2013). Using self-monitoring: Implementation of collaborative empiricism in cognitive-behavioral therapy. *Cognitive and Behavioral Practice, 20,* 419–428.

Dattilio, F. M., & Hanna, M. A. (2012). Collaboration in cognitive-behavioral therapy. *Journal of Clinical Psychology, 68,* 146–158.

Evans-Jones, C., Peters, E., & Barker, C. (2009). The therapeutic relationship in CBT for psychosis: Client, therapist and therapy factors. *Behavioural and Cognitive Psychotherapy, 37,* 527–540.

Hays, P. (2009). Integrative evidence-based practice, cognitive-behavior therapy, and multicultural therapy: Ten steps for culturally competent practice. *Professional Psychology: Research and Practice, 40,* 354–360.

Kazantzis, N., Beck, J. S., Dattilio, F. M., Dobson, K. S., & Rapee, R. M. (2013). Collaborative empiricism as the central therapeutic relationship element in CBT: An expert panel discussion at the 7th International Congress of Cognitive Psychotherapy. *International Journal of Cognitive Therapy, 6,* 386–400.

Kazdin, A. E., Marciano, P. L., & Whitley, M. K. (2005). The therapeutic alliance in cognitive-behavioral treatment of children referred for oppositional, aggressive, and antisocial behavior. *Journal of Consulting and Clinical Psychology, 73,* 726–730.

Keijsers, G. P., Schaap, C. P., & Hoogduin, C A. (2000). The impact of interpersonal patient and therapist behavior on outcome in cognitive-behavior therapy: A review of empirical studies. *Behavior Modification, 24,* 264–297.

Kivlighan, D. M., & Shaughnessy, P. (2000). Patterns of working alliance development: A typology of client's working alliance ratings. *Journal of Counseling Psychology, 47,* 362–371.

Klein, D. N., Schwartz, J. E., Santiago, N. J., Vivian, D., Vocisano, C., Castonguay, L. G., . . . Keller, M. B. (2003). Therapeutic alliance in depression treatment: Controlling for prior change and patient characteristics. *Journal of Consulting and Clinical Psychology, 71,* 997–1006.

Leahy, R. L. (2008). The therapeutic relationship in cognitive-behavioral therapy. *Behavioural and Cognitive Psychotherapy, 36,* 769–777.

Raue, P. J., Goldfried, M. R., & Barkham, M. (1997). The therapeutic alliance in psycho-dynamic-interpersonal and cognitive-behavioral therapy. *Journal of Consulting and Clinical Psychology, 65,* 582–587.

Rogers, C. R. (1959). A theory of therapy, personality, and interpersonal relationships, as developed in the client-centered framework. In S. Koch (Ed.), *Psychology: A study of science: Formulations and the social context* (Vol. 3, pp. 184–256). New York: McGraw-Hill.

Rogers, C. R. (1995). *On becoming a person: A therapist's view of psychotherapy.* New York: Houghton Mifflin.

Stiles, W. B., Glick, M. J., Osatuke, K., Hardy, G. E., Shapiro, D. A., Agnew-Davies, R., . . . Barkham, M. (2004). Patterns of alliance development and rupture-repair hypothesis: Are productive relationships U-shaped or V-shaped? *Journal of Counseling Psychology, 51,* 81–91.

Strong, S. R. (1968). Counseling: An interpersonal influence process. *Journal of Counseling Psychology, 15,* 215–224.

Wright, J. H., & Davis, D. (1994). The therapeutic relationship in cognitive-behavioral therapy: Patient perceptions and therapist responses. *Cognitive and Behavioral Practice, 1,* 25–45.

3

CBT Assessment, Case Formulation, and Treatment Planning

The assessment and case formulation process is vital for any CBT therapeutic approach. Unlike some theoretical orientations, CBT requires a purposeful process in determining the most effective treatment approach. Stated differently, before developing a formal case formulation, there needs to be an assessment process through a CBT lens. Additionally, true CBT treatment planning needs to be based off of a working and malleable CBT case formulation. Essentially, a CBT conceptualization will be the driving force for developing and testing hypotheses for understanding and treating client problems and symptoms.

This chapter is divided into four interconnected parts. First, intake interview basics are addressed with a primary focus on common client information that is gathered during the assessment process. Second, CBT assessment strategies that are necessary for the development of an accurate case formulation that will inform effective treatment planning are discussed. Third, the process of developing a working CBT case formulation based on the assessment process and continuous client interactions is addressed. Finally, how to develop a CBT treatment plan is discussed, including treatment goals and interventions informed by a CBT case formulation.

INTAKE INTERVIEW BASICS

Assessment often begins the first time you have contact with your client (at least face-to-face). The initial, formal assessment process is often referred to as an "intake" in most agencies. It is important to note here that although the focus of the first meeting is assessing the clients' presenting problems, collaborative empiricism begins here. With that said, it needs to be emphasized that the very first interactions between you and your clients have therapeutic relationship and treatment implications.

31

Pragmatically, almost all agencies that provide therapy will require a semistructured intake interview on first seeing a client. The format of such an interview can vary greatly by setting; however, there is a general consistency of content that is addressed. A semistructured interview includes specific questions that must be asked based on agency (and perhaps managed care) expectations and follow-up questions that you ask at your own discretion based on information provided by the client. Although the following content is not necessarily unique to CBT, it is essential to address these basic skills, as they are important to build off of when focusing on CBT-specific assessment information. Table 3.1 provides a summary of key areas of information that are typically gathered during a semistructured intake interview, excluding presenting problems and symptoms, which will be addressed in the section "CBT Assessment." Even though this section is addressed separately from CBT assessment, these two parts are not mutually exclusive and are often integrated.

Demographic and Background Information

This information is very basic but may provide helpful contextual data when conceptualizing the case formulation. These questions are often noninvasive and can be the initial steps for establishing therapeutic rapport. Additionally, the process of covering this basic content may also provide a preliminary perspective of how the client is functioning.

Primary Presenting Concern

This is often reported when a client calls an agency to schedule an intake; it is essentially what initially brings the client to therapy. What clients disclose from their perspective is a good starting point to help guide the direction of some of your intake questions. You will often find that what clients share as their primary presenting concern may be a little different from how you eventually conceptualize their distress. Sometimes, this is a good time to examine the client's other presenting problems (see the section "CBT Assessment").

Development and Life History

Even though CBT therapists are primarily present focused, it is still important to gather key historical information. Indeed, as already mentioned in Chapter 1 and discussed later in this chapter (and future chapters), core beliefs, which are often the driving force of most automatic thoughts, are initially developed due to past life events. Despite much of this information being rather basic, particular emphasis should be placed on both family relationships and significant life events. Relationships with close family members can shape the way people perceive themselves and interact within their world (Schermerhorn, Cummings, & Davies, 2008). This is not to say that family relationships fully dictate a client's presenting problems and symptoms (it is just one of many factors); rather, there is a

Table 3.1.   Common Intake Information Gathered

Demographic and background information	Name, date of birth (age), race/ethnicity, spiritual/religious background, level of education, current work/student status, economic status, current living arrangements
Primary presenting concern	What brings clients to therapy from their perspective
Development and life history	Developmental milestones, school adjustment and milestones, childhood relationships, internalizing/externalizing behaviors of concern, family relationships and dynamics (e.g., parents/caregivers, siblings, close relatives), significant life events
Medical and mental health history	Significant medical events/complications, past mental health, prescribed or nonprescribed medications, substance use and abuse, criminal history/current legal involvement, family medical and psychiatric history
Interpersonal relationships	Relationship (romantic) history, current relationship status (e.g., long-term relationship, casual, married, divorced), peer relationships, colleague relationships, family relationships, children
Current presentation	Physical appearance (e.g., dressed, groomed), motor activity (e.g., restless, sluggish, tics), attitude (e.g., standoffish, eager to please), speech (e.g., pressured, loquacious, slurred), memory (e.g., recent, remote, immediate), thought perception/content and concentration (e.g., coherent, tangential, disconnected, delusional, insightful), intellectual level (includes awareness of social events), orientation (aware of person, place, time), mood (e.g., agitated, depressed, anxious, apathetic, euthymic, euphoric), affect (e.g., full range, blunted, flat, inappropriate, labile)
Strengths/assets	What clients are good at doing or enjoy (e.g., exercise, music, writing), personality qualities (e.g., conscientious, compassionate, optimistic), anything (or person) in clients' lives that can be a protective factor (e.g., supportive family member, stable job, available social network), sociocultural factors (e.g., extended family, spirituality)
Contributing negative sociocultural factors	Poverty/homelessness, discrimination, immigration status, dangerous community

reasonable possibility that most core beliefs have been influenced by such relationships (Beck, 2011). Similarly, significant life events, especially those that are life changing (traumatic or not), can also shape core beliefs. Events that significantly impact people cognitively and/or emotionally tend to have a greater chance of being a "permanent" memory (Meng et al., 2017), even if inaccurate, and possibly influence our view of self and the world.

Medical and Mental Health History

Essentially, this section is a review of any current or past significant medical and mental health events. It is important to note any medical events that may influence the process of therapy. For example, traumatic brain injury can significantly impact cognitive, emotional, and behavioral functioning (e.g., memory, problem solving, concentration, aggression, impulsivity, or anxiety; Jennekens, de Casterle, & Dobbels, 2010). Furthermore, some symptoms that may present as mental health related may be medical (e.g., hypothyroidism is often associated with depressive-like symptoms, and persistent hypoglycemia can be mistaken for anxiety, depression, dementia, or schizophrenia). Although therapists are typically trained to look at mental health primarily through a cognitive and environmental lens for etiology, contributing medical and biological processes should also be considered. Relatedly, this is why family history, especially for mental health, needs to be reviewed due to biological and environmental contributing factors.

Similar to medical events, although therapists do not prescribe medications, it is important to be aware of the influence that such medications (including side effects) have on mental health and physical functioning. It is advisable that you maintain communication with the prescribing physician to monitor client impact, especially if the client is on medications for a specific mental health disorder.

Interpersonal Relationships

The quality of clients' interpersonal relationships has the potential to provide fruitful information on precipitating and maintaining factors for their presenting problems. Many mental health problems are often interpersonally related, either as a contributing factor or as an indicator of distress (Segrin, 2000). In other words, sometimes a difficult relationship with a colleague, family member, friend, or romantic partner may be a considerable source of distress even if it is not the "cause" of the presenting problems. In other cases, impairment of interpersonal relationships may be a consequence of mental health distress and presenting problems. Finally, the dynamics of clients' relationships can also be informative of how they interact with their social world, which can prove valuable to consider for case conceptualization and integration into treatment planning.

Current Presentation

How a client presents during the intake provides some preliminary information that can aid in therapeutic relationship building and treatment planning. Simply noting how clients appear, their motor activity, and their attitude toward you can be informative for initial case conceptualization impressions. Other examples to consider include speech, memory, mood (general presentation), affect (expression of emotion), and thought/perception content. These noted presentation observations are very similar to a mental status exam. Formal mental status exams are rarely necessary in most agencies unless working in a psychiatric hospital setting. However, there may be times when asking questions similar to those found in a mental status exam is necessary. There are some excellent resources that provide a good review of the full content and process for completing a formal mental status exam (e.g., Trzepacz & Baker, 1993).

Strengths and Assets

It is common for many therapeutic approaches to therapy to focus so much on the presenting problems and symptoms, as outlined in the *Diagnostic and Statistical Manual of Mental Disorders* (DSM), that the strengths and assets of clients often get overlooked. This is understandable considering that the focus of such approaches, like CBT, is to identify the symptoms and problems and alleviate distress. However, having too narrow of an assessment lens often results in overlooking client strengths and assets that can be effectively integrated into treatment goals. In fact, using client strengths and other available resources can enhance the collaborative process of treatment planning and facilitate intervention effectiveness.

Contributing Negative Sociocultural Factors

Just as client strengths can enhance the therapeutic process, contributing negative sociocultural factors can be inhibitive. Recognizing such sociocultural factors is important to consider because they may be directly contributing to clients' distress and presenting problems. In fact, in some cases, you should be cautious with providing certain diagnoses if there are legitimate, outside/external forces (often uncontrollable) affecting the client (e.g., minority groups experiencing "paranoia" over law enforcement officers threating their well-being). Not only should you consider relevant sociocultural factors in their case formulation, but you also need to be pragmatic in your goals and interventions. This does not mean that standards are lowered during treatment planning; rather, goals need to be more contextual to allow for greater flexibility of potential obstacles.

CBT ASSESSMENT

Although a pragmatic goal of assessment is often obtaining a formal DSM diagnosis for managed care, the focus should really be on the presenting problems for each client. Getting caught up in DSM-specific symptoms can result in missing many important contextual factors, especially for a CBT therapist. Thus, the CBT assessment process also includes understanding the precipitating and maintaining mechanisms of these problems. A well-done CBT assessment will set the stage for developing a working cognitive-behavioral hypothesis (case formulation) of the client's presenting problems and symptoms. Of course, a detailed and accurate case formulation allows the best chance for ameliorating client distress (treatment plan).

Table 3.2. Specific CBT Assessment Information

Compatibility with CBT	Ability to establish a CBT therapeutic alliance
	Ability to identify automatic thoughts and associated emotions
	Ability to work within a goal and problem-oriented focus
Presenting problems	Identification, frequency, duration, and intensity
	Impact on daily life
	Precipitating and maintaining factors
	Automatic thoughts, emotions, and associated behavioral responses
Motivation and responsibility to change	How much does the client actually want to change?
	What is the client's own perception of responsibility to change?
	What does the client expect to get out of therapy?
	Does the client have hope/optimism that change can happen?
Formal symptom measures	Formative assessment to continuously monitor treatment progress
	Assessment provides feedback to make any necessary therapeutic modifications
	Assessment can provide information that might not be stated verbally

When clients arrive for their intake session, they often do not truly know "what's wrong" with them. They just know that they are experiencing some type of distress beyond their level of comfort and ability to cope, and there may be external indicators that something is not right. Of course, there are some clients who do have a relatively sophisticated understanding of their distress, but they know that they need assistance in alleviating such distress. Regardless, it is up to you to help clients develop an understanding of their problems. Although the previously mentioned intake interview basics are important for gathering information, it is the CBT assessment process that truly provides a clearer understanding of what precipitates and maintains clients' presenting distress and problems. Although assessment is ever evolving throughout therapy, a thorough CBT assessment during intake allows for a higher-quality case formulation and corresponding treatment plan. Table 3.2 provides a summary of key content areas that are addressed specific to CBT assessment.

Compatibility with CBT

A client's compatibility with CBT deserves consideration when developing your case formulation and treatment plan. However, caution is warranted in not getting caught up in the notion that you have to be highly selective of who can receive CBT. In fact, this is contraindicative of CBT. There is a common myth that only high-cognitive-functioning individuals can benefit from CBT (see Chapter 12). This is not true. In fact, there are many modifications that can be—and have been—made, including those with below-average intelligence, young children, and those who are not "thinkers." It is best to look at compatibility with CBT on a continuum (i.e., low to high) to help inform your approach to psychoeducation and interventions. The following are a few compatibility considerations that may have at least some influence on therapeutic outcomes. Keep in mind that when you are assessing compatibility for CBT, this is more of an internal process as you observe your client and take into account background information during the intake and early sessions.

Ability to Establish a CBT Therapeutic Alliance

The therapist–client relationship is necessary for all therapeutic approaches, including the therapist–client alliance in CBT. Right from the very beginning, clients' expectations about therapy, including CBT, can impact the therapeutic alliance and outcomes (Dew & Bickman, 2005). This also includes first impressions, which puts the onus on you. In other words, your interactions and explanation of CBT during the first few sessions can significantly impact responsiveness to therapy. The key point here is that your clients' ability to establish a therapeutic relationship is as much your responsibility as it is their responsibility.

As touched on in Chapter 2, a vital specific factor for CBT is collaborative empiricism, which includes you and your clients working together toward mutually agreed-on goals. However, it is possible that you will come across a few clients who expect you to do at least the majority of the therapeutic work to "fix them." For example, they may have the expectation that you will give them life advice, independently develop treatment goals, and use interventions that can be passively learned. Although it is up to you to make sure that each client understands the process of CBT, having at least a basic sense of your clients' expectations can inform your approach in providing psychoeducation (e.g., explicitness, details, examples, and follow-ups) and therapeutic relationship development (e.g., empathy with language conveying client autonomy, eliciting client feedback, and proposing that the client engage in a mutual task). In the end, the issue is often not that clients are poor at establishing a therapeutic alliance and working collaboratively. Instead, it is up to you to make sure that your clients feel comfortable with CBT and have a clear understanding of the therapeutic expectations.

Ability to Identify Automatic Thoughts and Associated Emotions

How well clients can identity their automatic thoughts and emotions is understandably a salient consideration for CBT. It may be more helpful for you to look at this ability more as a potential strength than as a possible weakness. In other words, the more naturally clients can identify their thoughts and fluctuations in emotions, the more they may be naturally advanced in a particular CBT skill. However, unless a client has a significant inability to access thoughts (e.g., amnesia and some forms of dementia), this skill should be viewed on a continuum (i.e., low to high), as something that can be improved on over the course of therapy. Relatedly, some research indicates that those with extreme negative thoughts are more likely to have a poorer prognosis than those with less severe negative thoughts (Whisman, 1993). This is important information to know but should not be surprising. Clients with extreme negative thoughts are most likely very emotionally distressed with multiple life problems. It only makes sense that these individuals will be more therapeutically challenging. In many ways, it would be ironic to consider potential clients not suitable for CBT if their thought and emotion identification skills were poor and/or they had extreme negative thoughts—this is probably the very reason they need therapy! These clients have the potential to greatly benefit from well-implemented CBT.

Ability to Work Within a Goal- and Problem-Oriented Focus

As will soon be discussed in the "CBT Treatment Plan" section of this chapter (and throughout the rest of this book), the effectiveness of CBT is partially attributed to its goal-directed nature and use of purposeful problem solving. Similar to identifying thoughts and emotions, this ability should be viewed as a potential strength. Some clients already have good goal-setting and problem-solving skills. Admittedly, this is a great strength to have because research indicates that clients who think that problems have solutions and take action to problem solve respond positively to CBT (Burns, Rude, Simons, Bates, & Thase, 1994). Nevertheless, this is also a skill that can be taught and improved on throughout therapy. Explaining the expectation of goal- and problem-oriented focused therapy early, along with a collaborative approach during the treatment planning process, can dramatically improve therapeutic outcomes. Thus, although this is an important skill set to assess, having minimal and/or poor experience with these skills does not preclude potential clients from being compatible with CBT.

Presenting Problems

Assessing presenting problems is done essentially for all therapeutic approaches. However, how presenting problems are assessed can vary greatly across therapeutic approaches. For CBT therapists, assessing presenting problems through a cognitive-behavioral lens is essential for clear case formulation development and effective treatment planning. While the content of a client's presenting problems is important, the process of gathering such information is also significant. More specifically, the questions that are asked about problems (e.g., What were you thinking at that moment? What were the consequences for your behaviors?) begin to shape client expectations for the focus and course of CBT. The more clients know about the expectations and the process of therapy early in the therapeutic relationship, the better likelihood for positive client outcomes. The following provides a detailed description of the key steps necessary for assessing clients' presenting problems.

Problem Identification, Frequency, Duration, and Intensity

Although seemingly relatively simplistic, identifying relevant presenting problems and knowing how often a particular problem occurs (e.g., number of panic attacks), how long the problem lasts when it does occur (e.g., few minutes and quick recovery or 15 minutes and disoriented afterward), and how much distress the client experiences (e.g., severity rating on a 0–10 scale) can provide rich contextual information. Not all presenting problems can be assessed in this manner, but, when possible, this information can be the beginning of establishing baselines for specific problems. This information will be helpful in the future when developing objective and measurable goals.

Impact on Daily Life

Determining the impact that presenting problems have on daily life can be naturally addressed when assessing frequency, duration, and intensity. The impact of a client's problems on interpersonal relationships (e.g., friends, colleagues, family, or romantic partner) can be a strong indicator of problem severity and impairment. It can also include work/school productivity or simply the ability to initiate and complete daily tasks. How much a client's work/school and daily routine are affected by their problems, combined with any interpersonal distress, often strongly contributes to why therapy is sought. In other words, the more clients' lives are impacted by their presenting problems, the more likely they will recognize that "something is not right" and at least consider therapy as a viable option. This information can also be helpful in establishing current baselines. As much as decreasing symptom distress is important for treatment goals, so is improving quality of life through interpersonal relationships, work/school productivity, and daily tasks.

Precipitating and Maintaining Factors

A vital part of any CBT assessment is identifying what factors initiate/start the problem (precipitating) and what factors continue or exacerbate the problem (maintaining). For many clients, there are often certain triggers that initiate the problem. This can range from a single life event (e.g., a traumatic accident) to a series of daily stressors that "added up" over time (e.g., multiple work deadlines and constant arguing with a partner). Furthermore, clients will typically present with multiple problems. Thus, each problem may have its own trigger mechanisms. In some cases, the precipitating factors for the presenting problems may be intertwined. Identifying precipitating factors is key for any CBT formulation. Knowing how clients' distress and impairment began can offer initial insight into how they perceive life events and correspondingly respond and cope.

Once a problem has been triggered, sometimes it will naturally dissipate and resolve itself over time. This can include actions of the individual as a way to cope. However, if clients are presenting for therapy, they have at least a few problems that persisted over time due to certain maintaining factors. Thus, it is important to in-quire into how long each problem has been present in the clients' lives (e.g., just the past few weeks or many years). Relatedly, it is helpful to know what clients have done in the past to help ameliorate the problem. What has not worked or has made things worse and what has worked (at least in part) to cope with their distress and impair-ment can influence how interventions are implemented. General examples of clients' maintaining factors include cognitive distortions, escape/avoidance behaviors, and poor problem-solving skills. There may also be other factors that are more external to the client that are maintaining the problem (e.g., being laid off from work or recent death in the family). A deeper understanding of clients' maintaining factors provides initial insight into their automatic thoughts and associated behavioral tendencies and coping skills. Overall, precipitating and maintaining factors are naturally intercon-nected with understanding automatic thoughts and associated behaviors.

Automatic Thoughts, Emotions, and Associated Behavioral Responses

Discussion of the previously mentioned presenting problem sections will naturally touch on your clients' thoughts, emotions, and behaviors. The focus here is to ad-dress how to formally assess specific automatic thoughts during the intake. Typically when assessing automatic thoughts, information about associated emotions and physiological sensations can be naturally gathered. Thereafter, it is necessary to assess any corresponding behaviors and associated consequences (i.e., person–environment impact). Overall, this information will be vital for developing a solid case formula-tion and working hypothesis. Although more information will be gained continu-ously in future sessions, this information will help guide the direction of initial goals and interventions.

The fundamental focus during assessment is to at least ascertain a few common automatic thoughts that occur immediately after an event. It is often too early to ac-curately identify core beliefs during the intake, but it does not hurt to take any notes if they are observed. Getting started can be as simple as bringing up a specific event and asking clients what they are thinking. Ideally, these automatic thoughts should be representative of how clients think in relation to their problems. It is additionally valuable to obtain any associated emotions related to the event–thought connection. In fact, emotions may be easier to ascertain than thoughts because many clients often talk about their emotions (even when asked about thoughts) when processing spe-cific events. It will be up to you to put the initial event–thought–emotion sequence together, as redirecting clients about the difference between thoughts and emo-tions often occurs later in therapy. Within the context of emotions, it is commonly natural to fit in questions about how the client's body feels when distressed during these events. Similar to asking about thoughts, many times clients will naturally talk about their bodily sensations when asked about emotions. Again, this is fine at this stage of the therapeutic relationship as long as you are able to accurately connect the event–thought–emotion–physiological arousal sequence.

Once clients' automatic thoughts and associated emotions and physiological responses have been established, it is equally important to assess how clients behave during and after these events. More specifically, clients should be explicitly asked what they are doing when they are processing a specific event. Ideally, these behaviors should be representative of how clients respond to their thought–emotion–physiological sequence to specific events. In many ways, these behaviors may be maintaining factors through negative reinforcement. In other words, clients are avoiding and/ or escaping from negative stimuli, providing short-term relief from emotional and physiological distress and reinforcing the perceived validity of their negative automatic thoughts. Thus, due to the short-term relief and not learning alternative, more adaptive behaviors, their thinking and behavioral patterns continue. It is also just as important to ask clients about the outcomes or consequences of their behaviors. This includes the impact of the behavior not only on the clients but also possibly on other people. Often, behaviors of clients that affect other people will generate a reciprocal environment where they are indirectly impacted (e.g., a client who frequently acts irritable and annoyed with his colleagues may notice that they are less likely to socialize with him over time). Table 3.3 provides some examples of common questions to ask during the intake assessment that can elicit client information about thoughts, emotions, physiological arousal, behaviors, and outcomes/consequences. This table is by no means exhaustive. For a more extensive discussion on automatic thoughts and associated responses, see Chapter 7.

When gathering information about presenting problems, especially within the context of automatic thoughts, it is best to use specific examples. This approach has

Table 3.3. Basic Intake Questions to Assess Thoughts, Emotions, Physiological Arousal, and Behaviors

Thoughts

What just went through your mind?
What thought comes to mind about . . . ?
What were you thinking when you . . . ?

Emotions

What are you feeling right now? (after sharing a thought)
What was your emotional response after having those thoughts?
What were you were feeling when you . . . ?

Physiological Arousal

How does your body feel right now? (after sharing thoughts and emotions)
Is there any part of your body that feels different/uncomfortable when you
   think about . . . ?
What did your body feel like when you . . . ?

Behaviors

What did you do next?
How did you cope with your thought/emotion/physiological arousal?
What were the consequences of your actions?

been repeatedly shown to have an early therapeutic impact that has been linked to an increased likelihood of good client outcomes (Persons & Davidson, 2010). Even more helpful is to use specific examples that are prominent in the client's mind. Such examples tend to be more emotional in content. Examples that are emotionally laden are often ideal because they bring past events more into the present. This can provide some in-the-moment client distress and allow for emotional processing. Beck (2011) explains that these examples often provide the most therapeutically effective automatic thoughts. Even if a client's memory for some of the specific event details is inaccurate, this is not of great concern because the focus here is on attempting to assess cognitive-behavioral response patterns of stressful events. Sometimes, you can facilitate this process by attempting to get the client to talk in first-person, present-tense language.

The following are two vignettes from Video Case Examples PDA-1 and MDD-1 demonstrating CBT assessment of presenting problems. The first vignette focuses on problem identification, frequency, duration, and intensity; impact on daily life. The second vignette focuses on precipitating and maintaining factors; automatic thoughts, emotions, and behaviors. Following each vignette are discussion questions. There is also an activity after the second vignette.

VIDEO VIGNETTE 3.1

PDA-1: CBT Assessment—Presenting Problems

Therapist: So if you can, just generally describe to me what these panic attacks feel like. If you want you can start with how your body feels.

Client: Yeah, my chest gets really tight, and that's usually the first sign for me. Then my breathing becomes very labored.

Therapist: The breathing is fast and . . .

Client: Yeah, and just taking a deep breaths and I try to stay aware of those things, but then I feel my body shaking, I feel like I'm losing control.

———————————

Client: I just feel like I'm losing control. It's almost like I'm having an out-of-body experience. I can't control it, I feel like I'm dying . . .

Therapist: When you say "dying," are there any other types of thoughts that you have?

Client: No, it's just like I'm having a heart attack and I don't know what to do to make it stop.

Therapist: Okay. So, that can get pretty scary if you think you're having a heart attack, your chest is tight. . . . So, we have the thoughts of losing control, maybe having a heart attack. Those are some of the common symptoms of panic attacks.

———————————

Therapist: One thing I just want to check with you is how long have these panic attacks been going on?

Client: I would say throughout the past year and half. But it's gotten really bad in the last 6 to 8 months.

Therapist: The last 6 to 8 months it's gotten pretty bad, okay, and we'll get to that in a second as well. The past year and a half they've been going on. So, that's a good period of time. Now we're here to try to help you out with that. I know it has probably varied over the past year and a half, but do you know over the past couple of months how many of these panic attacks you've had in a week?

Client: Maybe two or three?

Therapist: Two or three. Okay. And, how long would you say, in minutes, that these panic attacks last?

Client: Oh gosh, they can be anywhere from 10 minutes to 25 minutes.

Therapist: I can see how that would feel very scary; a panic attack for 25 minutes.

Client: It just feels like it's never going to end.

Therapist: I understand. I know this is a bit of a subjective score and they can vary, but on the scale of 0 to 10, with 10 being the strongest and 0 "doesn't bother me," where would you rate your panic attacks right now?

Client: They always bother me. Um . . . I would say maybe . . . 7 to 10?

Therapist: So, they do get pretty high.

––––––––––––––

Therapist: You mentioned at the beginning that you've been struggling getting outside and doing things.

Client: Yeah.

Therapist: I'd like to flush that out a little bit more. Can you tell me what that's like for you?

Client: Well, I just feel safer at home in terms of knowing what my ritual is. So, say when a panic attack happens, it's like whenever I leave the house, I don't know when it's going to hit or how I'm going to respond to it. I just don't know. I don't like going anywhere without my husband. He's started doing a lot of the grocery shopping for me because it's an area I start to feel labored breathing and I can feel the onset of the panic attack.

Therapist: So, when you're in the grocery store, you can feel those panic attacks.

Client: Yes, yes.

Therapist: Does it feel a little bit of a relief that you don't have to now go to the grocery store?

Client: Absolutely. It's really taken a load off in that sense. Even something as simple as taking my dog for a walk. I can stick within just the immediate 1-mile radius of the house, but anything past that I really start to freak out, and I'm just so scared that I'm going to have another panic attack.

Therapist: Now you told me you can do a few things to go out . . .

Client: Yeah . . .

Therapist: But is that by yourself or is that with some help . . . sometimes you do go to restaurants and do things?

Client: Initially, I was okay on my own, but I just felt like the more these panic attacks happened then the more expected they are. I just don't know what to anticipate, so I do feel better when my husband's with me.

Therapist: Okay.

Client: I have my best friend.

Therapist: Do you feel like he makes you feel safe?

Client: Yeah . . .

Therapist: . . . and comfortable?

Client: Yeah . . .

———————————

Therapist: One of the key points I wanted to ask you a question about is how are these panic attacks and agoraphobia impacting your daily life. One of the things that you just mentioned is school. You said you're an MBA student?

Client: Yeah.

Therapist: You're working what you would call a near graduate-level full-time schedule. You told me how that's one area you've been doing well, but now it's starting to impact you there?

Client: Yeah, the only way I know how to describe it is that I'm so scared of having a panic attack in class. Even just knowing that the professor might call on me to answer a question . . . I get stressed out thinking about what happens if whenever I start to respond, I start to hyper-ventilate or something that's going to lead to a panic attack. But even beyond school, just going out to eat with my friends after class isn't even something I can do anymore.

Therapist: You can't even do that with them as a group?

Client: No, I just feel better with my husband or someone really close to me who knows how to respond. And it's embarrassing.

Therapist: So instead of going to eat with your friends after class, you just go home with your husband.

Client: Yeah, yeah.

Therapist: Okay.

Client: And there's been a couple of times that I might leave class a little bit early just to miss the traffic or . . . something, I mean kind of excuse myself or give other people excuses. But really it's just I start to get so scared of having another panic attack that now my grades are really suffering from it.

Therapist: Oh, okay. So it's not just in the classroom, in the moment, it's what I call a residual effect too as well. Is it hard to study, get the papers done, the exams done?

Client: Yeah, and then I'm missing material that's being taught in class, and . . .

Discussion Questions 3.1

- What information provided in the intake support that Lindsey is having panic attacks and agoraphobic behaviors?
- What additional information would you like to know about Lindsey's presenting problems?
- What are your concerns about how Lindsay's presenting problems are impacting her daily life?
- Are Lindsey's husband behaviors (e.g., going the grocery store) helpful to her? Explain.

VIDEO VIGNETTE 3.2

MDD-1: CBT Assessment—Presenting Problems

Therapist: You've had multiple episodes, right? And you feel like you're kind of stuck in a rut, right now. What I want to talk about is—it's not always clear, but sometimes there are patterns or triggers—is anything that comes to your mind when these depressive episodes happen?

Client: I think that one of the things is that I definitely feel really lonely, especially back in high school where I'd see my friends post something up on Facebook that I wasn't a part of . . . and I feel bad.

Therapist: Okay.

Client: I feel really lonely . . . and like, why wasn't I invited? Why wasn't I included in this? And I don't know, I think those were one of the first couple times that I definitely felt the little ruts. It was because I was really isolated, and I think that's one of the reasons why when I actually spend time with my friends, I felt better.

Therapist: Right. Makes sense in a lot of ways.

Client: Even thinking about it right now it makes sense to me. I think one of the things right now that has just really been tough for me is all the work that I do at work. I mean, it is a reflection of myself, but I take it really hard . . . and it just kind of keeps whacking me down that I feel awful when I'm not able to get a job posting up in time, when I'm not able to get someone hired in time when I need to fill a position that is essential.

Therapist: What I'd like to talk about is what you've done, either in the past or in the present, to help cope. For example, the loneliness, or the work, or the relationship, to see the details of how that plays into your depression.

Client: Yeah. I mean, I think one of the best things was spending time with people. I mean, when I was younger, that would always be my go-to way to snap out of a tough week—spend time with people. Most recently, spending time with my dog has been one of the most helpful things that lets me get out of the house. I'm not looking at the piles of clothes, the piles of dishes; I'm not getting into arguments with Melissa. It's just me and the dog walking. I think that's something that's helped me to kind of cope with some of the emotions I'm going through right now.

Therapist: It does sound like recently it's been tough to even get out with the dog.

Client: Yeah, it's walking him around the house as opposed to actually going to the dog park. And I made some friends when I was there. I had a couple good people.

Therapist: At the park, right.

Client: I don't even see them anymore. I feel like I can't quite cope that way anymore. I feel like I'm more kind of withdrawing . . . going upstairs and playing video games all night as opposed to actually trying to do something active. I'm just kind of secluding myself and just kind of shutting out the outside world.

Therapist: Okay. In one way, that is what we would say is positive coping . . . like you said more than a few times, go out and do something with your friend, your wife, your dog.

Client: Yeah.

Therapist: On the flip side is some of your other, for a lack of a better word, not so effective coping skills, has been more of like withdrawal.

Client: Yeah.

Therapist: I bet you it feels a little bit okay to play video games, but in the long term it's like, "I didn't go out with my wife or hang out with my friends" or "I didn't go to the park and socialize with other people."

Client: Yeah. And that was one of things to do during tough times . . . back in high school I was playing these games with my friends.

Therapist: Okay.

Client: I mean every once in a while I've been able to play with them and kind of keep in touch, but now it's more just kind of like you said, withdrawing and seclusion.

Therapist: I think in college when you were younger, people joke "video games blah, blah, blah," but you're socializing. It's what some guys do to socialize, but you don't have that option as much anymore.

Client: Yeah.

Therapist: What I'd like to do is talk about an event that's recently happened over the past couple of days. When we talked earlier you said it's been a rough couple of days.

Client: Yeah.

Therapist: It helps me a little bit to understand these thoughts, emotions, and behaviors. You may not be aware, but . . . even when you're not doing something is still an action, right?

Client: Yeah.

Therapist: An action is a choice. Can you give me that example of something that's happened in the past couple of days that's been, as you describe, eating away at you?

Client: What comes right to mind is I tried to hang out with my buddy George this weekend.

Therapist: Okay.

Client: Again, he's one of those guys from that group of elementary school friends that I've been friends with forever, but we've been kind of going our separate ways recently. I mean, he's really busy. He's an investment banker. I tried calling him the other day and I got him—typically sometimes it goes to voice mail—but he was short with me. I would think that if he had called me I would've been like, "Oh hey George! How's it going?" Instead all I got was like, "Hey Mark, I can't really talk too much right now. Is this important? Can I get back to you?" And that was really tough for me to hear. I wanted to ask him if he wanted to watch the latest HBO show. We love *Game of Thrones*. We love it. And, I was so down that he wouldn't even hear me out, to what I even wanted to talk about. It was, "I don't have enough time for this/you." That's what I heard.

Therapist: It's what he didn't say that's tough, right?

Client: He said he didn't have time right now . . .

Therapist: Okay.

Client: But, you're right. That's how I took it.

Therapist: Kind of personally. I noticed you also said, "Well, if it was me this is how I would've responded."

Client: Yeah.

Therapist: But it wasn't you. It was him, right?

Client: Yeah . . . yeah.

Therapist: One of the things we'll talk about is maybe some assumptions were made there.

Client: Yeah.

Therapist: I can definitely understand your emotions based upon how you perceived that event.

Client: Yeah.

Therapist: To give you some credit, it took you some courage . . .

Client: Yeah.

Therapist: It's been a while since you've hung out or done anything with him.

Client: Yeah . . . yeah.

Therapist: You finally got ahold of him on the phone and he says, "Ah, I'm too busy for you."

Client: Yeah.

Therapist: And so all these thoughts—I'm already noticing a little bit of a theme here in terms of when you're at work when you do the job postings—and you said it yourself, you personalize it/internalize it. Then, over here . . . was his name George?

Client: Yeah, George.

Therapist:	He's really busy.
Client:	Yeah.
Therapist:	He told you he was busy, but it was still tough for you. You really personalized it.
Client:	Yeah.
Therapist:	And you haven't heard back from him or anything like that?
Client:	Yeah, no. He said that he was going to call me the next day. He never did. And I never called him again because I took his word for it.
Therapist:	Right, right. It sounds like you fill in that ambiguity with your thoughts or perceptions?
Client:	Yeah . . . yeah.
Therapist:	In this case with your depressive episode, you're not only personalizing it, but also making a negative assumption of it.
Client:	Okay.
Therapist:	That's one thing that we can work on, as well as some of those assumptions of personalizing things, where you're assuming what one thinks when you don't really know.
Client:	Yeah.
Therapist:	Who knows, maybe he'll call you in a day or two and say, "Look Mark, I was really busy, let's do it."
Client:	Right . . . right.
Therapist:	But, in the moment you're not thinking that way at all.
Client:	Right.

Discussion Questions 3.2

- How do you conceptualize Mark's precipitating and maintaining factors in relation to his depression? In other words, what themes do you notice with his thoughts, emotions, and behaviors across contexts?
- What additional information would you like to know about Marks's presenting problems?
- What are your concerns about how Mark's presenting problems are impacting his daily life?
- What themes did you notice in Mark's negative automatic thoughts patterns (e.g., cognitive distortions and assumptions)?

ACTIVITY 3.1: CBT ASSESSMENT—PRESENTING PROBLEMS

With a partner, practice role-playing assessing a specific problem. Take a few minutes to make up a presenting problem (keep it simple) and then take turns asking questions related to CBT assessment: frequency, duration, intensity, impact on life, precipitating and maintaining factors, automatic thoughts, emotions, and behaviors. It is okay for the person with the problem to "make up" this information during the role play. At this point, do not worry about doing this perfectly—you will learn more specific skills in future chapters. For now, the focus here is for the interviewer to practice asking questions based on the information provided about the problem. Consider what is most challenging when asking questions about the problem. Notice if any particular types of questions are more effective than others. Do your best to connect events to thoughts to emotions to physiological arousal to behaviors to consequences (take notes!).

Motivation and Responsibility for Change

The concept of client motivation to change is not unique for most therapeutic approaches. However, formally assessing client motivation to change is not common when treating many disorders (the major exception here is substance abuse; Moyers & Houck, 2011). Research consistently shows that the more clients are motivated to change, including levels of hope and optimism, the better therapeutic outcomes they have relative to clients who are not motivated to change (DiClemente, Nidecker, & Bellack, 2008). Accordingly, it makes sense to consider the level of motivation clients have to change their maladaptive thinking and behavioral patterns early in therapy in order to make the necessary adjustments for treatment goals and determine how interventions are implemented.

It may seem odd that some clients attend therapy but are not motivated to change. However, there are a couple of things to consider. First, some clients may be attending because they have to complete therapy (e.g., mandated by court) or are attending reluctantly (e.g., ultimatum from significant other). Second, some clients are attending therapy fully on their own volition, but their expectations are that they are not responsible for their own change. Their reasons can range from expecting that the therapist should be responsible for their change to a strong adherence to the medical model (e.g., chemical imbalance). In either scenario, there is a theme of external responsibility for change.

When asking questions about motivation, consider these three key domains: (a) How much does the client actually want to change (i.e., motivation)? (b) What does the client expect to get out of therapy? (c) What is the client's own perception of responsibility for change (i.e., internal vs. external)? (d) Does the client have any hope or optimism that therapy will help? In sum, the more you know about a client's motivation to change, the more you can confidently make any necessary therapeutic relationship and treatment planning adjustments for optimum effectiveness.

The following are two vignettes from Video Case Examples PDA-2 and MDD-2 demonstrating CBT assessment of motivation to change. Following the vignettes are discussion questions.

VIDEO VIGNETTE 3.3

PDA-2: CBT Assessment—Motivation to Change

Therapist: I want to talk about what you would like to get out of therapy.

Client: Well, I just want to get my life back.

Therapist: In what way? What would that look like?

Client: Just the quality of life. Being able to . . . like, take my dog on a hike again. Maybe go grocery shopping.

Therapist: Start going out and doing those things that you can't do anymore. Maybe alone too?

Client: Yeah.

Therapist: To some degree. And your panic attack symptoms—what would they look to you if they started to improve?

Client: I mean, if we have any say in it, they wouldn't exist. They would go away.

Therapist: So, have those panic attacks gone and no more agoraphobia, right? That would be the perfect scenario?

Client: That would be ideal, yes.

Therapist: What I can tell you is that although we can't promise or guarantee anything in therapy that way, there a lot of the techniques and interventions that we'll start using in future sessions that have been very successful in helping clients get better.

Client: Okay.

———————————————

Therapist: What are your thoughts about therapy being able to help you? Are you hopeful or optimistic? What are you thinking right now as you sit here?

Client: I think that this is probably one of the better opportunities I've been given because nothing I've tried in the past has worked yet.

Therapist: You've tried going to the hospitals . . . the medical doctors . . .

Client: Yeah.

Therapist: I see a little bit of trepidation but I understand that. We've just met and we're talking about these things for the first time. I'm glad that at least there's a little bit of hope there that we can work on this. That's very helpful for us.

Client: Absolutely. I'm willing to do anything at this point.

Therapist: Right. And like we mentioned earlier, you already started doing something. It may not seem like much, but being able to make the call to come here, walking here, and sitting here for the first session is really a big start. And for what it's worth, I'm pretty hopeful, too.

———————————————

Therapist: What are your thoughts about having to start working on changing the way you think and behave in terms of your role in therapy?

Client: Will you help me through that process?

Therapist: Oh, I definitely will be there with you, yeah.

Client: Okay.

Therapist:	Especially in the beginning. I'll be leading the way to some degree and later on, you may find yourself taking the charge of that as well.
Client:	Okay.
Therapist:	So I'll always be there working with you as well.
Client:	As long as I have some help, I'm absolutely willing.
Therapist:	Right, a lot of it is what we call a collaborative relationship.
Client:	Okay.

VIDEO VIGNETTE 3.4

MDD-2: CBT Assessment—Motivation to Change

Therapist:	Mark, what you would like to get out of therapy?
Client:	I think one of the obvious things is I want to stop being so depressed. I mean I think that's kind of obvious. I'd like to be able to spend maybe some more time with my friends, my dog, and my girlfriend. I think getting my life back in those areas and then the work life will follow.
Therapist:	Your priorities—you feel comfortable the work life will follow? But especially focus on you your friends and your wife.
Client:	Yeah. I think especially those relationships are something that I really want to get back to working on.
Therapist:	Okay. That makes sense. And also too, maybe not necessarily a priority, but getting stuff done; some of those tasks.
Client:	Yes.
Therapist:	I only say that because it seems to also play a role in your relationship with your wife, at least at home; chores and tasks.
Client:	Yeah.

Therapist:	How do you see your role as we work toward helping you be less depressed?
Client:	I think part of it is I wish it were as easy as just snapping my fingers and making it go away. I understand that that's not something that you can do. But, I'm not quite sure how much work I'm actually going to have to do. So, I think that's something that I need to figure out or kind of work through.
Therapist:	Yeah, and I think that's something that you'll learn between the rest of today and the next couple of sessions is that our roles will be a collaborative process.
Client:	Okay.
Therapist:	Sometimes it depends on other people's past experiences with therapy. And, as you said, it's not just therapy. It doesn't just magically get better.
Client:	Yeah.
Therapist:	Therapy can definitely help initially. What you'll find is I'm going to be there to support and guide and direct us initially. But as we progress and as you start to feel a little bit better, some of the role will become more and more your responsibility as well.

Client:	Okay. Alright. It sounds . . .
Therapist:	A little daunting at first?
Client:	Yeah. I mean, I'm not quite sure like how much I'm actually going to be capable of.
Therapist:	And, that's okay. Like I said, it will be on my shoulders to make the clinical judgments.
Client:	Okay.
Therapist:	And I always will check in and get your feedback, and we'll bounce it back and forth.
Client:	Okay.
Therapist:	This is down the road, but the ultimate goal is eventually when you're feeling a little bit better, that you'll feel like you're more in control of your life in general and have more autonomy.

Therapist:	How would you consider now your hope or motivation to change?
Client:	I'm sitting in here today. I definitely feel a little bit of hope.
Therapist:	Okay.
Client:	I mean I feel a little proud that I at least I came here and made the appointment. I'm in here meeting with you. I guess Melissa asked me to do it, so I at least feel good that I'm in here. But as far as the long-term outlook, I'm not quite sure yet.
Therapist:	Yeah, right.
Client:	I mean things have been rough for a while now, and they've just been getting tougher, so it's going to take a while before things get better, so I'm just not sure.
Therapist:	No, and you're absolutely right about taking a while before things get better. Like you alluded to earlier, it's not a quick fix.
Client:	Yeah.
Therapist:	I give you a lot of credit for you coming here, and I agree. Thinking long term, it's kind of hard, especially with some of the level of depression you've been describing.
Client:	Yeah.
Therapist:	For what it's worth, we can't guarantee any outcome, but I sincerely mean it when I tell you that I'm pretty hopeful too.
Client:	Yeah, okay.
Therapist:	The way you've been able to come in here and articulate some of your thoughts and feelings, you seem to have a pretty good insight.
Client:	Yeah.
Therapist:	You know, of course there's stuff to work on and the fact that you're able to at least verbalize a little bit of hope, that's very helpful.

Discussion Questions 3.3

Discuss the similarities and differences between the two clients about the following:

- Their motivation to change
- What they want to get out of therapy
- Their perception of responsibility to change (i.e., internal vs. external)
- What hope or optimism they have that therapy will help

Formal Symptom Measures and Formative Assessment

Although many therapists use formal symptom assessments, their use is especially important for CBT therapists, as they can provide a relatively objective means to assess symptom distress over time. In other words, not only are these assessments helpful during the intake, but they should also be used continuously to monitor treatment progress. In fact, therapists who continuously assess client symptom distress have better client outcomes compared to therapists who do not (Lambert et al., 2003; Reese, Norsworthy, & Rowlands, 2009). In many ways, it is surprising that more therapists do not continuously use assessments considering how many are available that are easy to administer and score, time efficient, and well validated. Assessment in therapy is not a summative, "one-shot" event at the beginning and end of therapy. Rather, a good CBT therapist understands that assessment is a formative process where monitoring client progress is continuous with ongoing feedback. This process provides information for the therapist and the client for any necessary therapeutic modifications that need to be made during therapy instead of finding out at the end of therapy (which is often too late).

Clients may reveal significantly meaningful information that might not otherwise be revealed face-to-face, especially during the intake and initial sessions of therapy, when the therapeutic alliances is in the early stage of development. For example, a client might verbally deny abusing alcohol during the intake assessment but endorsed a few self-report items indicating high frequency of drinking alcohol and concerns from others. Thus, sometimes it is helpful to review responder to individual assessment questions. This information can then be used for sensitive follow-up inquires for clarification.

As for when formal assessments should be administered, it is often best to do so right before the intake session starts. Most symptom assessments are client self-report (or caregiver) measures that typically do not take much time to complete. These assessments are also relatively easy to score and interpret. Thus, feedback can be provided to the client soon after being completed with immediate information that can be used in session concurrently. For assessments that take longer to complete and/or score, it is best to use them less frequently and allow time between sessions to interpret and provide feedback.

For any assessment that you plan to use during the intake and for future sessions, you should know how to administer and score them correctly. Additionally, you must know how to interpret the score and its clinical utility. This also includes knowing how to provide feedback to clients in a clear and meaningful way.

The following are two vignettes from Video Case Examples PDA-3 and MDD-3 demonstrating CBT assessment with formal symptom assessments. Following the vignettes are discussion questions and an activity.

VIDEO VIGNETTE 3.5

PDA-3: CBT Assessment—Measures

Therapist: Earlier, when we met you filled out some intake information. Because you told me a little about your panic symptoms and agoraphobia I had you fill out a couple scales. One of them is the Panic Disorder Severity Scale. It doesn't take too long for me to score and look them over, and I just wanted to go over those today with you. So, what I have here is the Panic Disorder Severity Scale. Before I go through this a little bit, I want to ask you what was it like filling out this assessment?

Client: I just think that it really raised a lot of awareness. Some of the stuff I've been avoiding.

Therapist: So, when you had to go through and circle all these symptoms it brought it to the surface a little bit for you?

Client: Yeah, it kind of caught me off guard. I didn't realize how many things I had been avoiding.

Therapist: Yeah. And so, what we have here are the panic symptoms . . . and, when I was just going through here they seemed to match what we were discussing earlier, which is good. You mentioned the pounding heart, the sweating, the shaking, the difficulty breathing, and even the chest pain discomfort. And, you even mentioned a little bit of chills and hot flushes. And we talked a few times this—the fear of losing control or going crazy and fear of dying.

Client: Yeah.

Therapist: Now, the scale is "only" seven questions, right? But they're pretty in depth and are helpful. What this scale does is it actually gives a score, which gives me a frame of reference of what's going on here. This scale here has a score range of 0 to 28. You scored a 21. This is considered markedly distressed. What does that mean? Basically, it means you're scoring on the pretty high end of being anxious for panic symptoms.

Client: Yeah.

Therapist: It sounds not too surprising?

Client: No, I'm not surprised at all.

Therapist: No, especially once you started filling out those initial questions with the symptoms, right?

Client: Yeah.

Therapist: Now the reason why we fill this out is because it is very helpful for me to track your symptoms. Even though you did a really good job telling me about your panic symptoms and your agoraphobia it's helpful to have objective measures to help track your symptoms. To me it's a good sign that what you told me verbally is also matching what you filled out. Does that make sense?

Client: Yes.

Therapist: The other thing is you're probably going to see these again in the future, meaning this assessment and the agoraphobia scale. Because one way of tracking effectiveness of treatment is to give continuous assessment over time. So, every couple of sessions or so I'll have you fill these out. They don't take too long. Right now, you're probably thinking "jeez, 21 out of 28," right? But, who knows, maybe over a few weeks down the line we can track and see that score decrease.

Client: Okay.

VIDEO VIGNETTE 3.6

MDD-3: CBT Assessment—Measures

Therapist: You already explained a little bit of your reaction to a couple questions on the depression scale. I went through them as well and when I was scoring it I highlighted a few of them.

Client: Yeah.

Therapist: You took this before we spoke, but after the intake and now looking at this it makes sense.

Client: Yeah.

Therapist: For "self-dislike" you chose "I am disappointed in myself."

Client: Yeah.

Therapist: What was your initial reaction to that question?

Client: Well, I think those were kind of some of the tougher questions for me to answer; especially with everything that's been going on at work, we've been having a lot of turnover lately and I've been having to look for a lot new people to hire. And, when I fail at that it really hits me hard.

Therapist: Yeah.

Client: I think that by putting it on paper made me realize how upset I am with myself when I don't do something successfully. It's upsetting to me and I blame myself . . . I'm really not worthy of the job. I'm not doing a good enough job. I'm not helping the company and I'm just holding people back.

Therapist: It's funny you say that. When I read this I immediately thought of your job and your work—really being critical of yourself for your faults. I think that this is helpful for us, not just the overall score. Even for our treatment goals and interventions I think you'll probably agree that working on your self-worth in relation to your job can be helpful; and I'm sure this may translate to your relationships. You seem pretty hard on yourself.

Client: Yeah.

Therapist: There are a couple questions here I wanted to look a little bit into for the hopelessness scale. One here you wrote down '"True. I might as well give up because there's nothing I can do about making things better for myself." What does that mean?

Client: It's one of those things where this has been going on for a while and I'm really wondering if I'm going to be able to make the changes necessary. I just kind of . . . that seed of doubt where . . . is this going to kind of all be worth it in the end? Is it going to be worth my time? Is it going to be something I'm going to be capable of doing? There's that doubt.

Therapist: That doubt.

Client: It's just always there.

Therapist: As soon as you said that word I was thinking the same thing—you kind of have that self-doubt if things are going to change or get better.

Client: Yeah.

Therapist: And to some degree, I understand where you're coming from. It's been 10, 12, 13 years since your first depressive episode and they've been getting progressively longer and more intense.

Client: Yeah.

Therapist: I can't promise anything, but I can assure that we're going to do our best. You're here and I hope to see you again in the weeks to come. We're going to try to work on this more.

Client: Okay.

Therapist: I think what's helpful with therapy, especially with behavior activation, is when you start to eventually experience that change for yourself. If you're willing to at least give it a shot each week with me hopefully that can show you it's possible that you can make these changes.

Client: Okay.

Discussion Questions 3.4

- How would you describe each client's response and receptiveness to reviewing the assessments?
- How can information from theses assessments be helpful so early in therapy for each client?
- What are some potential benefits to explaining and providing feedback about these assessments to each client?
- How is providing an overall symptoms score helpful to the client or treatment?
- Why is it helpful to review responses to individual questions from assessments?

ACTIVITY 3.2: CBT ASSESSMENT—MEASURES

Administer a symptom measure to yourself. Read the administration instructions and score it as instructed. Without discussing individual scores, you can share the experience or process of completing the assessment with your peers. Does this experience influence/change how you would respond to your clients after completing an assessment? You can also practice administering an assessment and providing feedback on scores and responses. Carefully consider what information is worth reviewing and how it is communicated.

CBT CASE FORMULATION

The CBT case formulation typically follows soon after the intake assessment and is vital for purposeful, efficient, and effective treatment planning (Kuyken, Padesky, & Dudley, 2009; Persons, 2008). Your CBT case formulation is essentially a cognitive-behavioral conceptualization of the presenting problems, associated symptoms, and contributing factors. This process begins with your first meetings with clients and continues to be modified throughout treatment as new information is gathered and they make progress toward their goals. All of the relevant information gathered in the preceding "Intake Interview Basics" and "CBT Assessment" sections should be integrated into your case formulation. Any additional information about clients' automatic thoughts, emotions, and behaviors can be especially helpful in developing an initial conceptualization that considers the interaction between their symptoms, problems, and environment. There are a variety of ways in which a case formulation can be developed, often depending on your agency. The following sections are based on the case conceptualization guidelines established by the Academy of Cognitive Therapy (http://www.academyofct.org). Even if the agency you serve has a different template, you can still integrate the following information in a manner that fits a true CBT case formulation.

Before moving forward, it is important to remember one of the key themes from Chapter 2 about the collaborative nature of CBT. The working alliance between therapist and client begins during the intake process, including case formulation and treatment plan development. There should always be some level of input and involvement from the client when developing these two documents. Making it a joined activity will not only provide added insight for the development but also model the importance of CBT collaboration. Furthermore, clients who play a role in developing a conceptualization of their distress and symptoms, along with assisting in what and how problems are treated, may be more likely to be motivated and hopeful for change than clients who are not involved in the process (Persons, 2008).

Precipitating and Maintaining Factors Summary

This section is relatively straightforward if you collected the necessary information in the "Presenting Problems" section. Here, precipitants are considered significant life events that have contributed to the development of the client's current distress. These precipitants can be psychosocial and/or biological. Activating situations are small-scale events (i.e., typical day-to-day activities) that incite clients' preexisting dysfunctional thoughts, emotions, and behaviors. For maintaining factors, focus on key actions or events that continue or exacerbate the effect of the precipitants. More specifically, it is typically most effective to focus on what the client has done to cope when experiencing distress related to the precipitants: both effective and ineffective strategies. Of course, any environmental factors that are maintaining the problems should also be included.

Cross-Sectional View of Cognitions, Emotions, and Behaviors

The cross-sectional view includes looking at current ("here and now") patterns of precipitants and activating situations that incite maladaptive automatic thoughts, emotions, physiological sensations, and behaviors. This approach focuses on the automatic thought patterns typically identified during the intake and early sessions. The information gathered in the "Presenting Problems" section fits well here. (Underlying core beliefs are part of the longitudinal view.) Thus, early in therapy, the cross-sectional view will have the most practical utility, as it can provide an initial—but flexible—cognitive-behavioral conceptualization of clients' distress and presenting problems.

Longitudinal View of Cognitions, Emotions, and Behaviors

The longitudinal view takes into account developmental events and other possible life-shaping influences. This approach develops more fully as therapy proceeds as underlying core beliefs begin to become more salient and understood by both you and your clients. This can also include enduring patterns of maladaptive behaviors that have mostly been reinforcing and/or maintaining distress. Remember, the information you may have to include in your longitudinal view part of your CBT case formulation may be minimal soon after the client intake. However, this section is still included here because your case formulation will evolve over time with more in-depth knowledge of your client; in turn, this section will considerably expand.

Working Hypothesis

Your working hypothesis is an overall summary for your CBT case formulation. In some ways it can be looked at as a "CBT story" of how clients came to their current distress. Of course, the primary focus of your working hypothesis will be on the development of the clients' present problems and symptoms. However, it is also strongly advised to integrate clients' strengths and assets, as these factors can significantly enhance treatment motivation, engagement, and effectiveness. Additionally, following the cognitive model, if you have enough information, hypothesizing on how clients see themselves, others, the world, and their future can provide added value in understanding their maladaptive thought patterns. Although the information in all sections of the case formulation is important, the working hypothesis will have a direct influence on the development of your treatment goals and interventions. Of course, this section will be ever evolving as more information is obtained during therapy and as clients work toward their goals. As the word "hypothesis" implies, this is a tentative understanding of your clients' symptoms and distress. Scientifically, hypotheses are made to be tested and are sometimes disproved. It is important to keep an open mind that what you might think you know about your client will change over time. This is okay. In fact, this is to be expected. What is key is that your working hypothesis is well informed by the current information but is also flexible enough to be modified when new and/or contradicting information is presented. Remember, the quality of your treatment plan is only as good as the quality of your CBT case formulation, and the working hypothesis is its driving force.

DSM Diagnosis

At some point toward the end of your case formulation, a diagnosis needs to be provided. At the very least, a diagnosis will be required for your agency and for reimbursement from managed care. A formal DSM diagnosis has its value; it helps provide clarity for sources of distress through consolidating multiple symptoms. It can also provide general guidance in treatment direction. Ultimately, the focus of your treatment should go beyond formal diagnostic symptoms and also include problems and level of distress negatively impacting daily functioning. Considering symptoms, problems, and distress is most pragmatic for clinical reasons. First, clients with the "same diagnosis" will present very differently in their problems and level of distress. Also, clients with the same diagnosis can even present with different symptoms according to DSM criteria (e.g., must have five of nine possible symptoms for major depressive disorder). Second, many clients receiving therapy have multiple diagnoses. In other words, this comorbidity means that there are multiple sources of distress across multiple diagnoses. Thus, focusing on key, or primary, overlapping symptoms and problems can often be the most effective means to treat client distress. In fact, this is now commonly referred to as a transdiagnostic approach to treatment. This topic is beyond the scope of this book, but there are some excellent sources available that specifically address transdiagnostic treatment approaches (Barlow et al., 2010; Frank & Davidson, 2014).

Sample Form 3.1 is a sample template for a CBT case formulation and treatment plan. Note that in addition to CBT-related information from assessment, common intake information (case history) should also be included. All case formulations will vary by your agency. The emphasis here is to highlight key case formulation components that are integral for conceptualizing clients' symptoms, problems, and distress through a CBT lens. The CBT treatment plan portion of Sample Form 3.1 is discussed in the next section.

CBT Case Formulation and Treatment Plan Template

CASE HISTORY

<u>**Demographic and Background Information**</u>

Name:	**DOB:**
Gender:	**Race/Ethnicity:**
Relationship Status:	
Therapist:	**Date:**

<u>**Primary Presenting Concern**</u>

<u>**Development and Life History**</u>

<u>**Medical and Mental Health History**</u>

<u>**Interpersonal Relationships**</u>

<u>**Current Presentation**</u>

<u>**Strengths and Assets**</u>

<u>**Contributing Negative Sociocultural Factors**</u>

CBT ASSESSMENT

<u>**Compatibility with CBT**</u>

<u>**Presenting Problems**</u>

1.

2.

3.

(Etc.)

<u>**Motivation and Responsibility to Change**</u>

<u>**Formal Symptom Measures**</u>

CBT CASE FORMULATION

Precipitating and Maintaining Factors Summary

Cross-Sectional View

Longitudinal View

Working Hypothesis

DSM Diagnosis

CBT TREATMENT PLAN

Problem List

1.

2.

3.

(Etc.)

Treatment Goals and Interventions

Goal 1:

Intervention 1:

Intervention 2:

Goal 2: (Etc.)

Anticipated Obstacles

CBT TREATMENT PLAN

Once your case formulation is complete, it is time to develop your treatment plan. As it was stated a few times earlier in this chapter, the information gathered from your CBT assessment and integrated into your CBT case formulation becomes the foundation and driving force for your CBT treatment plan. Typically, most agencies will require a completed treatment plan within the first few weeks of the intake. Thus, the quality of your assessment information and case formulation is important for developing a treatment plan that best meets the needs of your client. Naturally, modifications will be made to the treatment plan over the course of treatment. However, when these modifications are made, they should be based on clients making therapeutic progress and an evolving case formulation. This process ensures that each treatment goal and intervention is purposeful and is within the context of the CBT model. Similar to case formulations, your agency will most likely have a preferred template for treatment plans. Nevertheless, the following sections are generally common across all agencies. Overall, it is essential to have consistency across your case formulation and treatment plan while integrating empirically based interventions.

Problem List

You will notice that this section is similar to the "Presenting Problems" section. However, for your treatment plan, this is a list with a brief description of any significant problems identified by you and your client to be of primary focus during treatment. These problems can occur across multiple domains: mental health symptoms (including substance use/abuse), medical, interpersonal, occupational, daily routine, leisure, sociocultural, financial, and legal/criminal. There is no "ideal" minimum or maximum number; it all depends on the clients' distress and needs. Generally, most lists will have three to six problems. The basic purpose of the problem list is to provide brief, key highlights of your clients' most significant problems. In turn, this list should also act as anchor for your proceeding treatment goals and interventions.

Treatment Goals and Interventions

There should be a logical connection between each treatment goal, the problem list, and the case formulation. Simply put, treatment goals are desired outcomes for the client. These desired outcomes should also be indicators of therapeutic progress by way of reduced symptom distress and improved quality of life. Because these goals are meant to be therapeutic indictors, it is best to make them as objective and measurable possible. These qualities allow you to more accurately track treatment progress for both your client and managed care. For example, for a depressed client, instead of "be less sad," a better goal is "will demonstrate reduced symptoms of depression as indicated by Beck Depression Inventory scores." Instead of "be more social," a better goal is "will engage in at least two social activities per week." Notice

Table 3.4. Treatment Goals: Poor Versus Better

Poor Goals	Better Goals
Will be less sad	Client will demonstrate reduced symptoms of depression as indicated by Beck Depression Inventory scores. *If appropriate, can give specific cutoff scores.
Be more social	Client will engage in at least two social activities per week.
Stop having anger tantrums	Client will reduce tantrums at home by learning and using emotion-focused coping skills, as evidenced by no more than one reported tantrum per week from parents.
Stop being aggressive	Client will learn and implement three problem-focused coping skills to manage confrontations with peers, as evidenced by no acts of aggression reported by school administration.
Talk about thoughts and feelings	Client will identify at least three negative automatic thoughts with associated emotions and behaviors.
Reduce panic attacks by 50%	Client will reduce panic attacks from eight times per week currently to four or fewer times per week.

how the initial goal statements sound like desired outcomes (and in some ways they are), but they are nearly impossible to measure and track due to their subjectivity and resulting lack of measurability. Although such wording may seem like semantics or as being too concrete, it really does make a difference how goals are worded in order to truly monitor progress and provide client feedback. Recall that frequent and accurate assessment of client progress corresponds with treatment effectiveness. Also, the reality is that you will almost always have to demonstrate to managed care that progress is being (or was) made. Using the above examples, simply saying that a client is now "less sad" or "more social" does not allow for enough objective data to be collected and monitored. Table 3.4 provides a simple two-column list of "poor goals" and "better goals" to help demonstrate how to make goals objective and measureable.

If goals are desired client outcomes, then interventions are the processes to achieve these outcomes. In other words, interventions indicate what needs to be done in order to meet each goal. One of the more effective means to provide a clear and succinct treatment plan is to link interventions to each goal. There obviously needs to be at least one intervention per goal, but there is no maximum number. Generally, most goals will have two to four interventions. One of the most important elements for interventions is that they are client specific and at least briefly describe the process. These qualities will provide a clear perspective, or picture, of how therapy will progress for both you and your client. For example, for a depressed client, instead of "cognitive restructuring," a better intervention is "cognitive restructuring for self-defeating, dichotomous automatic thoughts (e.g., I probably did that task wrong; I always let my friends down)." Instead of "behavioral activation," a better intervention is "behavioral activation for morning routine (e.g., getting out of bed by a certain time or completing morning hygiene) and pleasurable activities (e.g., playing favorite music instrument)." Notice how the initial intervention statements may sound appropriate, but they are very generic and still do not describe the process. If an intervention reads as if it can

Table 3.5. Treatment Interventions: Poor Versus Better

Poor Interventions	Better Interventions
Psychoeducation	Psychoeducation of panic attacks (e.g., fight-or-flight response) and the protective and motivating utility of anxiety (e.g., anxiety levels on a continuum). *Then connect to client's specific panic attack symptoms and possible initial triggering false alarm(s) and current learned alarms.
Behavioral activation	Behavioral activation for morning routine (e.g., getting out of bed by a certain time or completing morning hygiene) and pleasurable activities (e.g., playing favorite music instrument). *Then explain the steps to introduce behavioral activation and necessary modifications to the weekly activity monitoring log and daily activity schedule.
Cognitive restructuring	Cognitive restructuring for self-defeating, dichotomous automatic thoughts (e.g., "I probably did that task wrong" or "I always not my friends down."). *Then describe how cognitive restructuring will be done specific to the client (e.g., any particular Socratic questioning techniques).
Hierarchy of feared situations	Provide rational for hierarchy of feared situations, identify and rank feared situations, and identify unhelpful coping strategies. *Then describe how the hierarchy for exposure will be developed specific to your client's fears (and note if imaginal or in vivo exposure).

simply be applied to any client with depression, anxiety, and so on, then it is probably not client specific and descriptive enough. It is also helpful to provide a brief description of how each intervention will be applied. Using the two examples above, describing how cognitive restructuring or behavioral activation will be applied provides greater client specificity. Similar to the previous discussion on goals, Table 3.5 provides a simple two-column list of "poor interventions" and "better interventions" to help demonstrate how to make interventions client specific and descriptive.

Anticipated Obstacles

This section can include any possible difficulties that might arise in the therapeutic relationship or other aspects of treatment. This part of the treatment plan is not meant to be negative or pessimistic but rather to prepare for and anticipate potential factors that might impede the therapeutic process. Stated differently, this is largely a preventive approach.

Therapeutic Relationship Considerations

This section simply notes the nature and quality of the current therapeutic relationship. Many times, this section may be only one or two sentences if it is a "typical" therapeutic relationship and the client appears to be at least moderately engaged and motivated to change. However, there may be times when there are current or potential problems that could hinder the therapeutic relationship. If so, it is best to note these problems immediately and be sure that they are monitored and addressed. If possible, you can indicate possible problem-focused and/or interpersonal approaches that can be used to help repair the relationship or avoid future damage to the relationship. Recall from Chapter 2 that it is vital to maintain a working collaborative alliance for effective CBT. A poor therapeutic relationship significantly increases the chances for poor therapeutic outcomes. There are many contributing relationship factors that you cannot change (e.g., race/ethnicity, gender, and lifestyle), but this does not preclude you from putting forth a concerted effort in establishing and maintaining a collaborative working alliance.

Client-Specific Factors

Beyond the therapeutic relationship, there may be client-specific factors that hinder therapy effectiveness. Although key problems for clients should already be addressed through the problem list and corresponding treatment goals and interventions, there may be particular elements of their distress that may require additional attention than typically necessary. For example, a client who has social phobia, by definition, has a fear of social evaluation by others. However, if this fear of social evaluation is especially strong in particular contexts, it can be helpful to make note of this to be sure that appropriate therapeutic accommodations are made. In other cases, a client-specific factor may be more of a general trait/disposition of the client. For example, a client who has generalized anxiety disorder may have an exceptionally perfectionistic personality trait. Although perfectionism is not uncommon in clients with anxiety disorders, awareness of such strong personality characteristics can aid in making necessary modifications in the collaborative working alliance (e.g., trust), which may influence how certain interventions are implemented.

External Factors

There also may be factors that are external to the client but are potential obstacles to achieving treatment goals. In other words, sometimes there are external factors that are outside of control of the therapist–client therapeutic relationship. Nevertheless, the external nature of such factors does not preclude you from taking the necessary steps to minimize the impact of these factors through problem-solving and coping skills. For example, a client recently found out that there will be layoffs at his job due to budget cuts. Although this is most likely bad news with potential financial repercussions, there are still options for the therapist and client to problem solve in response to this life stressor (e.g., financial planning or job searching). There can also be external factors that may be more sociocultural. For example, a client is experiencing racial discrimination in her community from her neighbors. It may not be possible to immediately change the situation (e.g., move), but there are still options to cope with the associated stressors (e.g., assertiveness, empowerment, or advocacy).

See Sample Form 3.1 again to review the CBT treatment plan. Similar to your case formulation, all treatment plans will vary by your agency. The emphasis here is to recognize that each goal should have at least one intervention "connected" to it. Also recognize that a problem list should be developed before goals and interventions. This problem list comes from your CBT case formulation. All problems contributing to your clients' distress should be addressed through your treatment goals and interventions. This is also space to note any anticipated obstacles to your treatment.

ACTIVITY 3.3: CBT CASE FORMULATION AND TREATMENT PLAN

Watch the full Video Case Examples for CBT Assessment (PDA-1–3 and MDD-1–3). For each case, use Sample Form 3.1 to fill in as much information as possible from the assessment to develop a tentative CBT case formulation. Of course, you will not have all information available to fully complete each section. If you want, you can make an educated hypothesis for any missing information. Then use Sample Form 3.1 to develop a tentative CBT treatment plan based on your CBT case formulation. Again, you do not have all client information available to you, but you can still work on appropriate wording of treatment goals linking relevant interventions. If you are not familiar with appropriate treatment for major depressive disorder or panic disorder and agoraphobia, you can research appropriate resources. When complete, discuss with your peers the similarities and differences between your case formulations and treatment plans. Consider: Can your care formulation and treatment plans be different but potentially equally effective?

COMMON CHALLENGES FOR CBT ASSESSMENT, CASE FORMULATION, AND TREATMENT PLANNING

Table 3.6 provides some common examples of challenges that can be experienced with CBT assessment or developing a CBT case formulation and treatment plan. The theme for many of the possible considerations for responses is being sure enough information has been gathered, that the client has been involved in the process, and that you are flexible in your approach.

Table 3.6. Common Challenges for CBT Assessment, Case Formulation, and Treatment Planning

Challenge	Possible Considerations
Client might have low compatibility for CBT	Consider possible concerns (i.e., therapeutic alliance, identifying automatic thoughts and associated emotions, or working within a goal and problem-oriented focus). Determine the reasons for your concern and make necessary adjustments. May require more psychoeducation, time, and patience. Remember that such individuals can benefit the most from CBT.
Difficulty developing a conceptual understanding of the presenting problems	Was enough case history gathered from the intake? Was enough information about presenting problems gathered (e.g., frequency, duration, intensity, or impact on daily life; precipitating and maintaining factors; automatic thoughts, emotions, and associated behavioral responses; and data from formal assessments)? Determine what domains of information are lacking and follow up with the client. Draw a visual diagram that connects life history, current problems, automatic thoughts (core beliefs), emotions, behaviors/consequences, and significant sociocultural and environmental factors.
Difficulty effectively providing feedback for formal symptom measures	Review the manual for interpretation of scoring and communicating with clients. Take the assessment yourself and interpret your own scores—consider what feedback would be most helpful to you. Clearly communicate the relationship between assessment scores, presenting problems, and treatment goals.
Poor agreement on case formulation and/or treatment plan	Was there collaborative development from the beginning? Provide clarification of expectations for therapy. Request feedback for changes in a nondefensive manner. Show a clear relationship between presenting problems, conceptualization, and treatment goals.
Treatment plan appears to not be effective	Was enough time given to apply interventions for each goal? Is there a good goal/intervention match? Consider timing of goals/interventions. Are goals realistic—proximal and possible? Is the client engaged and motivated? Are appropriate problems identified? Be flexible and make adjustments to how interventions are implemented while considering the context of the client's presenting problems. Consider if client is fearful of negative evaluation.

REFERENCES

Barlow, D. H., Farchione, T. J., Fairholme, C. P., Ellard, K. K., Boisseau, C. L., Allen, L. B., et al. (2010). *Unified protocol for transdiagnostic treatment of emotional disorders: Therapist guide*. New York: Oxford University Press

Beck, J. S. (2011). *Cognitive behavior therapy: Basics and beyond* (2nd ed.). New York: Guilford Press.

Burns, D. D., Rude, S., Simons, A. D., Bates, M. A., & Thase, M. E. (1994). Does learned resourcefulness predict the response to cognitive behavioral therapy for depression? *Cognitive Therapy and Research, 18,* 277–291.

Dew, S., & Bickman, L. (2005). Client expectancies about therapy. *Mental Health Services Research, 71,* 21–33.

DiClemente, C. C., Nidecker, M., & Bellack, A. (2008). Motivation and the stages of change among individuals with severe mental illness and substance abuse disorders. *Journal of Substance Abuse Treatment, 34,* 25–35.

Frank, R. I., & Davidson, J. (2014). *The transdiagnostic road map to case formulation and treatment planning*. Oakland, CA: New Harbinger Publications.

Jennekens, N., de Casterle, B. D., & Dobbels, F. (2010). A systematic review of care needs of people with traumatic brain injury (TBI) on a cognitive, emotional, and behavioral level. *Journal of Clinical Nursing, 19,* 1198–1206.

Kuyken, W., Padesky, C. A., & Dudley, R. (2009). *Collaborative case conceptualization: Working effectively with clients in cognitive behavioral therapy*. New York: Guilford Press.

Lambert, M., Whipple, J., Hawkins, E., Vermeersch, D., Nielsen, S., & Smart. D. (2003). Is it time for clinicians to routinely track patient outcome? A meta-analysis. *Clinical Psychology: Science and Practice, 10,* 288–301.

Meng, X., Zhang, L., Liu, W., Ding, X., Li, H., Yang, J., & Yuan, J. (2017). The impact of emotion intensity on recognition memory: Valence polarity matters. *International Journal of Psychophysiology, 116,* 16–25.

Moyers, T. B., & Houck, J. (2011). Combining motivational interviewing with cognitive-behavioral treatments for substance abuse: Lessons from the COMBINE research project. *Cognitive and Behavioral Practice, 18,* 38–45.

Persons, J. B. (2008). *The case formulation approach to cognitive-behavior therapy*. New York: Guilford Press.

Persons, J. B., & Davidson, J. (2010). Cognitive-behavioral case formulation. In K. S. Dobson (Ed.), *Handbook of cognitive-behavioral therapy* (3rd ed., pp. 172–193). New York: Guilford Press.

Reese, R. J., Norsworthy, L. A., & Rowlands, S. R. (2009). Does a continuous feedback system improve psychotherapy outcome? *Psychotherapy: Theory, Research, Practice, Training, 46,* 418–431.

Schermerhorn, A. C., Cummings, E. M., & Davies, P. T. (2008). Children's representations of multiple family relationships: Organizational structure and development in early childhood. *Journal of Family Structure, 22,* 89–101.

Segrin, C. (2000). Interpersonal relationships and mental health problems. In K. Dindia & S. Duck (Eds.), *Communication and personal relationships* (pp. 95–111). New York: Wiley.

Trzepacz, P. T., & Baker, R. W. (1993). *The psychiatric mental status examination*. New York: Oxford University Press.

Whisman, M. A. (1993). Mediators and moderators of change in cognitive therapy of depression. *Psychological Bulletin, 114,* 248–265.

4

CBT Session Structure

Purposeful and Flexible

A key feature of CBT is structure from the first session all the way through to the final session. All the CBT skills addressed in the proceeding chapters will have little to no value if the directionality and focus that are afforded in structured sessions are lacking. CBT provides more session structure than many other therapeutic approaches (Dobson & Dobson, 2013), some of which there is minimal to no planning or purposeful direction for. Therapy is not just talking about the stressor "du jour" over the past week; this is not helpful. Ultimately, most clients want and need structure. Clients are clearly attending therapy because they are feeling distressed. Additionally, some clients may still be unsure if therapy is a viable option. Simply put, many clients feel vulnerable at the onset of therapy. Structure from the first session instills comfort and hope that therapy might actually be able to provide some relief to their distress. It also demonstrates your expertness, trustworthiness, and attractiveness as a therapist—important factors for developing a therapeutic alliance.

Consistent session structure essentially socializes clients to CBT. This includes naturally modeling how to approach and solve problems related to client distress. More specifically, session structure allows you to model the collaborative nature of CBT, ranging from conceptualizing clients' problems and identifying appropriate goals to receiving feedback and making necessary treatment modifications. Ultimately, session structure provides direction for both you and the client. As much as clients require guidance in maneuvering each session, so do the most experienced therapists. The difference, at least to start, is that you are responsible for this structure.

Furthermore, session structure within the CBT context enhances therapeutic efficiency by facilitating organized therapy that stays focused on the problems of most relevance and the corresponding goals and interventions. Efficient therapy is important for not extending client distress any longer than necessary. If two approaches to therapy both alleviate client distress but one does so in half the time, is it not logical to pursue the approach that improves client quality of life more efficiently? Also, efficient use of sessions is important when working with managed care systems that put a limit on the number sessions you have with your clients. Thus, you will need to make the best of the time that you do have.

How much structure is necessary for your clients will vary, often depending on the current phase of therapy discussed in Chapter 2. Obviously, early phase therapy will require significantly more structure and guidance by the therapist compared to late phase therapy. Not only are clients generally more distressed and less hopeful during the early phase of therapy, but they also do not yet have the CBT skills necessary to independently guide therapy and cope with some of their problems. By late phase therapy, clients should be less distressed, experienced in independently utilizing CBT skills, and able to self-solve many of many their problems. Eventually, clients should take more responsibility for how their own therapy progresses over time. This process is ideal because it mirrors the expected client autonomy for maintaining and generalizing therapeutic gains after termination of therapy.

Although the ebb and flow of session structure can fluctuate over time, it is helpful to break down each session into four stages: pre-session, early session, middle session, and late session. The components of each stage do not necessarily have to be followed exactly step-by-step; this will depend on the needs of your client and the current nature of the therapeutic alliance. However, using these stages as an initial template to structure your sessions will provide guidance in ensuring that there is a purposeful nature to each session while also being flexible enough to be responsive to client needs. Table 4.1 highlights each stage and its associated components to help you prepare for executing structured and purposeful sessions.

PRE-SESSION STAGE

Technically, this is actually not a stage that takes place during a session. Yet, in many ways, this stage is probably the most critical because how you prepare before your session will influence the effectiveness of the following three session stages. Ironically, as important as this stage is, it can often be overlooked or minimized. This is unfortunate because preparing for the next session typically takes only 5 to 10 minutes and can prove invaluable once the session begins. The two key components of this stage are reviewing client information to prepare for the session and any possible formal assessments.

Sample Form 4.1 is a Therapy Session Worksheet that can help make sure you review and prep for both content and process during the pre-session stage. After entering the client's name, date, and session number, there is space to fill in the client's most recent assessment scores and previous assessment scores. There is also a spot

Table 4.1. Therapy Session Stages

Pre-Session Stage	
Review client information	A few minutes reviewing client information before session can increase therapy efficiency and effectiveness; includes therapeutic notes from previous session and recent life events.
Pre-session formal assessment	Take time to have assessment completed right before session starts or early in session; provide immediate feedback.
Early Session Stage	
Check-in	Personalize greeting by remembering any recent relevant events between sessions; try to elicit positive experiences.
Mood and symptom check	Ask open-ended questions to elicit emotions to recent events; can rate symptom distress severity; option to provide feedback on pre-session assessments; follow up on medications.
Set agenda	Agenda items guide direction of session; should be tentatively planned before session starts and collaboratively reviewed with client; as therapy progresses, clients have a more direct role in developing agenda.
Review homework	Must be integrated into each session; reviewing the previous sessions' homework provides an opportunity to assess client progress and focus on current goals and interventions.
Middle Session Stage	
Review problem	Focus on a specific agenda item; most problems are contributing to client distress or an extension of client distress; focus should still be tied to specific goals and interventions.
Problem solving	Collaboratively decide on appropriate cognitive-behavioral techniques to approach the problem; need to ensure that intervention approach matches clients' needs and treatment goals.
Feedback and summarize	Provide periodic feedback of encouragement and redirection; should be a continuous and reciprocal process; can assess current symptom distress; summarize key points related to the agenda, including rationale for approach, what was learned, relation to treatment goal, and steps moving forward.
Late Session Stage	
Summarize session	Focus is on summarizing the overall theme of the session; integrates cognitive-behavioral model in relation to interventions; demonstrates to client progress made toward symptom distress; clients can take lead as therapy progresses.
Assign homework	Should be based on current session content and relevant to the next session's content; the more clients understand, the more likely they are to complete homework.
Final questions and feedback	Formally ask what client thinks about the overall experience of therapy; if positive, consider what is effective; if negative, consider what can change.

to include any relevant information for the current session, which generally comes from your notes during the previous session. This information helps plan for what goals and interventions will receive primary focus during the session. Also, initial thoughts about session agenda items should be recorded. The remaining sections are for assigning homework and recording any in-session thoughts or observations that may be relevant for the next session (i.e., pre-session preparation) and/or the case formulation and treatment plan. Relevant Sample Form 4.1 information that is typically gathered at each session stage is addressed in its corresponding section.

SAMPLE FORM 4.1

Therapy Session Worksheet

Client's Name:
Date:
Session #:

Most Recent Assessment Scores & Previous Assessment Scores

Relevant Information for Today's Session (e.g., notes from previous session, other sources)

Session Focus: Treatment Goals, Interventions, & Process Objective

Goal 1 {Working towards change} –

    Intervention 1 {What to do} –

        Process Objective 1 {How to do it} –

        Process Objective 2 –

    Intervention 2 –

Goal 2 –

    Intervention 1 –

        Process Objective 1 –

        Process Objective 2 –

    Intervention 2 –

Goal 3 –

    Intervention 1 –

        Process Objective 1 –

        Process Objective 2 –

    Intervention 2 –

Collaborative Agenda

Item 1 – Review last session homework:

Item 2 –

Item 3 –

Item 4 –

Session Highlights/Themes/Observations

Homework for Next Session

Next Session Thoughts

Case Formulation & Treatment Plan Thoughts

Some therapists do not like or do not think it is necessary to take notes during sessions. Although it does take time to practice taking notes and remain engaged with the client (e.g., eye contact, head nods, and knowing when to stop note taking during a client's emotional state), this skill is invaluable for effective therapy. Research shows that therapists' perception of what they remember from a recent session is often inaccurate (Wynne, Susman, Ries, Birringer, & Katz, 1994). Furthermore, effective CBT often also involves clients taking notes as well (to be discussed later in this chapter). Therefore, over time, in-session note taking will not feel awkward because the therapy norms will include both therapist and client note taking.

Review Client Information

This is truly the pre-session preparation stage where any pertinent client information should be reviewed in order to facilitate structure and direction for the upcoming session. Some therapists, especially those with many years of experience, may think it is "silly" and not worth the time (typically only 5 to 10 minutes!), or their time is limited (e.g., too many clients or back-to-back clients). However, the few minutes spent in the short term can save a lot of time in the long run when revising case formulations, treatment goals, and interventions. It is easy to lose track of important information when seeing multiple clients and/or much time has passed between sessions. Thus, reviewing client information also improves overall therapy efficiency and effectiveness by way of having a purposeful direction for each session. Finally, simply coming into session and being able to recall basic life information about your client (e.g., recent weekend vacation, favorite hobby, or grade on recent exam) can go a long way toward building a strong therapeutic alliance.

Sources of information include recent progress notes, your Therapy Session Worksheet from the last session (see Sample Form 4.1), and your client's therapy notes (see Sample Form 4.2, discussed later). At this time, it is also helpful to review your client's case formulation and treatment plan, including goals and interventions. The Therapy Session Worksheet includes space to write down any of this information that will be of primary relevance for your upcoming session. This is also a good time to take any side notes for future consideration in modifying your case formulation or treatment plan as therapy progresses.

Although setting the agenda for the upcoming session is discussed during the early session stage because it involves collaboration with your client, you should still note in advance what you believe should be covered in session. You will want some flexibility in your agenda to allow input from your client, but the direction and purpose of the session should be clear. This process involves highlighting goals from your treatment plan that will be of primary focus and corresponding interventions that you will utilize in order to work toward these goals. It can also help to supplement your treatment goals and interventions with what is called "process objectives." Process objectives are what you actually have to do to achieve a larger goal. In therapy, an intervention is a statement of *what* will be done to work toward a goal (e.g., cognitive restructuring), while a process objective states *how* it will actually be done (e.g., complete thought record with focus on dichotomous thinking). Often, knowing what to do comes rather easily, but knowing how to do it within the context of each client's presenting symptoms and problems can be a bigger challenge. Process objectives do not necessarily have to be linked to a specific goal/intervention. For example, you might want to work on building your therapeutic alliance even though this may not be a formal treatment goal. Thus, your process objective could simply be "validate feelings about recent breakup with partner using nonverbal language and highlighting strengths." Overall, linking process objectives to treatment goals/interventions provides another layer to help you stay focused and purposeful with each statement and action you make in therapy. In the back of your mind, you should always be asking yourself questions like, "Why am I saying this? What is my purpose in doing this activity?" If you are not able to answer these questions, it may be worth reviewing the content of your Therapy Session Worksheet, especially your process objectives.

Pre-Session Formal Assessment

As stated in Chapter 3, ideally you want to give any client self-report assessments right before the session begins. It usually takes only 5 to 10 minutes to complete most assessments. If possible, ask your client to arrive about 10 to 15 minutes early. If this is not possible, on occasion it is okay to have the assessments completed during the first 5 minutes or so of the session. If your client does arrive a few minutes early, you should have time to also score and interpret the assessments before the session starts. In this way, you can give relatively immediate feedback by the early stage of the session. You can also use the Therapy Session Worksheet to compare the current assessment scores with previous assessment scores.

EARLY SESSION STAGE

Once you have prepared the necessary pre-session information, you are ready to meet with your client. There are many "small" parts to cover in this stage, but they will shape and influence the direction of your agenda items by the middle stage. A good portion of this stage focuses on checking in on your clients' well-being since your last session. This can range from recent activities to current mood states and symptoms. Thereafter, there is a shift to setting the agenda collaboratively for the session and reviewing any homework assignments.

Check-In

The start of the early session stage begins during the first interaction with your client. Like many relationships, it is common to greet each other and ask how each other is feeling. The difference here is that the focus of the check-in is on the clients' status through your greeting and asking purposeful follow-up questions based on previous interactions. This also continues the rapport building process by showing sincere interest in your clients and possibly remembering any recent relevant events between sessions. Thus, when possible, personalize your greeting. For example, "How was your weekend vacation?" "Did you get a chance to visit your mother over the past week?" "How are you feeling since last session? I realize we ended last session on a sensitive topic about your best friend." Also, if possible, try to elicit any positive experiences (e.g., "You stated last week you were looking forward to your daughter's birthday party. How did it go?"). Sometimes, clients experiencing severe distress may have difficulty independently reporting recent positive events and/or associated thoughts and feelings. If you are able to elicit at least a minimally positive experience, this can provide them a good start to the session and possibly a little more hope or optimism. Overall, such questions during your check-in will typically elicit responses that provide an initial informal assessment of your clients' current functioning while also helping them settle in and eventually transition to "deeper" therapeutic content.

Sometimes, the information revealed during the check-in may be relevant enough to inform and possibly modify your agenda. Even though the agenda will be formally addressed a little later, it is good to note any significant events or problems that should at least be reviewed as a possible agenda item. If possible, it is helpful to see if the presenting problems can fit naturally within your tentative agenda items. Many times, problems that clients present with immediately at the start of the session are indicative of their broader source of distress.

Mood and Symptom Check

Checking in with your clients' mood can easily flow from your initial check-in. Asking clients how they feel at this point is more purposeful in nature in order to assess not only their current mood but also their emotions over the past week (or since the last session). This process builds on your therapeutic rapport by showing concern for your clients' feelings and allows you to naturally monitor their treatment progress. Often, asking open-ended questions about their previous week (either in general or specific events, if known) will elicit recent emotions. Ideally, eliciting "fresh" emotions to recent events will be the most useful, as it can have a more "here-and-now" effect, giving you the opportunity to incorporate any themes into your agenda.

Depending on the phase of therapy you are in with your clients, you may be able to do symptom checks that are a little more formal. For example, you can ask your clients to rate their level of depression or anxiety on a 0–10 scale, where 0 is no distress and 10 is the highest level of distress. Other examples include number of binges, substance use (frequency and amount), aggressive/violent incidents (verbal or physical), self-harm, or panic attacks (number and severity). Typically, if you are at this point in therapy, this information will often be related to the information reported in their homework assignments. In fact, although homework is addressed at the end of this stage, it may be appropriate to review any cognitive-behavioral monitoring forms at this point, especially if the emphasis of these forms is on their current symptoms and distress. Although somewhat subjective, using such scales provides you substantive information to estimate their current cognitive and emotional functioning. Of course, this information can also be helpful in moving forward with your agenda. However, this information also affords you the opportunity to integrate and reinforce the cognitive model. This is often done by assessing your clients' awareness of how their perceptions of events influence their thoughts, emotions, and corresponding behaviors.

Another source of information comes from any pre-session assessments you may have given. If the assessment can be easily scored, now is a good time to provide feedback to your client. You can also review any formal assessments that were given in previous sessions that are now scored. (If determined to be more clinically appropriate, you can choose to review assessment scores later in the session as one of your agenda items.) If possible, you can also compare assessment scores from previous sessions as a way to track progress. If you do have multiple assessment data points, it is helpful to visually plot their changes on a graph for some clients. Although formal symptom scores are not all-telling, they do provide a valid source of insight into targeted areas of symptom change. Clients tend to be responsive to self-report objective data that are relevant to their own distress. Thus, the information provided by these assessments not only helps you track progress but also allows for clients to explain possible reasons for their progress within the framework of the cognitive-behavioral model to help facilitate insight into their therapeutic progress. Even if there has not been much progress/symptom reduction recently, this information should still be processed. There is still much value in asking clients if they have any insight into why they are not improving. This may be an opportunity to formally discuss what clients think about the effectiveness of therapy. If warranted, changes in interventions (both what and how) should be considered. It may also be a good time to review the cognitive model, emphasizing key parts the client is struggling with.

Using formal assessments to focus on overall symptom change is not the only way to track client progress. Sometimes, it is helpful to focus on individual items on the assessments. This allows you to recognize if there are specific domains of concern that are "red flags" (e.g., suicidal ideation) or have been inconsistent in the past (e.g., interpersonal relations). It can be further confirming if what your clients are self-reporting is consistent with the formal assessment. This also demonstrates that your clients' insight and self-awareness of well-being is consistent. However, there may be times when there are discrepancies between self-report and individual items on a formal assessment. These contradictions should be addressed as soon as possible. Reasons for such inconsistencies can range from not understanding the assessment question to poor insight of their own thoughts, emotions, and/or behaviors. Simply asking a question such as, "You said to me during our check-in that you haven't had any thoughts of suicide over the past week, but I've noticed that you selected 'sometimes' for thoughts of suicide on the suicide scale. What are your thoughts about this difference?" You do not want to be too confrontational, but you should still be direct and clear in noting any inconsistencies. Not only does your follow-up question provide clarification of your clients' reported symptom distress, but the reason for the inconsistency (e.g., did not understand the question, did not feel comfortable about reporting the information directly to you, or was not aware that what was being said was different from actual thoughts/behaviors) can inform both your session agenda and interventions later in therapy.

Finally, if your client is on psychiatric medications, it is prudent to follow up on possible side effects, adherence, and any related problems or questions. You are not the prescribing health care provider, but you should maintain open communication with this individual to keep each other updated on both mental health and relevant medical information. Your questions for medication adherence should be as specific as possible. For example, simply asking your clients if they have taken their medications is not enough. A more appropriate question could be, "How many times did you take your medication over the past week?" The type of questions asked will vary based on your clients' needs. What is important is being specific enough to have information that is measurable and trackable.

Set Agenda

If treatment planning sets the stage for the course of therapy, then agenda setting sets the stage for the course of each session. Similarly, just like treatment plans require modifications as therapy progresses, agendas should also be flexible in response to events within a session. However, if appropriately planned in advance during the pre-session stage, your agenda should be the driving force for the direction of therapy for the remainder of the session. The most effective agendas contain items that are directly connected to the goals of your treatment plan. Just like your treatment goals, it is best to keep your agenda items specific and measurable. Also, you want make sure that your interventions, including your process objectives, allow for the opportunity for the client to experience some level of progress and success (i.e., achievable) by the end of the session, including skill development and symptom distress.

Clients need structure when they first start therapy. During the early phases of therapy, it is generally best to initially present a tentative agenda with your plans for the session and then elicit feedback from the client. Then you can collaborate with your client, with guidance, on what agenda items to prioritize. By the first or second session, perhaps as part of pyschoeducation (see Chapter 5), you should explain the purpose, process, and value that come with agenda setting. Presenting an agenda sets explicit expectations for CBT: it is purposeful and flexible and requires effort from both the therapist and the client. Even during the early phase of therapy, it is essential that your agenda not be too rigid in order to model collaboration and build a therapeutic alliance. Too much structure may also inhibit adaptability and spontaneity to unpredictable events (e.g., life outside of therapy), which can result in missed "therapeutic moments" to enhance client skills across multiple contexts and within multiple domains. This can possibly result in increased client distress due to the fact that life outside the therapy office truly is unpredictable. You are essentially socializing clients to the agenda-setting process, especially on how to identify and prioritize specific problems. Effective agenda setting also implicitly demonstrates your expertness and confidence in your ability to effectively treat your client, which can instill hope, optimism, and motivation to change.

As you approach the middle phase and especially by the late phase of therapy, you can still have a template in mind for the agenda, but it is best for the client to have more of a role in developing the session agenda. This can begin by providing your clients with some choice in what agenda items to address and eventually taking the lead in setting specific agenda items for their problems and even particular interventions (i.e., both what and how). This is a key skill for your client to eventually obtain because this process facilitates solving problems independently (i.e., client does not need the therapist) and eventually maintaining treatment gains after the therapeutic relationship is over. The key skill for you in agenda setting is knowing how to balance the transition from the teacher–student relationship to the mentor–protégé relationship. Client autonomy is a must for the generalization and maintenance of client therapeutic gains.

At some point during the early phase of therapy (second or third session), you should introduce clients to taking their own notes within sessions. Sample Form 4.2 is a Client Therapy Notes Worksheet that can be used by clients to help monitor their thoughts/emotions, reflect on homework, focus on their identified problems and positive experiences, note progress on learning new skills, and reflect on experiences during session and outside of session. If your clients have been introduced to this technique, asking them to review and share their notes at this time can be a helpful contribution to the session agenda. Without this worksheet, many clients may not be able to spontaneously state their problems, skills still in need of improvement, and even progress. Having clients establish a routine of writing down therapy-related content "in the moment" enhances preparedness to both collaborate and take responsibility for their therapeutic progress.

SAMPLE FORM 4.2

Client Therapy Notes Worksheet

How am I feeling?

What am I thinking?

What did I do for homework? What worked? What was challenging?

What happened since last session (positive and negative)?

What do I want to put on today's agenda?
(e.g., problems, negative thoughts/emotions, recent pleasure or accomplishment experiences)

Session Highlights
(e.g., What did I learn? What was challenging?)

What are my thoughts and feelings about today's session?

What is my homework (between now and next session)?

Any thoughts/experiences to share before end of session?

Any thoughts/experiences to share for next session?

Regardless of the phase of therapy, the information gained during your check-in, mood and symptom check, or review of client therapy notes may result in some modifications to your agenda. Nevertheless, if your agenda (or your clients' agenda later in therapy) targets your clients' primary problems and corresponding treatment goals, your modifications will typically be only small shifts in a particular direction (i.e., the context may fluctuate, but the process is generally consistent). Relatedly, you may need to prioritize agenda items based on available session time and your clients' immediate needs and level of distress. There is nothing wrong with "triaging" agenda items in order to focus on what is most important in the present and saving others for future sessions. Additionally, there may be times when an agenda item in session may need to be changed or modified if it is not addressing a key problem effectively as initially anticipated. An in-session shift with a particular agenda item models awareness of ineffective problem-solving strategies and making necessary adaptations.

Review Homework

Homework is such an important topic that Chapter 10 is specifically dedicated to how to assign, monitor, and review clients' homework. Here, the focus is simply to highlight the importance and integration of homework within the structure of the session. Sometimes, reviewing homework can be brief; other times, it may be the main focus of the session. Regardless, reviewing your clients' homework is a must. If you neglect this important part of therapy, clients will eventually stop doing it because it is no longer perceived as important. Not reviewing homework may also damage your therapeutic alliance—it is a "turnoff" to assign work to be completed the previous session and never acknowledge it the next session. Most important, CBT without homework can negatively impact client outcomes (Kazantzis, Whittington, & Dattilio, 2010; LeBeau, Davies, Culver, & Craske, 2013).

Reviewing homework is another great opportunity to provide structure to therapy and bridge content and themes from the previous session. Typically, homework assigned follows at least one session of learning and practicing a new skill. Clients then practice these newly learned skills between sessions (outside of the office and independently) and process what worked and what did not work during the next session. The purpose of homework is for clients to build on their CBT skills in order to manage their problems outside of therapy (i.e., generalize skills to the "real world"). Thus, reviewing the previous week's homework assignment provides another occasion to assess client progress and remain focused on current goals and interventions. This information will also partially influence moving forward with your agenda. For example, perhaps you need to spend more time reviewing a particular skill with your client, or maybe your client is ready to move on to learn the next skill (or work on another goal). Even if a client does not complete a homework assignment, it is still beneficial to discuss possible reasons (e.g., the client did not understand the assignment, the assignment was too difficult, or the client lacked motivation). Again, this information can result in modifications to your agenda and future homework assignments (e.g., review the skills and instructions for the assignment, reduce difficulty by breaking it into small steps, or shift to motivational techniques).

The following are three vignettes from Video Case Examples MDD-6, MDD-13, and MDD-18 demonstrating the early session stage across all three phases of therapy with the same client. Following the vignettes are discussion questions and an activity. (Note: See Video Vignettes 4.2 (MDD-13), 6.2 (MDD-6), and 8.6 (MDD-18) demonstrating reviewing homework during the early session stage across all three phases of therapy with the same client.)

VIDEO VIGNETTE 4.1

MDD-6: Early Session Stage—Early Phase Therapy

Therapist:	Hi, Mark, how you doing?
Client:	Not too bad.
Therapist:	Not too bad?
Client:	Can't really complain too much.
Therapist:	Can't complain. So, kind of okay?
Client:	Yeah, I mean a little "meh." The week . . . there were some good spots, but the overall trend—it was kind of a tough week.
Therapist:	Okay.
Client:	But there definitely were . . . watching the Patriots game was fun. So, there was a couple good moments.
Therapist:	Okay. The Patriots game was one thing we just talked about last session. You did get a chance to watch it and it went well?
Client:	Yeah, it was a good game. They won. So, I was pretty happy.
Therapist:	By a lot?
Client:	Uh, yeah.
Therapist:	One of the things we talked about is you wanted to make sure you followed through with your scheduled date with Melissa.
Client:	Yeah, it wasn't set in stone, but we were able to throw something together last minute on Friday.
Therapist:	Okay.
Client:	It started off a little tough . . . kind of a little late getting started. It took a while to find a parking spot. The little stressors . . . was just in a funk in the beginning. But by the time we got our food and a couple drinks I was feeling a little bit better.
Therapist:	Okay, yeah.
Client:	Relaxing and being past the point of getting ready for the date night . . . because it really seemed like getting going for it was just one of the hard parts.
Therapist:	Okay. Maybe that'll be something, if it's okay with you, we can talk a little bit later in more detail.
Client:	Yeah.

Therapist: Maybe it fits into your activity schedule there. I want to do a brief mood check as well.

Client: Yup.

Therapist: How's it been the last couple of days?

Client: I don't know. I mean, things have been going okay. . . . Obviously not quite where I want them to be, but I mean . . . fine?

Therapist: How would you rate your depression 0 to 10, then?

Client: Maybe some days like a 6, but I think right now maybe like a 7.

Therapist: Okay, 6 or 7.

———————————————

Therapist: It seems like you're kind of doing okay, but obviously there are things we need to talk about, to work on.

Client: Yeah.

Therapist: My agenda for us today—and let me know what you think about it—is I think the first thing we should do is obviously talk about your weekly activity monitoring log.

Client: Yeah.

Therapist: And you did get a chance to fill out the hopelessness scale before you came in. I want to take a few minutes to score and process your level of hope and motivation.

Client: Yeah.

Therapist: One thing that wasn't on the agenda initially—not that it was horrible or bad—I want us to spend more time teasing out some of the themes about your date with Melissa.

Client: Yeah.

Therapist: It seems like they start off with some friction. I think that it might be related to some automatic thoughts that we've only briefly talked about.

Client: Yeah.

Therapist: And then, lastly, what we'll do if your weekly monitoring log goes well—it looks like you did a decent job filling it out—we'll talk about scheduling activities within the next week or two.

Therapist: How does that sound to you?

Client: Yeah, that sounds pretty good.

VIDEO VIGNETTE 4.2

MDD-13: Early Session Stage—Middle Phase Therapy

Therapist: How are you doing Mark?

Client: I'm doing pretty good, actually.

Therapist: Good. How was your visit with George over the last couple of days? You said you were going to meet with him and do a few things and hang out.

Client:	Yeah. We hung out the other night. We actually grabbed some sushi. It was a really good night. It actually reminded me why . . . when I was younger, I actually just like felt so much better after hanging out with friends. It kind of really takes the weight off. I'm able to kick back and talk about just some things. I don't really feel quite as stressed. I'm actually talking about doing things with someone like George. It was a really nice night.
Therapist:	It sounds like you took some time to reflect after the night out?
Client:	Yeah.
Therapist:	That's good. You're seeing the benefits of taking the time to make the effort and follow through with your friends.
Client:	Yeah.
Therapist:	I want to ask—how would you say your mood's been overall over the past week?
Client:	I can definitely see that it's starting to get better. I'm definitely not feeling quite as down. I don't know . . . if I had to rate it, maybe like a 5?
Therapist:	So, depression you would rate from a five out of 0 to 10?
Client:	Yeah.
Therapist:	Okay. That's better than before.
Client:	Yeah.
Therapist:	This is kind of related to what we're going to talk about today for our agenda.
Client:	Yup.
Therapist:	The first thing is, you have there is your first formal homework assignment for a thought record.
Client:	Yeah.
Therapist:	We've been talking a lot about it but this is the first time I've had you go home and spend some time doing a couple of these. We'll definitely address this.
Client:	Yeah.
Therapist:	Related to your mood and depression, as you know you've been filling out the BDIs every 1 or 2 weeks, and we've been talking about them. I was able to put together some of the data over the last few weeks, and I want to take a look at that and get your feelings on how you think you're doing . . .
Client:	Okay.
Therapist:	I want to see if there's anything else that you wanted to put on our agenda for today. We've been making some good progress and you've been taking more of a lead.
Client:	I've been having a little bit of trouble with a couple of thoughts that I've been having.
Therapist:	Okay.
Client:	I just want more practice with the thought record. That's what I would like to focus on.

Therapist: That makes perfect sense. We'll start with your homework assignment—thought record—follow up with the BDI scores, and you're telling me you want to do a little more practice with the thought records in session.

Client: Yeah.

VIDEO VIGNETTE 4.3

MDD-18: Early Session Stage—Late Phase Therapy

Therapist: Mark, are how you doing?

Client: I'm doing pretty well, actually.

Therapist: Good. How did the plan go with doing that couple date with your colleagues?

Client: I'm even just kind of thinking over here . . . it went better than I expected. So, pretty good.

Therapist: It was better than you expected, good.

Client: Yeah.

Therapist: I can't wait to talk about that.

Client: Yeah.

Therapist: It seems like overall you're feeling good and looking good. How would you rate your depression on 0 to 10 right now?

Client: I'm definitely doing better. There are still some moments that it's a little bit of a tough time here and there, but I'd say it's more like a 3. I'm kind of around there.

Therapist: Okay. That's pretty good. For the agenda, and you've been slowly taking over more in control, as long as we stay within the realm we want to work, I want to get from you what you would like to start off with here.

Client: Obviously, I want to start with the homework. I'm actually kind of proud of how it went. So, I definitely want to start with that.

Therapist: Good.

Client: And then, like I said, I've still been having a hard time with a couple things. Those feelings of worthlessness have been popping up every once in a while. So, I'd like to talk about that and the thoughts that are associated with them. I still think maybe . . . I really like that core belief worksheet that we did.

Therapist: Okay.

Client: The one where you actually challenged me. At first it was kind of difficult, but . . . just kind of doing more and more of those have been really helpful in terms of even getting myself to challenge myself when we're outside.

Therapist: All right, that makes sense. I think that's probably more than enough today.

Client: Yeah.

Therapist: So, we'll review in a moment here your homework assignment. It looks like you've done a pretty good job of filling it out and moving forward with that. Then what we'll do, like you said, is explore your thoughts of worthlessness and see what other automatic thoughts are related to it.

Client:	Yeah.
Therapist:	And I do believe the core belief flow chart would be helpful.
Client:	Yeah.
Therapist:	What I might also add onto it, depending on what we're doing, is maybe the downward arrow technique as well.
Client:	Yup.
Therapist:	Again, sometimes when you already know the core belief it can still be helpful; perhaps unlikeable . . . processing that as well.
Client:	Yeah
Therapist:	Does that sound okay?
Client:	Yeah, I really like that.

Discussion Questions 4.1

- How does the client's check-in and mood and symptom check change from early phase therapy to late phase therapy?
- How does the role of client–therapist shift during agenda setting from early phase therapy to late phase therapy (i.e., teacher–student to mentor–protégé)?
- How did the content of the agenda items shift from early phase therapy to late phase therapy?

ACTIVITY 4.1: EARLY SESSION STAGE

With another peer, practice role-playing the early session stage, focusing on check-ins, mood and symptom checks, and agenda setting. Try each phase of therapy and make the necessary adjustments to the questions you ask and how you lead the conversation. How did your questions evolve across phases? What did you do therapeutically to allow your "client" to have a greater role (e.g., participation or contribution) across phases?

MIDDLE SESSION STAGE

Once you have prioritized your session agenda items, you are ready to focus on your first agenda item. The number of agenda items per session will vary depending on your clients' needs. Sometimes, you may be able to complete two or three agenda items; other times, you may need a full session (or more) for one agenda item. How much of a lead you or your clients take in initiating and moving forward with the agenda item will depend on the phase of therapy and the type of problem. The structure of this part of the session is relatively straightforward, but both the content and the process can vary greatly for each client depending on presenting problems, goals, and corresponding interventions. Because of this, the following sections serve as only a general template to ensure that key components are covered for each agenda item.

Review Problem

You and your client may already have a general understanding of the problem in order for it to get on the list of agenda items. However, be sure to gather as much information about the problem as possible. Consider these questions: What were the precipitating factors? How is the problem contributing to the client's current distress? What did the client do that worked or did not work? What other factors are currently contributing (i.e., maintaining) to the problem? How much control does the client have over the problem? Additionally, it is often best to use a problem or an event that is recent (a few days to a week) so that it has strong emotional content and accurate recall. Accurately recalled emotional events have a better chance to elicit a sense of immediacy and engagement. When possible, also try to add an objective and a measurable element to the problem (e.g., typically two or three verbal arguments with significant other per week or missed bill payments about two times per month). Not all problems will lend themselves to this type of measurement, but when possible, this allows for easier tracking to assess progress.

At this time, it is best to conceptualize the problem in how it fits within your overall case formulation, including the cognitive-behavioral model. You will find that most clients' agenda item problems are an extension or a part of their distress, either as a contributing factor or as an outcome. Therefore, even though you may be focusing on a "micro" problem (relatively speaking), your approach should still be tied into specific goals ("macro") and interventions. This strategy allows you to use daily, common life events that are contributing to their distress to teach broad skills for eventual generalization and maintenance of change.

Problem-Solving Strategies

Once you and your client have a clear conceptualization of the problem, the next step is to collaboratively decide on how you will focus on the problem using the cognitive-behavioral model: psychoeducation of specific CBT skills, basic problem-solving strategies, behavioral activation, emotion and thought identification, modification of automatic thoughts and core beliefs, relaxation techniques, and exposure. Of course, these techniques are not mutually exclusive; many times, you will use these sequentially and/or simultaneously. Each of these approaches requires your CBT knowledge and skill in application, which are addressed in great detail in the upcoming chapters. The focus here is to provide a guide in determining possible intervention options to solve the presenting problem. This is also the time to consider your process objectives. Regardless of your intervention strategy, you need to make sure that its implementation appropriately matches your clients' needs and treatment goals to maximize effectiveness in reducing distress and learning new skills.

Additionally, this is also an ideal time to use your Therapy Session Worksheet and for your clients to take notes for their Client Therapy Notes Worksheet. Reviewing this information both during and after a session can inform strategies and process objectives for future interventions.

Feedback and Summarize

As you work on your agenda item, you should provide periodic feedback of encouragement and redirection when necessary. This communicates to your clients what they are doing well and other areas in need of improvement. It is also ideal for you to encourage and elicit feedback from your clients about what is and is not working for them. Overall, feedback should be a continuous, reciprocal process. Additionally, this is a good time to ask clients to rate their current symptom distress. It may not be practical to use any formal assessments at this point, but following through with any relevant subjective self-report 0–10 scales (e.g., anxiety or depression) is appropriate. Client feedback and self-report of distress will allow you to more accurately assess the effectiveness of your interventions and possibly make any necessary modifications. Again, this is where your process objectives and your Therapy Session Worksheet can be beneficial. Many times, the intervention will be appropriate, but you may need to change how it is being implemented.

On conclusion of working on the agenda item, make sure that a summary is provided, highlighting the rationale for the approach, what skill was learned/used, how it can be applied to other problems, its relation to a particular treatment goal, what was helpful and not helpful, and the next steps in moving forward. Depending on the phase of therapy, either you or your clients can provide the summary. If you provide the summary, be sure that your clients understand the key points and be open for any follow-up questions. When your clients provide their summary, this is a good opportunity to assess their understanding of the problem and how the interventions were helpful, including their current level of distress. If their summary is inaccurate, this simply provides another learning opportunity to process any content in need of clarification. Overall, the progress made with each agenda item and the feedback received from the summaries will inform future session agendas and homework assignments.

LATE SESSION STAGE

With about 5 to 10 minutes left in the session, you should transition to the late session stage to ensure that you have enough time to adequately close the session without rushing or overlooking any key points or themes. This stage is often only a few minutes but is just as essential as the other stages because it provides an opportunity to integrate key conceptual themes and review what was learned during the session. Putting this capstone to your session is also the beginning of your bridge for the next session. The most formal way to continue this bridge is through assigning homework, which provides additional opportunity to track symptoms and practice skills learned outside of therapy. These homework assignments will then be reviewed during the next session.

Summarize Session

This part of the stage is similar to the summarization process for agendas discussed above. However, the major focus here is broader because you want to focus on the overall themes that were covered. This means providing a summary that explicitly integrates the cognitive-behavioral model relevant to the interventions (and process objectives) implemented. Ideally, you should try to integrate the overall conceptualization of the clients' distress and treatment plan. The rationale for this approach is that it keeps you focused as a therapist on the "big picture" and also demonstrates to your client that the work done during the session was purposeful toward overall symptom distress reduction and improved quality of life. Also similar to the agenda summaries, if your clients are ready, it can be therapeutic for them to summarize the session. Unlike summarizing an agenda item that is typically more problem focused, a session summary for clients can be a great opportunity to integrate and modify their own conceptualization of distress. If there is time, you can also ask them to reflect not only on the content that they learned but also on the process of the experience This can provide greater personal meaning and autonomy in improving their own well-being

This is also a good time to highlight any symptom relief. Although you may have been doing this periodically while working on each agenda item, concluding the session with any client self-report of distress reduction will reinforce the effectiveness of the learned skills and interventions. Being able to connect what clients have done in session to how they currently think and feel can be very powerful for developing and enhancing hope and motivation to change.

Assign Homework for Next Session

You can assign the next homework assignment either before or after your summary, depending on your clinical judgment where it best fits. Sometimes, it is best to transition from your last agenda item to the related homework for the next session. Other times, you may want to wait until after the session has been summarized and you have received feedback, as this information may influence the direction for the next homework assignment. Either way, your homework assignment should be based on current session content while also keeping in mind your focus for next session. Be sure to give yourself enough time to explain the homework and answer any possible questions. Finally, provide a clear rationale for the homework assignment and convey the role it will have during your next session. The more clients understand why they are completing an assignment and know that the information they provide will influence the next session, the greater the chance they will complete it with effort. When reasonable, you can also initiate the homework assigment during your explanation. It is easier to finish a task that is already started.

Final Questions and Feedback

Before the session is over, consider asking your clients to review their Client Therapy Notes Worksheet and elicit questions or feedback they may have about any part of the session. You can also remind them to take any final notes that may be worthy to review before the next session. This is a good strategy to use periodically throughout the session, but it is also beneficial to follow up one more time toward the end of the session as it is being fully processed. At this time, you can ask them what they think about the overall experience of therapy. If their response is positive, you can ask them what they attribute for this experience and what they have found most effective thus far. Even then, you can still ask if anything could be done differently to improve their therapeutic experience. If clients have negative feedback or questions of concern, it is important to be self-aware and nondefensive. If anything, you should positively reinforce them for their honesty and being proactive in ensuring that they are receiving the most from their therapy. Follow up with clients on what they think can be done to improve their therapeutic experience. It is important to remember that a significant contributing factor to effective therapy is receiving constant feedback from clients. This provides you with the opportunity to adapt to your client. In fact, for some clients, this is a good example of assertiveness and empowerment. For others, this shows that they are developing their own autonomy as they take more control over their therapy. Occasional negative or constructive feedback is typically not a major concern, especially if it is something that can be worked through with minimal disruption to therapy. However, if this occurs on a more frequent basis, this may be a concern for the therapeutic alliance and should be formally addressed.

Finally, as soon as the session ends, take down any final notes on your Therapy Session Worksheet. If you wait too long, you may not remember an important thought or observation. Simply noting client progress toward treatment goals, what worked or did not work, and thoughts on how to move forward will be invaluable the next time you look at your notes during the pre-session stage for the next session.

The following are three vignettes from Video Case Examples PDA-5, PDA-8, and PDA-10 demonstrating the late session stage across all three phases of therapy with the same client. (Note: The interventions discussed in these Video Vignettes are addressed in Chapter 9, and assigning homework is addressed in Chapter 10.) Following the vignettes are discussion questions and an activity.

VIDEO VIGNETTE 4.4

PDA-5: Late Session Stage—Early Phase Therapy

Therapist: Okay, Lindsey, our time is almost up. What I want to do is summarize some of the key points that we discussed, just to make sure we're all on the same page before we leave. I also want to assign our first assignments for you to take home. Does that make sense?

Client: Yeah.

Therapist: Okay. So, one thing that we talked about today, just to remind us, was the therapy expectations—how CBT works and the therapeutic relationship. One of the bigger things we talked about is called collaborative empiricism. We talked about working together. We're going to generate hypotheses and test them. . . . Also, how we can provide feedback and set goals with each other. And homework, which we'll assign today. Overall, knowing that with CBT there's a lot of challenging of thoughts and behaviors . . . and sometimes, not always . . . there may be moments where we have increased distress, but then eventually it becomes reduced over time as well. The other thing too, which I think you had a pretty good grasp on, was we talked about the cognitive model and we also addressed that with the psychoeducation of panic disorder and agoraphobia. We talked about the triggering events, like what starts these events, getting us aroused. What are the automatic thoughts are, or images that we have. What are your emotions and physiological arousal, which is largely anxiety related. Then, what are those behaviors that we do. And even some of the consequences, whether they're real or perceived. Do you have any questions about that?

Client: No.

Therapist: Does that fit with what we discussed today.

Client: Yeah, that makes sense.

Therapist: Okay, good. So, what I want to do is discuss our homework assignment for today. I know we've been talking about them and now we get one of our first ones to do.

Client: Okay.

Therapist: It's relatively simple, and it follows along with what we've been talking about. If you recall, lately we've been talking about the importance of assessment, where we talked about the panic anxiety scale. We also talked about the agoraphobia scale. In CBT, and especially when we talk about panic attacks and agoraphobia, is we want to track our symptoms between sessions. You will only see me for about 50 to 60 minutes, but obviously a good portion of your life takes place in between. And it's one thing to come to therapy and talk about those symptoms, where we reflect on the past, which is still very helpful and you've done a great job with that, but it's another thing where in the moment, or soon after the moment, we can write down how you're feeling or thinking, etc. Does that make sense?

Client: Yes.

Therapist: I'm not going to just send out the door and say, "here you go give it a shot." I want to walk you through one. So, let's walk through completing this panic attack record together.

Client: Okay.

_____

Therapist: There's a spot here for triggers. Do you remember what was being said or done that started this?

Client:	Well, the professor was talking about some assignments that were due and an upcoming midterm.
Therapist:	Okay. So I'm going to write down assignments and midterm?
Client:	Okay.
Therapist:	When he started talking about the assignments that are due is that when it started happening?
Client:	Yeah . . .
Therapist:	Was this expected or unexpected? In the moment . . . ?
Client:	Well, actually . . . it was very unexpected.
Therapist:	Okay. I know now it seems like looking back that you didn't see that coming at all; it was very surprising. Okay, We've used a scale before earlier. This is a maximum fear scale for in the moment. At its worst moment—we're going talk about the symptoms in a second—from 0 to 10, where would you put it?
Client:	Probably rank it an 8.
Therapist:	Okay. So what I'm going to do here is check off an 8 like that.
Client:	Okay.
Therapist:	I know it's a relatively subjective scale. What's important is what it is to you.
Client:	Okay.
Therapist:	When we do a bunch of these over time we can compare what the score and symptoms mean to you. Does that make sense?
Client:	Okay, yeah.
Therapist:	Now again, obviously you won't be doing this in the middle of the panic attack, but you would have this available afterwards. What we want to do here is just check off the symptoms of the particular panic attack. So, did you have chest pains or discomfort?
Client:	Yes.
Therapist:	Yes, right. Did you have any sweating?
Client:	Yes.
Therapist:	Yes. Heart racing?
Client:	Yes.

Therapist:	This is just one example. I'll let you take this home to practice this. I have a bunch of copies of these that I can give you.
Client:	Okay.
Therapist:	You may have no panic attacks this week . . .
Client:	That would be great.
Therapist:	Or you might have a couple of them.
Client:	Okay.
Therapist:	You can carry this on your person however you think is best. You can fill it out right after the event; the sooner the better, but I know you have to relax and collect yourself. Just do what I did just there. It only takes a few minutes.
Client:	Okay.

Therapist:	Fill that out the best you can. If you have any questions when you're filling this out just write it down to follow up. What we will do when we meet next is review your homework assignment. Do your best to complete it, even if it's only partially done that's okay. We'll go through them and process that, okay?
Client:	Okay.
Therapist:	That information will be very helpful for me and for us to eventually develop some more specific treatment goals and what type of interventions we're going to use. Does that sound good?
Client:	It does sound good. It makes sense.
Therapist:	Good. As you look at this homework assignment and your therapy notes, do you have any other questions for me about today's session to clarify anything before we go?
Client:	No, I mean everything that you've explained really does make a lot of sense.
Therapist:	Great. As you know, of course, in the future you can always ask questions to clarify. I think, today's session was pretty clear. How do you overall feel about today's session? From when you came in a couple sessions ago and where we are now?
Client:	I feel hopeful.
Therapist:	Okay, good.
Client:	I just feel like things are definitely . . . I have a chance of really getting better.
Therapist:	Good. And I'm feeling hopeful, too. You seem to be understanding this stuff pretty well. I'm optimistic that we can really work through this and help you feel a little bit better. Okay?
Client:	Good.
Therapist:	So, there's one last thing. I just like to check in with my clients and see how they're feeling. Do you have any feedback or any other questions before moving on for next week?
Client:	No.
Therapist:	Okay, good. I just wanted to clarify that. You'll find as we move forward in therapy there might be some constructive feedback you might have for me, like "do a little bit of this," "a little less of that," or "I find this helpful, this not as much helpful." I wanted to clarify and put that out there. You're more than welcome to provide feedback because the more you tell me how things are going, the more we can adapt together and make changes to be even more efficient as we go through therapy.
Client:	Okay.
Therapist:	Does that make sense?
Client:	It does.

VIDEO VIGNETTE 4.5

PDA-8: Late Session Stage—Middle Phase Therapy

Therapist: Al right, Lindsey. Our session's almost done. We've just got a few more minutes. I want to summarize some of the key points today—talk about our homework assignment, and just briefly check in if you've got any questions. Does that sound good?

Client: Yeah.

Therapist: Well . . . we really focused on negative automatic thoughts, and we also talked about how you have a tendency for one particular negative automatic thought or cognitive distortion—catastrophizing. This time instead of me highlighting and summarizing all the key points, I want you to take a turn and let me know what you remember about what we talked about, from negative automatic thoughts and catastrophic thinking.

Client: Sure.

Therapist: Okay.

Client: Well, you said negative thoughts are like a cognitive reflex.

Therapist: Yes, and what does that mean?

Client: That it just kind of comes out of nowhere and that it's really brief, and that we kind of feel it as an emotion. You just don't even think about it. We experience it as an emotion. We believe that it's real. It's just a thought. It's real and usually based on some kind of past experience.

Therapist: Yeah. That's pretty good actually. We covered a lot of key points, but you pretty much highlighted the majority of them. With regard to the thoughts, like you said, we often believe that they're fact; that they're valid. Because they happen so fast we don't really recognize that maybe they're not as accurate as we think they are. I realize as we were talking in session they feel very real for you when you have some of these thoughts. The other component too, as you mentioned as well, is they're based on past experiences.

Client: Yes.

Therapist: Sometimes they can be based upon even childhood or adolescent experiences. But that doesn't mean they can't be based upon experiences as adults as well.

Client: Okay.

Therapist: I think overall that's a really good summary . . .

Therapist: For your homework, this is a negative automatic thought tracking worksheet. It's relatively simple. We've actually done some versions of these earlier. I'll give you a couple copies of these to take home as well. What you see here is the event. As you can tell, verbally we have done a lot of these, right?

Client: Yes.

Therapist: What's the thought? What are you feeling? And then, what does your body feel like?

Client: Okay.
Therapist: I know you understand this to some degree, so let's do one now.
Client: Okay.
Therapist: What was the most recent event? Was it the trip to the ER room?
Client: Well, whenever I went to the grocery store with my husband.
Therapist: Okay. We can do that one.
Client: Yeah.
Therapist: That's good. I'm just going to put down grocery store and your husband?
Client: Okay.
Therapist: What would just be one or two examples of thoughts that you had there?
Client: I was thinking I was going to have a panic attack.
Therapist: Okay. I'll put that down.
Client: And then I also thought that if I had that panic attack I wouldn't have anywhere to go. Where I could get help or be safe.
Therapist: Nowhere to go . . . get help . . . be safe. Do you notice here with the space, you can put multiple thoughts down here as well?
Client: Yeah.

Therapist: For right now, I want you to focus on the next week. Whenever you have a particular moment where you feel anxious try to fill it out. After the event go back and fill in the blanks. I think I already have a good picture of what's going on here, but this information will be helpful for when we do future thought records and we start doing some exposure techniques.
Client: Okay.
Therapist: Any questions or comments or feedback before we end?
Client: I would say the main thing is that, for me, I think that it's more about the physiological effects rather than . . . I don't really think about the emotions because for me it feels like my body's telling me that something's not right.
Therapist: Right. I noticed that, too, when the last time you immediately went to the bodily sensations.
Client: Yes.
Therapist: So, if I understand you correctly, it's easier for you to think event, thought, and then the physiological sensations.
Client: Yeah.
Therapist: The emotions are important, but . . .
Client: They're kind of an afterthought.
Therapist: Yeah. Okay. I'll keep that in mind as well when we come back next week. I can even tweak this a little bit in how we do that.
Client: Okay.

Therapist:	Both how I process with you verbally and even some of the other work-sheets I have. I can maybe put a little bit more emphasis on the bodily sensations. We'll still acknowledge the emotions, of course, but we'll flag the bodily sensations.
Client:	Okay.
Therapist:	Even though the form here that you're taking home today is like this. . . . You can fill this out any way you want. So, don't worry too much about the order. Just do what works best for you.
Client:	Okay.
Therapist:	Does that sound good?
Client:	It does.

VIDEO VIGNETTE 4.6

PDA-10: Late Session Stage—Late Phase Therapy

<outside after completing in vivo exposure exercise>

Therapist:	Well, you look excited. How did it go?
Client:	I am excited. I'm so proud of myself. I not only got a menu, but I got today's specials as well.
Therapist:	Wow. I see something else in your hand too. What's that?
Client:	Yeah, I ended up meeting Val, and she's manager, she owns this place. We talked for a few minutes. It was great.
Therapist:	Wow. That seems really good. Do recall what your anxiety rating was before you went in?
Client:	It was like a 7 or an 8.
Therapist:	Yeah. How would you say your feel right now?
Client:	A lot closer to like a 2.
Therapist:	Okay. So, you feel much better, right?
Client:	Yeah.
Therapist:	Do you recall what your prediction was going in? Before we started this, you told me what?
Client:	Well, I didn't think I'd make it as far into the restaurant as I did, no less come out with all of these things.
Therapist:	You told me you're afraid that once you take a couple steps into the door you're going to come running back out.
Client:	Yeah, that's what I thought.
Therapist:	Yeah, that's what I thought too maybe, because you seemed pretty strong about that thought. But, I wanted to give you a chance and see how it went. I was thinking to myself, you disappeared for a few minutes . . . but it was because you took some time to get the menus and chat it up with manager a little bit.
Client:	<laughs>
Therapist:	<laughs>
Client:	Yeah.
Therapist:	That's really good. Would you say that your prediction before was accurate?

Client:	I don't think it was accurate at all in hindsight.
Therapist:	Yeah. It sounds like it went a lot better than you thought it would, right?
Client:	It did.
Therapist:	So, we've done a few other exposure techniques, but this one seems to have been really effective. Instead of talking too much about it, we said when we got here let's just go and do it and see how it goes, right?
Client:	Yeah.
Therapist:	What are your thoughts right now? Your thinking? You have had those catastrophic thoughts that we've talked about.
Client:	No, I don't have those right now . . .
Therapist:	No, okay.
Client:	I feel like I had them leading up to going inside, but now, I feel really good.
Therapist:	Okay.
Client:	I just want to know, like . . . what's next?
Therapist:	<laughing> One of the things that we talked about . . . I want you to take the lead on trying a few of these approaches.
Client:	Yeah.
Therapist:	I want to ask you, what do you think would be a good thing for you to practice between now and next session?
Client:	Well, I think that I can do this again, but on my own.
Therapist:	Okay.
Client:	I'd like to try this without you and without my husband.
Therapist:	Okay.
Client:	I just want to go into another restaurant and do it by myself.
Therapist:	I think that's a really good plan. Just to briefly summarize . . . the last couple of times you've done this, I didn't go in with you, but I stood out here. The very first time, a few weeks ago, we went in together, but this was by yourself. One of the things you're saying is, eventually you want to be able to do this all by yourself. Maybe it feels a little safe having me standing here, or your husband. And I think that's a perfect thing to do. The only thing I want to remind you to do, just write down on a piece of paper—you don't have to do too much, because you're making good progress—still write down your anxiety before you go in. Make sure you write it down, the 0 to 10, when you come back. Also, write down your prediction, like we've done before, and then when you come back write down how accurate that prediction was or not.
Client:	Okay.
Therapist:	For our next session, what we're going to try is work on one of your top rakings on your hierarchy, which is going into the grocery store.
Client:	<laughs>
Therapist:	<laughing> Right?
Client:	I don't know.
Therapist:	Ah, come on, let's feed off of some of that optimism, right?
Client:	Okay.

Therapist: It's understandable to be anxious. For next session we're going to meet at my office first.

Client: Okay.

Therapist: We'll prep for it a little bit more and we both have a little bit of homework to do to prepare for that for next week.

Client: Okay.

Therapist: I think we know what we're going to do. We'll come to my office, talk about the expectations, how it's going to work . . . and then we'll leave together to the grocery store. Because this is toward the top, and you did a great job with the restaurant, there's going to be a lot more people. So, the first couple of rounds I'll come with you and coach you through the grocery store.

Client: Okay, good.

Therapist: We'll then go from there.

Client: Okay.

Therapist: Does that sound good?

Client: Yeah.

Therapist: Alright, you've done a great job. I'm really proud of you.

Client: Thank you so much.

Discussion Questions 4.2

- How does the session summary change from early phase therapy to late phase therapy (i.e., teacher–student to mentor–protégé)?
- How do the content and process of assigning homework change from early phase therapy to late phase therapy?
- How do the final questions and feedback change from early phase therapy to late phase therapy?
- What makes the late phase therapy a little different from other "typical" sessions during this stage and phase? How did this change the content and process of the late session stage?

ACTIVITY 4.2: LATE SESSION STAGE

Similar to Activity 4.1 for the early session stage, with another peer practice role-playing the late session stage, focusing on summarizing, reviewing homework, and questions and feedback. Try each phase of therapy and make the necessary adjustments to the questions you ask and how you lead the conversation. How did your questions evolve across phases? What did you do therapeutically to allow your "client" to have a greater role (e.g., participation or contribution) across phases?

COMMON CHALLENGES FOR CBT SESSION STRUCTURE

Table 4.2 provides some common examples of challenges that can be experienced with CBT session structure. You will notice that a significant theme for these challenges centers on the pacing of the session and setting a collaborative agenda that is consistently followed.

Table 4.2. Common Challenges for CBT Session Structure

Challenge	*Possible Considerations*
Too busy to follow through on the pre-session stage (reviewing client information and pre-session assessment)	Try to formally schedule at least a small part of your day to review client information, even it is not before every single session.
	Even just taking a couple minutes to read last week's progress notes is better than nothing.
	Schedule at least some time during the week to score and interpret assessments, then review during next session.
Difficulty with pacing throughout the session (i.e., appropriate amount of time for each part of the session)	To some degree, this improves with increasing therapy experience.
	If necessary, it can be helpful to portion out time to be spent for each part before the session begins (but this can reduce flexibility; do not do this long term).
	Be self-ware that relevant information is being addressed (i.e., minimize tangential distractions).
	If the client is having difficulty staying on task, you will need to be clear in your redirection.
	Be sure that agenda items are clearly prioritized.
Too rigid with structure	More common with beginning therapists—so focused on "doing it right" that flexibility is lost.
	Try to focus on the broader conceptualization of the client's distress—thinking in themes allows for flexibility—for example, a topic that may seem "not relevant" may actually be related to the client's distress.
	Remember that although most parts of the session structure must be covered, it does not always have to have the same sequence and be explicitly noted.
Difficulty collaboratively agreeing on agenda topics	Be clear in demonstrating that good agenda items are related to the treatment plan, which in turn is related to the conceptualization.
	Is the client engaged or hesitant to put relevant problems on the agenda?
	Some clients truly do not know what to put on the list; be sure to model early in therapy appropriate topics to put on the agenda.

Challenge	Possible Considerations
	Some clients may avoid certain problems that are especially distressing; in this case, take some time to process their thoughts and feelings about what they think it would be like to address the problem; client may not be ready or may need to process the experience first.
	Some clients want to address too many problems at once; try to summarize problems into themes (i.e., condense) and have them choose the problem(s) they think is most important; "bench" the other problems for future sessions.
	Some clients frequently present "in crisis" with a problem (at least perceived) that is very pressing; many times, this is a reflection of the client's distress tolerance and problem-solving strategies—this can be an agenda item or treatment goal itself; sometimes adding the problem later on the agenda list can deescalate the immediacy and reduces distress while other problems are addressed.
Client distress at end of session	This is largely due to timing of agenda items.
	Try to prioritize the most distressing agenda item first to allow time for you to help deescalate the client before heading into the late session stage.
	Increase frequency of check-ins to continuously monitor client distress and active coping skills.

REFERENCES

Dobson, D. J., & Dobson, K. S. (2013). In-session structure and collaborative empiricism. *Cognitive and Behavioral Practice, 20,* 410–418.

Kazantzis, N., Whittington, C., & Dattilio, F. (2010). Meta-analysis of homework effects in cognitive and behavioral therapy: A replication and extension. *Clinical Psychology: Science and Practice, 17,* 144–156.

LeBeau, R. T., Davies, C. D., Culver, N. C., & Craske, M. G. (2013). Homework compliance counts in cognitive-behavioral-therapy. *Cognitive Behaviour Therapy, 42,* 171–179.

Wynne, M. E., Susman, M., Ries, S., Birringer, J., & Katz, L. (1994). A method for assessing therapists' recall of in-session events. *Journal of Counseling Psychology, 41,* 53–57.

5

Psychoeducation

Teaching, Supporting, and Motivating

Psychoeducation in CBT is a key specific factor that is absolutely necessary for the progression of therapy. A major tenet of CBT is that clients will need to learn new skills as they collaboratively participate in their own therapy (Beck, 2011). Generally, this includes insight into their diagnosis and distress, identifying and modifying their negative automatic thoughts and core beliefs, making changes to their maladaptive behavior patterns, and learning any necessary skills specific to their presenting problems. Another major tenet of CBT is to provide clients with the knowledge and ability to effectively apply cognitive-behavioral skills autonomously (Beck, 2011). The goal is to ultimately have clients be their own CBT therapists where they can independently solve their life problems long after therapy is over. If done successfully, this can reduce the risk of future relapse and, it is hoped, improve their overall quality of life. In sum, your therapeutic effectiveness is strongly influenced by your psychoeducation skills.

For some therapists, especially those early in their careers, psychoeducation is viewed with disdain as something that is not worth the time and that has little value. This perception may due to feeling vulnerable to be in the expert role (e.g., must know the CBT model really well) or a strong desire to immediately begin specific steps to reduce client distress (i.e., focused more on the outcome than the process). Ironically, minimizing psychoeducation in therapy may compromise being perceived as competent by your clients and reduce the pace and effectiveness of therapy. Like most therapeutic skills, the more practice and experience you have in psychoeducation, the more natural it will feel and foster confidence in your role as a competent therapist.

It should also be noted here that psychoeducation is helpful in establishing therapeutic rapport. If done effectively, psychoeducation can be a learning process for both you and your client. While providing psychoeducation, you need to make sure your clients are actively involved. In other words, you should not be lecturing to your client. Rather, you should be continuously asking questions and eliciting feedback. Not only does this help you assess if your clients comprehend the material/concepts you are reviewing, but it also provides another opportunity to learn more information about their presenting problems. This information can also inform your evolving case conceptualization. Overall, the psychoeducation process is another way to model for your clients the collaborative role in their own treatment, which can also facilitate motivation to change and treatment retention (Delgadillo & Groom, 2017).

Without psychoeducation, CBT cannot move forward, as it has a continuous role through all phases of therapy. Psychoeducation at the beginning of therapy is more of a formal process where general expectations for therapy and information related to your clients' diagnosis and problems must be addressed by the first couple of sessions. As therapy progresses, there will still be multiple opportunities for psychoeducation where a new skill needs to be taught and practiced. With this in mind, this chapter is divided into two main parts: early phase CBT psychoeducation and CBT skill psychoeducation.

EARLY PHASE CBT PSYCHOEDUCATION

The psychoeducation content reviewed in this section takes place during the early phase of therapy. If fact, soon after the intake session (and in some cases during the intake), you will need to discuss what clients should expect while participating in CBT. This discussion should also include the cognitive model, including its relation to their presenting problems and diagnoses. Additionally, within a few sessions into therapy, it also advised to review your case formulation and treatment plan with your clients.

As stated earlier, psychoeducation provides a great opportunity to continue building therapeutic rapport. This is especially true during the first few sessions of therapy. Most of the initial psychoeducation content is relatively nonthreatening (i.e., CBT expectations and the cognitive model). This process allows clients to naturally acclimate to the therapeutic experience instead of being put immediately on the spot by being asked a deeply personal question or expected to engage in a new behavioral routine. During this time, you can also use psychoeducation as a foundation for building optimism and motivation. It is not unusual to have clients who are frustrated with their current distress and hopeless that their situation has minimal chance for improving. Some of these clients may have found enough motivation to initiate therapy, but they are still "testing out" the prospects of therapy; they are not fully committed to therapy. Educating clients about their specific condition (i.e., diagnosis) and how CBT has legitimate potential to reduce their distress and improve their quality of life can be just enough to remain in therapy in order to "give it a chance." Reviewing your case formulation and treatment plan can often be a relief to many clients, as it demonstrates your competence and dedication to your clients' well-being and provides direction in how therapy will progress.

The topics covered in this section will require substantial knowledge of how to conduct CBT, the cognitive model, and a variety of disorders. Therefore, you should prepare in advance before educating your clients on specific topics. Furthermore, knowledge of these topics is one thing; it is another to know how to communicate this information in a way that clients can both understand and be engaged. Thus, the more practice and knowledge you have, the better you can naturally integrate this information into your early sessions. Although beginning therapists may have limited clinical experience, it is still important to at least know basic information related to the early phase of CBT. If you come off as unsure or unclear about these topics and/ or have minimal client interactions due to being rigid or scripted, your therapeutic rapport could be damaged, or, worse, your client may terminate prematurely.

Table 5.1 is an Early Phase Psychoeducation Worksheet. This worksheet can be helpful in providing you a template to ensure that certain information is addressed with your clients soon after your intakes. In general, the Early Phase Psychoeducation Worksheet may seem a little generic because certain information has to be covered for every client. However, a brief description of relevant content is provided for each topic, and there is space available for your own client-specific notes to assist you in effectively conveying certain information.

Therapy Expectations

Either at some point during the intake session or soon after, clients should be provided a detailed description of what therapy will look like, including the expectations and role for both the therapist and the client. In many ways, this is like setting a broad agenda for therapy as a whole rather than for just one session. Some clients may have absolutely no expectations for therapy, while others may have a good idea of what to expect. Either way, a review of what to anticipate while receiving CBT is necessary. For those with no expectations, explaining CBT can provide some comfort by minimizing the mystery of therapy and setting structure. For others, their expectations and/or previous therapeutic experiences may not be similar to how CBT actually works. Thus, you might be in the position to adjust their expectations or even "retrain" their role as a client, especially if they have received a form of non-directive therapy in the past. Overall, the more you are up front about the expectations for CBT during the early phase of therapy, the less surprised clients will be as therapy progresses. This often results in clients who are more prone to be engaged and motivated throughout therapy, even when challenged to think and behave in ways that are new and different to them.

At this point in therapy, it is generally best to be brief and simple in your explanation of therapy expectations (there will be more time later in therapy). Spending too much time on this topic and/or using too much CBT jargon (i.e., terms they do not know yet) has the potential to intimidate and overwhelm clients. Therefore, you

Table 5.1. Early Phase Psychoeducation Worksheet

Therapy Expectations	Example Content	Client-Specific Notes
Collaboration	Clients will do work; feedback goes both ways; questions are encouraged to be asked.	
Session structure	Symptom review; setting agenda; reviewing homework; problem solving; summarize.	
Goal directed	Although there can be flexibility, therapy will have a clear purpose and direction.	
Taking notes	Encouraged throughout therapy; should refer to notes.	
Homework	Much practice and learning takes place between sessions; always reviewed next session.	
Challenging ways of thinking and behaving	Will take time with practice; learn news ways to think and behave to reduce distress.	
Increased distress before reduced	Sometimes experience distress (not always) when challenging "old" thoughts and behaviors.	
Autonomy	Rely less on therapist as therapy progresses; generalize and maintain change.	
Cognitive model	Explain relationship between triggering events, automatic thoughts, emotional and physiological responses, behaviors, and outcomes; reciprocal determinism.	
Diagnosis, case formulation, and treatment plan	Explain common symptoms, incidence/prevalence rates, etiological factors; refer to cognitive model; normalize while recognizing unique experience; open to feedback about case formulation and make modifications; connect case formulation to treatment plan.	

want to provide just enough information to effectively move forward with therapy but also trust that they will learn how CBT works once therapy begins. There will be many opportunities to provide psychoeducation about specific topics and skills throughout therapy. Obviously, this is a great opportunity to elicit questions from clients and to share their concerns. This models the collaborative nature of CBT, contributes to building a therapeutic alliance, and helps you assess their understanding of therapy expectations.

Information that should be addressed while discussing therapy expectations include collaboration, session structure, being goal directed, taking notes, homework, challenging ways of thinking and behaving, possible moments of increased distress before reduced, and autonomy. All of these topics have already been discussed or will be discussed in this book. However, Table 5.1 also provides some examples of content to be addressed for each topic. Remember, what information you focus on and how you present it will vary by your clients' presenting problems and personality traits (i.e., match to your clients' needs).

Cognitive Model

It is a good time to segue into providing some psychoeducation for the cognitive model after reviewing expectations for CBT. This information must be reviewed early in therapy because it sets the foundation for how clients' problems are conceptualized and treated. Again, similar to CBT expectations, you do not want to get caught up in using too much jargon too soon. However, this is the time to begin introducing key cognitive model terms and their meanings. Learning the cognitive model is sort of like learning a new language for some clients. Using CBT language naturally provides a new and different lens in how the self, others, and world are viewed.

Much of the content during your cognitive model discussion is similar to what was discussed in Chapter 1. Of course, however, you want to convey it in a manner that can be easily understood by your clients. A key theme that should always be covered is explaining the relationship between triggering events, automatic thoughts, emotional and physiological responses, behaviors, and associated outcomes. You can also include a review of reciprocal determinism if you think your client has poor awareness between how thoughts, emotions, and behaviors influence the environment, which in turn precipitates and exacerbates your clients' distress. This is a good place to provide visual examples of the Reciprocal Cognitive-Behavioral Model (see Figure 1.1) with handouts or using a whiteboard in your office. You can make your own modifications so that they are more appropriate to your clients' needs. In fact, using an example specific to your clients' presenting problems is often most effective because it is more relevant to their own distress.

The following is a vignette from Video Case Example MDD-4 demonstrating psychoeducation of therapy expectations and the cognitive model. Discussion questions and an activity will follow Video Vignette 5.2 (psychoeducation of diagnosis).

VIDEO VIGNETTE 5.1

MDD-4: Psychoeducation—Therapy Expectations and the Cognitive Model

Therapist:	Mark, what I'd like to do next is talk about therapy expectations.
Client:	Okay.
Therapist:	We talked a little bit about a few things but I want to clarify what CBT looks like in session. I also want to go over the cognitive model.
Client:	Okay.
Therapist:	One of the things that we hinted a little bit earlier is that CBT is collaborative in nature.
Client:	Yes.
Therapist:	We use the fancy word sometimes—collaborative empiricism—collaborative relationship. Basically what that means is not only are we going to work together in terms of the relationship, but we're also going to use the evidence that we have; whether it's measurements or having you tracking your thoughts and feelings between weeks.
Client:	Yeah.
Therapist:	We'll use that information and then do what we call mini-experiments or tests.
Client:	Okay.
Therapist:	And the key part is that we're going to be working together with that. Okay? The other thing too is that we're going to have some structure to our sessions.
Client:	Yeah.
Therapist:	Of course there's flexibility, but I will always come in with a part of an agenda, but I'll always ask for your input. There may come a time where you're the one setting the agenda.
Client:	Okay.

Therapist:	One thing I've already hinted at as well—some people don't like this word, but we can use a different word if you want—is homework. What it comes down to is you and I only meet for an hour a week.
Client:	Yeah.
Therapist:	There are many hours between sessions. The goal is essentially for you to be able to start doing some of the stuff we do in session between sessions.
Client:	Okay.
Therapist:	Okay? To give you time and opportunity to practice a lot of things.
Client:	Okay.
Therapist:	How are we doing so far?
Client:	Yeah. I mean, as long as I'm not graded on it. <laughs>
Therapist:	<laughing> No, no grading or anything like that.
Client:	Okay.
Therapist:	And those homework assignments will always be reviewed the next session.

Client:	Okay.
Therapist:	And I won't grade . . . but we'll give each other some feedback on how they went. It's not about . . . good or bad. It's more of what was done and what can we do to work on it.
Client:	Okay.
Therapist:	The other thing is to start gently identify and challenging some thoughts and behaviors; that's a key component.
Client:	Yeah.
Therapist:	What we're going to be doing soon is activity monitoring.
Client:	Yeah.
Therapist:	You know, scheduling activities and changing some behavioral patterns.
Client:	Okay.
Therapist:	And later on, as I'll explain on the whiteboard as well, we'll talk about changing some of those thoughts.
Client:	Okay.

Therapist:	I want to show you a visual of a basic version of the cognitive model that we talked about, but we haven't really fully teased it out. I'll just put "B" for behaviors. <using whiteboard>
Client:	Okay.
Therapist:	The event that we recently spoke last week with your friend George.
Client:	Yeah.
Therapist:	And we talked about how—to give you some credit—you got the courage to make the phone call.
Client:	Yeah.
Therapist:	You called him, right?
Client:	Yeah.
Therapist:	Those can be considered behaviors.
Client:	Yeah.
Therapist:	But what ended up happening is from your perspective he didn't want to talk to you.
Client:	Yeah.
Therapist:	Then there were other behaviors, right? The withdrawal . . . and then the I'll put "T" for thought.
Client:	Yeah.
Therapist:	Let me just put over here too, this little square. This is just the event itself.
Client:	Okay.

Therapist:	I know some time has passed, do you remember what you were feeling or thinking at that time?

Client:	I mean, besides like hurt? I was thinking that maybe he doesn't want to be friends with me. Maybe he doesn't like me anymore because I would think that if we were such good friends, he wouldn't just say, "Hey I'll call you back," and not call me back.
Therapist:	Yes.
Client:	So, I think that was one of the biggest things that I was just kind of thinking—he doesn't like me. That's what's tough for me. I was sad . . . I don't know about any other emotions. I think really the sadness was one of the biggest ones.
Therapist:	Yeah.
Client:	That kind of hurt . . .
Therapist:	You mentioned how you cried a little bit afterwards as well.
Client:	Yeah.
Therapist:	I put "cried" here, but that can also play a role too as a behavioral piece as well.
Client:	A behavior, okay.
Therapist:	So I wrote down hurt and sad. The other things you mentioned are actually more in the thought area.
Client:	Yeah.
Therapist:	"He doesn't like me."
Client:	Yeah.
Therapist:	Or "doesn't like me anymore."
Client:	Yeah.
Therapist:	"He doesn't want to be friends with me anymore." There are a couple things here. I would actually call these thoughts.
Client:	Yeah.
Therapist:	And the reason why is because these are what's called automatic thoughts. They're very quick, and they're fast, and we believe them to be true.
Client:	Yeah.
Therapist:	I think that's why in this case you probably felt—and maybe even now you feel like—he doesn't want to be your friend and doesn't like you. The fact of the matter is . . . this is a little challenge here . . . we don't know that for sure yet.
Client:	Okay.
Therapist:	It may not be "valid." One thing we'll do later on is challenge some of those thoughts. Right here we can also call this kind of thought jumping to conclusions. You don't have to answer this now, this is more of a rhetorical question, but what is the evidence for that thought? Now you could say, "Well, he didn't call me back."
Client:	Yeah.
Therapist:	But we could also look at other scenarios where we could dispute that thought and show where he does like you and still wants to be your friend.
Client:	Yeah.

Diagnosis, Case Formulation, and Treatment Plan

Although your case conceptualization is continuously evolving, within the first few sessions you will most likely need to have a diagnosis along with some initial hypotheses of presenting problems development and associated distress. Thus, at some point in the early phase of therapy, you will have the opportunity to provide some psychoeducation for your clients' diagnoses and associated problems interfering with their daily functioning. Obviously, the specific content of psychoeducation here will vary greatly across your clients. However, regardless of most diagnoses and problems, there should still be a consistent cognitive-behavioral model theme in your explanation. This also provides an ideal opportunity to transition into sharing your initial case conceptualization and thoughts for treatment planning.

Most clients often feel at least some relief when informed of their diagnosis because it is a step closer to understanding their distress. Psychoeducation on common symptoms, incidence/prevalence rates, and possible etiological factors of associated problems can help normalize their experiences. Although you cannot ethically guarantee that therapy will fully "cure" them, it is also prudent to assure your clients that you have treated other people with similar diagnoses and problems with positive outcomes. Clients are often relieved to hear that you do not think they are "crazy" and that many other people have similar experiences. This process can help build rapport by demonstrating your expertise of the problem and optimism that their well-being can be improved with treatment. An important note here is to be careful with balancing normalizing clients' diagnoses and problems and not minimizing their own unique experiences related to their distress. If you overcompensate with normalizing, this can actually hurt rapport ("I'm just another depressed client.") and possibly communicate that treatment is not necessary ("If so many other people have what I have, why bother?").

Similar to your psychoeducation of the cognitive model, it can be helpful to provide or draw a diagram of the CBT model specific to your clients' diagnoses. Using the general cognitive model as a foundational concept, you can use a whiteboard to explain the specific diagnostic components related to the interaction of their thoughts, emotions, physiological sensations, behaviors, and environmental influences. If using a recent client-specific example, as you draw each component of the model, you can ask clients how it applies to them. Your response to your clients can vary depending on their level of understanding of the cognitive model and awareness of their own thought and behavior patterns. Accordingly, using both praise and reviewing concepts is common. Overall, this information can be helpful in assessing your clients' understanding of the cognitive model and further developing your conceptualization.

Psychoeducation and discussion of your clients' diagnoses and problems provides a natural opportunity to segue into presenting your initial case formulation. Although you may have already touched on parts of your case formulation earlier, you can use your CBT model psychoeducation of diagnoses and problems as a backdrop to explain your conceptualization of your clients' distress. Be sure to be open to client feedback and not present your case formulation as infallible; it will evolve over time. The clearer and more accurate your case formulation, the greater the chance that your clients will feel validated that their experiences are understood and hopeful that improvement is possible. Even if your client has some questions and believes part of your case formulation is inaccurate, this is a great opportunity to gather additional insight and make any necessary modifications. This not only models the collaborative process but also demonstrates that client input is valued.

If there is at least some general consensus for the conceptualization of your client's distress, then you can move forward with the treatment plan. The more clients agree with your case formulation, the more apt they are to be "on board" with your suggested treatment goals and interventions. The chances for treatment compliance are significantly higher when there is a collaborative understanding and mutual agreement of the precipitating and maintaining factors for client distress and an understanding for why specific interventions will be used.

The following is a vignette from Video Case Example PDA-4 demonstrating psychoeducation of diagnosis. Following the vignette are discussion questions and an activity.

VIDEO VIGNETTE 5.2

PDA-4: Psychoeducation—Diagnosis

Therapist: Okay, Lindsey. Well, it seems it's clear that you have what's called panic disorder and agoraphobia. I want to do something that we call psychoeducation to understand what we're dealing with. Now, this may sound a little silly but guess what? Anxiety . . . it's not that bad.

Client: Are you sure? <laughs>

Therapist: <laughs> Yes, I am. Believe it or not, anxiety is a normal experience that all of us have. In fact, in a lot of ways it's evolutionary. Anxiety is a good thing because it protects us from actual threats. In other words, if something harmful is going to happen—a legitimate harmful experience—we start to experience those symptoms, and that helps protect us. Believe it or not, it also motivates us. It can enhance our performance when we're engaging in tasks. For example, when we're studying for an exam we feel a little bit of anxiety, as we get closer to that date. In some ways that's kind of a good thing, right? . . . Where anxiety becomes a problem is where it can really vary in severity and frequency. If we have too many moments in our lives with extreme anxiety, that can result in poor task performance. I think that's what's going on using the classroom example where you start to feel really anxious—now that it's too high, instead of that middle optimal range, our task performance tends to decrease. So, when we're talking about panic disorder this is when we start to experience anxiety as a threat. Now this feels like, "I'm feeling these physical symptoms, I'm having these thoughts, I'm having these behaviors like avoiding something or fleeing a situation . . . and now it feels like something really bad is going to happen." But, maybe it isn't that bad, but you don't know until after the fact. One thing that you might be familiar with is the sympathetic system. You maybe have heard of that before in high school or college?

Client: Right.

Therapist: You are a little bit familiar with that?

Client: Yes.

Therapist: Some of us just call it the flight or fight. It's either we're going stand our ground and fight, or we get the heck out of there.

Therapist: It does make complete sense the way you're physiological response responds to some of these thoughts. We call these initial responses false alarms because probably afterwards, when you reflect back, you're thinking, "Well, no I probably wasn't going to die or nothing catastrophic was going to happen, but in the moment it feels very real." Eventually these false alarms become what we call learned alarms, where you start to fear some of these bodily sensations. You talked about how your hands start to shake and you start to feel flushed before everything else starts. These are what we call interoceptive cues. We'll actually work on exposing you to your racing heart and that sense of dizziness. What you're doing with these interoceptive cues is you're misappraising bodily sensations . . . and eventually that results in feeling like you're losing control and thinking you're dying. The sensations are real, but the way you think about them in the moment tend to get exaggerated.

Client: Right.

Therapist: You also get thoughts of "I'm going to die." . . . We're going to try to treat these thoughts as guesses, or information without a whole lot of facts. Does that make sense?

Client: Yeah . . . maybe . . . I guess.

Therapist: Basically what's going on here are these thoughts, even though they feel very real to you in the moment, there's not much evidence for that, right? So, I know class isn't going well, but have you dropped out of class yet and failed the program?

Client: No.

Therapist: No. You might be thinking, "Well, not yet," right? <laughs>

Client: <laughs> Right, exactly, pretty much, yeah.

Therapist: And have you had a heart attack yet?

Client: No. Not yet <laughs>

Therapist: <laughs> That's a good start. That's what we're going work on in our other sessions.

Client: Okay.

Therapist: We're actually going to evaluate the evidence. Like, what is the evidence for this bad situation that's going to happen? What is the evidence of this really bad situation that's not going to happen? Eventually what's going to happen, if we have the breathing skills, some other coping skills, some new thinking strategies . . . then we'll be ready to eventually start going into these situations and saying, "All right, I think I have the tools here. What can I do now to not only break the cycle here with the thoughts, but also break the cycle here with some of these behaviors."

Client: Okay.

Therapist: How does that sound to you?

Client: I'm willing to give a try. It actually seems to make a lot more sense than I initially thought.

Discussion Questions 5.1

- How can you adjust psychoeducation of therapy expectations and the cognitive model based on a client's distress and presenting problems? That is, what can be said differently, and how can it be done differently?
- For psychoeducation of specific disorders, what are some ways you can "normalize" each client's experience without alienating him or her or coming off as lacking empathy?
- What are your thoughts about your largely "dominating" the conversation during psychoeducation? Can anything be done (or said) differently?
- What are your thoughts about using a whiteboard (or similar device) to aid in your psychoeducation?
- Do you think it is okay to use notes (i.e., a "cheat sheet") when providing this type of psychoeducation? Explain.

ACTIVITY 5.1: PSYCHOEDUCATION

Practice trying to remember key points for psychoeducation of therapy expectations and the cognitive model. You can also practice psychoeducation of disorders that you are knowledgeable about. Include rehearsing content out loud to yourself or in front of a peer. Try to balance communicating key psychoeducation content while also being engaging (i.e., not boring!). Discuss any anxiety or concerns about being able to remember important content for therapy expectations and the cognitive model. Discuss possible challenges in trying to balance providing enough information without providing too much where the client feels overwhelmed and/or disinterested.

CBT SKILL PSYCHOEDUCATION

Psychoeducation does not stop after the early phase in CBT. Although what is discussed during the early phase is necessary for effective CBT, there will be many moments of psychoeducation during essentially every session throughout the remainder of therapy. While there is much general overlap for the type of psychoeducation during the early phase of therapy, there is significantly greater variation during the middle and late phases of therapy, depending on your clients' type of distress and severity. More specifically, there are a variety of client-specific skills that will need to be taught in order to both relieve current distress and minimize future distress long after therapy is over. These new skills can range from problem solving in session to exposure between sessions. Assigning readings (i.e., bibliotherapy) and the use of technology can also facilitate new skill development. CBT skill psychoeducation is discussed in general terms in the following sections. Psychoeducation of specific skills is addressed in the upcoming chapters.

Teaching New Skills: In-Session Practice to Between-Session Application

Throughout therapy, you will find yourself providing many "mini-lessons" of new skills for your clients. By themselves, these mini-lessons may not seem like much, but over time you are helping your clients build a skill set to increasingly improve their overall quality of life. In fact, these mini-lessons will accumulate into some very "big" and necessary cognitive-behavioral skills essential not only for relieving immediate distress but also for building autonomy and changing many long-standing maladaptive cognitive-emotional-behavioral patterns.

A common and effective way to teach new CBT skills is to provide an example of a completed exercise through a worksheet or on a whiteboard. This example can aid both you and your client in explaining and understanding how to apply a new skill. When possible, it is also advisable to use an additional example specific to your clients' presenting problems. You should scaffold your clients through each step of the exercise. Providing a real-life example and guidance often provides a nice balance of immediacy and moving at pace that is not too fast. Many of these skills will be used both in session and between sessions. Therefore, providing a copy of the completed exercise or a photo of the whiteboard can be used as template for the client to study and use outside of session. For some clients, a therapy notebook can be used to organize these completed exercises. Additional information to be saved in the therapy notebook include homework assignments, handouts, client therapy notes worksheets, and any self-report measures. This information can help track progress and reinforce learning and memory of specific skills between sessions and, it is hoped, well after therapy ends.

There will also be opportunities where is it most appropriate for clients to practice and apply their new skills beyond written exercises. These exercises can range from behavioral activation of returning to basic day-to-day activities to exposure of anxiety-provoking situations. Similar to written exercises, you will want to first practice these new skills in session because they can sometimes be distress provoking for some clients. It also allows you to provide direct feedback to ensure that the skills are being applied appropriately. Successful application of these skills outside of session is a strong indicator of clients making progress toward their goals and eventual readiness for the termination of therapy. Like completing worksheets, clients can track their progress to integrate into future sessions, including associated thoughts and emotions, in their therapy notebook.

Bibliotherapy and Technology

There are many self-help books and related materials available through multiple avenues of technology (e.g., professional mental health websites, computer programs/games, or smartphone applications). Initially, this may seem like a valuable option for clients in distress. However, without appropriate professional assistance, many of these resources do not provide long-term effective change and in some cases can cause more harm. With that said, there are many great CBT resources that can be used in conjunction with therapy and that greatly facilitate learning outside of sessions. Your role as a therapist is to make sure that you are judicious in what CBT materials are assigned to your clients and continuously monitor their impact on therapy. Chapter 11 discusses in great detail appropriate options to integrate technology with therapy.

When using bibliotherapy or technology resources, you need to make sure that there is an appropriate fit for the phase of therapy. Assigning resources that are too advanced or too simple can significantly reduce motivation and inhibit the effectiveness of in-session work. Similarly, consider your clients' level of intelligence, cognitive and emotional sophistication, and psychological self-awareness. Of course, you should only provide resources that are specific to your clients' needs, including diagnosis and associated symptoms, level of distress, and specific skill deficits. Furthermore, you should read and review any resources you assign to your clients in advance. You must understand the content in order to determine appropriateness and monitor clients' use.

Your assigned resources will be most effective in providing desired outcomes if they are purposefully integrated into your treatment plan. This means that what clients are reading and using outside of session matches what is being covered in session. In fact, some of the content of these resources should be explicitly integrated into your sessions when appropriate. Thus, any assigned materials are typically used as an adjunct to therapy in order to reiterate and reinforce key interventions and associated skills. Similar to other psychoeducation exercises, clients should be strongly encouraged to use their Client Therapy Notes Worksheet to write down any thoughts or questions they may have about the reading content and related exercises. Reviewing this information is helpful in monitoring progress and to make any necessary modifications to your treatment approach.

COMMON CHALLENGES FOR PSYCHOEDUCATION

Table 5.2 provides some common examples of challenges that can be experienced with CBT psychoeducation. The two most common themes for challenges tend to be therapists' confidence and ability to provide clear communication and clients' ability to understand key information.

Table 5.2. Common Challenges for CBT Psychoeducation

Challenge	Possible Considerations
Not confident/comfortable with knowledge about specific psychoeducation content	Practice really does help; audio record yourself and/or role-play with a peer.
	Okay to use notes or whiteboard; handouts are also helpful.
	Educate yourself more by reading relevant additional material; the more you know the content, the more "automatic" it will be.
Too scripted; not engaging	Avoid trying to memorize specific lines of dialogue.
	Focus on remembering key themes (i.e., bullet points)—this will ensure that you remember key points, but you will be more natural in your explanation.
	Increase pauses by asking clients if they understand or have any questions—your response will most likely be more natural, as it was not prepared for in advance.
Client struggles understanding cognitive model	Keep it simple; may have provided too much information at once.
	At the very least, provide the basics—will at least need to know relationship between events, thoughts, emotions, and behaviors.
	Integrate visual aids through using handouts and a whiteboard.
	Be patient—not everything has to be learned in the first session; much of the content can be frequently reviewed in future sessions.
	Accept that some clients will not understand the model as well as others.
	It is helpful to know if a client struggles now rather than later; can take into consideration when developing interventions for treatment goals.
Client struggles accepting diagnosis	Clarify that it does not define the client but rather is something that the client has.
	While still validating the individuality of the client, provide some normalization and basic facts about the diagnosis.

(continued)

Table 5.2. *Continued*

Challenge	Possible Considerations
	Frame within the context that it does not have to be used as a label, but it at least helps provides clarity and informs treatment goals and interventions. Ultimately, do not focus on the diagnosis; rather, focus on the symptoms and distress.
Client struggles learning particular CBT skills	Be sure that your psychoeducation was clear and understood; ask for feedback. Is the client therapeutically ready to learn the skill (i.e., moving too fast)? Is this skill too complicated for the client? If so, consider ways to modify skill implementation.

REFERENCES

Beck, J. S. (2011). *Cognitive behavior therapy: Basics and beyond* (2nd ed.). New York: Guilford Press.

Delgadillo, J., & Groom, M. (2017). Using psychoeducation and role induction to improve completion rates in cognitive behavioural therapy. *Behavioural and Cognitive Psychotherapy, 45,* 170–184.

6

Behavioral Activation

Monitoring, Scheduling, Moving, and Getting Things Done

Ferster (1973) and Lewinsohn and colleagues (Lewinsohn & Graf, 1973; Lewinsohn & Libet, 1972) are largely credited with initially developing the general behavioral concepts that are applied to current treatment approaches for depression (either as specific interventions or as an independent theoretical approach). Following the basic principles of behaviorism, depression is viewed as a result of a learning history where clients' actions (i.e., behaviors) do not result in receiving positive reinforcement from the environment and/or the actions are negatively reinforced by allowing the client to escape or avoid an aversive environment. Eventually, behaviors that would typically provide positive consequences no longer do so. This often results in clients putting less effort into seeking positive reinforcement from the environment and relying on their own internal state. Correspondingly, depressed clients can develop passive/inactive behavioral patterns that become precipitating and maintaining factors for their emotional distress.

Beck, Shaw, Rush, and Emery (1979) included behavioral activation, through "activity scheduling" (first developed by Lewinsohn and known as "pleasant events scheduling"), as a key CBT-specific factor for the treatment of depression. The primary goal of behavioral activation in CBT is to reduce negative reinforcing behavior patterns (e.g., social isolation or a reduction in daily routines) while increasing positive reinforcing behavior patterns (e.g., spending time with friends/family or completing chores). Helping clients be more active increases their sources of reward by engaging in previously avoided daily tasks and pleasurable activities. In fact, research supports behavioral activation as an effective treatment for increasing depressed clients' level of activity and reducing their levels of distress and depression (Cuijpers, van Straten, & Wamerdam, 2007; Mazzucchelli, Kane, & Rees, 2009). Even if not depressed, behavioral activation can help clients who have difficulty getting things done by problem solving to break down large tasks into smaller, achievable tasks while also setting therapeutic goals (Martell, Dimidjian, Herman-Dunn, & Lewinsohn, 2010).

Behavioral activation techniques are typically the first interventions used during the early phase of therapy, especially the first few sessions. Later, additional behavioral and cognitive strategies are applied during the middle phase of therapy. However, behavioral activation techniques can be used throughout all phases of therapy, especially for more chronic issues and generalization and maintenance of change. It is important to note here that behavioral activation is different from behavioral exposure, the latter of which is typically used for anxiety disorders after some initial cognitive work (with some exceptions; see Chapter 9).

The CBT theoretical rationale for behavioral activation is that many clients who are significantly distressed tend to have low levels of energy and negative automatic thoughts (e.g., "I never have the energy to get things done." or "Why bother trying? There is just too much for me to do."), which results in negative emotions (e.g., sadness, hopelessness, or guilt). In turn, this interaction of negative automatic thoughts and emotions makes it hard for them to initiate (i.e., inactive) and complete (i.e., active but do not finish) what used to be basic daily tasks and activities. Additionally, the clients' ability to experience a sense of accomplishment and pleasure is also greatly reduced (often called anhedonia in depressed individuals), resulting in low self-efficacy. Concurrently and subsequently, their negative automatic thoughts and emotions begin to perpetuate because they are not getting things done (e.g., not paying bills), not meeting basic needs (e.g., not getting out of bed), and not socially engaged (e.g., spending less time with friends). This vicious cycle perpetuates and solidifies the clients' maladaptive cognitive-emotional-behavioral patterns as their new baseline. Ultimately, clients feel "stuck" or "in a rut" to the point where they perceive there is nothing they can do to relieve their distress (recall: no positive reinforcement from environment and active negative reinforcement to escape/avoid aversive environment). Figure 6.1 provides a visual depiction of how behavioral inactivity and low accomplishment and pleasure develop into distressing maladaptive cognitive and behavioral patterns.

With behavioral activation, the ultimate goal is to get clients moving in the "opposite direction" of their current course in order to break their maladaptive cognitive-emotional-behavioral patterns. Due to their distressing negative automatic thoughts and emotions, many clients have little to no motivation or optimism for change. With that said, most clients generally want to experience at least some improvement sooner rather than later; they just need some help to get "unstuck." Behavioral activation provides something relatively simple and tangible that can be used soon in therapy. Therefore, most clients will be receptive to your suggestion to "immediately" start making some changes. What is somewhat unique about behavioral activation relative to many other CBT techniques is that the initial primary target area in the cognitive-emotional-behavioral pattern consists of the behaviors, not the thoughts. It is important to have at least some working rapport before initiating behavioral activation techniques because this will be considered a significant challenge to many clients in the early phase of therapy. The shared experience of "therapeutic successes"

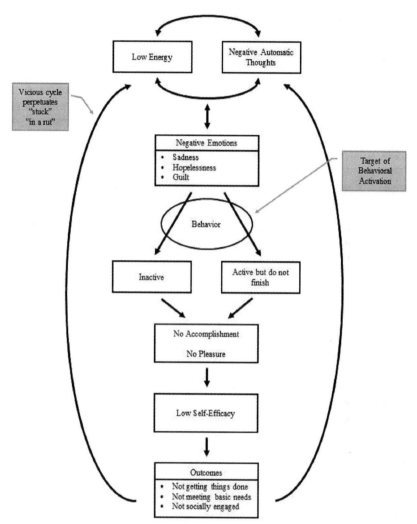

Figure 6.1.   Behavioral Inactivity and Distress

often gradually contributes to reduced distress, improved mood, and increasing levels of motivation and hope for change, including the development of future "bigger" tasks and goals. Additionally, effective behavioral activation can naturally reinforce the therapeutic expectation of the collaborative nature of CBT to be actively involved in therapy. In sum, if behavioral activation is effectively implemented, maladaptive behavioral patterns are slowly transformed into a lifestyle where accomplishment and pleasure are experienced and self-efficacy is developed.

The following sections focus on two of the most common and effective forms of behavioral activation: activity monitoring and scheduling and graded task assignments.

Both of these sections outline the rationale and specific interventions that can be used to break maladaptive behavior patterns maintaining distress. It should be emphasized here that these behavioral strategies are not mutually exclusive of cognitive strategies. Although initially behavioral, these interventions also include cognitive strategies and natural modification of thoughts, which are often required for long-term change for clients who are experiencing significant distress.

ACTIVITY MONITORING AND SCHEDULING

Activity monitoring and scheduling can be considered a single technique. However, for the purpose of explaining this technique in adequate detail, it is broken down into three stages. This approach also emulates the natural progression of this technique with most clients.

Psychoeducation and Assigning Weekly Activity Monitoring Logs

In many ways, the process of monitoring activities is one of the first formal interventions with your clients. Furthermore, this will also likely be your clients' first formal homework assignment, as their own self-assessment will need to take place between sessions. Therefore, it is imperative that you have a good collaborative relationship with your clients and that they are motivated to change. Poor initial therapist–client collaboration and/or low levels of client motivation to change have the potential to set up your first attempt at behavioral activation to fail. This can significantly damage the therapeutic alliance, as there are most likely no prior intervention "successes" to fall back on and it provides a poor "first impression" of intervention effectiveness. On the other hand, if successfully implemented, this intervention will most likely further develop your collaborative relationship and increase motivation to change.

If you do not believe that there is at least the beginnings of a developing collaborative relationship, it is best to reassess your approach to psychoeducation of CBT to make sure that collaboration was clearly reviewed and understood by your client. Additionally, be sure that you have an accurate assessment of your clients' motivation to change. At this time, some clients may be too distressed and/or have very low energy levels. If this is the case, it is probably best to temporarily defer this intervention and consider alternative "smaller" steps (see the section "Graded Task Assignments" later in this chapter) or motivational interviewing techniques to increase levels of readiness to change. Again, it is always important to make sure that clients are ready before moving on to any new intervention. However, the importance is heightened during the early phase of therapy due to the developing nature of the therapeutic alliance and first collaborative intervention.

If you believe there is a collaborative relationship and there is at least some motivation to change, most clients will be receptive to behavioral activation. Providing

Table 6.1.   Psychoeducation for Activity Monitoring and Scheduling

Behavioral Inactivity and Distress

Distressed individuals tend to have low levels of energy and negative automatic thoughts, resulting in negative emotions.

Interaction of negative automatic thoughts and emotions makes it hard to initiate and complete basic daily tasks and activities.

Ability to experience accomplishment and pleasure is reduced.

Engage in behaviors that maintain or increase current distress.

Vicious cycle develops when maladaptive behaviors reinforce negative automatic thoughts and emotions.

Feel "stuck" or "in a rut," where it feels like nothing can be done to relieve distress.

Behavioral Activation

Will help to move in the "opposite" direction by breaking the vicious cycle and be "unstuck."

Has the potential to provide some immediate short-term relief.

Will first focus on behavior patterns before thoughts—initially less invasive.

Will return to completing daily tasks and activities with a sense of accomplishment and pleasure.

---

initial psychoeducation on the purpose of activity monitoring and scheduling, based on the introduction of this chapter, naturally highlights the attractiveness of behavior activation because it is relatively simple to follow, is nonthreatening, and can provide some immediate distress relief (i.e., something tangible to further build hope for change). In addition to psychoeducation, simply asking your clients a few questions about their behavior patterns (e.g., "What daily behavior would you like to increase or decrease?") and how it would affect them if they could change that behavior pattern (e.g., "How do you think you would feel if you could change behavior X?") often provides a convincing perspective to move forward with behavioral activation. Table 6.1 provides key points that should be addressed when initiating psychoeducation for activity monitoring and scheduling. If you think it will be helpful for some clients, you can use Figure 6.1 as a supplement to your psychoeducation.

Before jumping into changing your clients' daily activities, you first need to assess their current baseline in order to know where to focus on specific target behavior patterns for change. Although this can be initially done while in session as part of psychoeducation, this is not a practical option by itself. Clients experiencing significant distress tend to view their themselves, others, and the world through a cloudy lens. In other words, they tend to focus on and generalize negative experiences, in both frequency and intensity, while at the same time minimizing positive experiences. Additionally, it can be hard for anyone to recall multiple daily events (including thoughts and feelings) over the past week during a therapy session, let alone someone who is experiencing significant life distress. Activity monitoring is a self-assessment that truly needs to be done for at least 1 week between sessions.

Table 6.2 is a Weekly Activity Monitoring Log that tracks what particular activities are completed at specific times during the day. The log is relatively simple in

Table 6.2. Weekly Activity Monitoring Log

	Sunday	Monday	Tuesday	Wednesday	Thursday	Friday	Saturday
6:00 a.m.							
7:00							
8:00							
9:00							
10:00							
11:00							
12:00 p.m.							
1:00							
2:00							

3:00						
4:00						
5:00						
6:00						
7:00						
8:00						
9:00						
10:00						

Include all activities for each hour of the day. Also rate you level of pleasure and accomplishment for each activity (0–10).

Thoughts: _____

Emotions: _____

design; it includes space for each day of the week to write down what activity was completed at 1-hour intervals. The instructions also state to rate levels of pleasure and accomplishment on a 0–10 scale. These ratings do not have to be used, especially for the first week. However, this may become a viable option later in therapy (see the section "Reviewing Completed Activity Monitoring Logs and Scheduling Activities" for a more detailed explanation). There is also space at the bottom to record any thoughts or emotions. Of course, the log should be explained and reviewed in session to ensure that clients understand how to accurately and fully complete the form. An honest self-assessment for just 1 to 2 weeks can provide a clearer picture of what behaviors to modify, at what day/time, and in what context—a true behavioral baseline. Review with your clients to actively monitor what activities they engage in each day, including the time. You may notice that certain maladaptive or adaptive behavioral patterns are more likely to occur during certain days or times of the week. They should begin this log the day of the session and continue until the next session. Emphasize that they do their best to record every activity they engage in, including what they may perceive as very mundane tasks (e.g., waking up, taking a shower, chores, meals, work activities, interactions with others, or going to sleep). In many ways, the mundane tasks are some of the best indicators of distress severity. Although at this point in therapy you most likely have not had an extensive discussion about thoughts and emotions (beyond your psychoeducation of CBT), this is an appropriate time to also have them record any thoughts or emotions they have while completing the log. At this time, it is not necessary to focus too much on "automatic thoughts" and "core beliefs." Rather, casually suggest to your clients to write down any thoughts or feelings they may be experiencing at the bottom of the log. This information can be taken into consideration for future behavioral activation tasks. Finally, remind them of the importance of completing this activity log over the next week, as it will be the primary focus for the next session.

The following is a vignette from Video Case Example MDD-5 demonstrating psychoeducation of behavioral activation and introducing a Weekly Activity Monitoring Log. Following the vignette are discussion questions and an activity.

VIDEO VIGNETTE 6.1

MDD-5: Behavioral Activation—Psychoeducation and Introducing Weekly Activity Monitoring Log

Therapist: What's fairly common for individuals who are depressed like you is we want to change some of your behavior patterns throughout the day. We're still monitoring your thoughts, but also looking at those behaviors. What we're going to do first is what's called activity monitoring.

Client: Okay.

Therapist: Before we leave we'll go through it and practice it and see what I'm talking about

Client: Okay.

Therapist:	What generally happens, and you'll probably agree with this, is that when people are depressed they have low energy levels. Right?
Client:	Yeah.
Therapist:	That's one of the reasons why you're here.
Client:	Yeah.
Therapist:	So this makes it hard to complete some daily activities whether it's at work or at home. It doesn't mean you're not completing any of them. You either don't get it done, or if you do get it done, it's usually kind of a chore.
Client:	Yeah, it's hard.
Therapist:	It's hard. Also, we've noticed your enjoyment in some of these activities tend to have been reduced; not completely for all, but for some of them . . . not much.
Client:	Yeah, yeah.
Therapist:	Also, you might also be engaging in some behaviors that might be maintaining this distress.
Client:	Yeah.
Therapist:	In some cases, it might be increasing your distress. For example, maybe you have a moment this week like you did the last couple weeks with withdrawing.
Client:	Yeah. That's what I was thinking about . . .
Therapist:	There's nothing wrong or bad about that, but it is important to write it down because it helps us to look at it and say, "Okay, this isn't helping."
Client:	Yeah.

Therapist:	How do you think you would feel if you could change some of your behaviors?
Client:	I'd feel pretty good, I think.
Therapist:	Okay.
Client:	I mean, if I was able to change like for instance, the withdrawal. If the withdrawal was gone I think I'd feel better.
Therapist:	Yes. And if you were a little less hard on yourself doing stuff at work?
Client:	Yeah.
Therapist:	Those are the two things that popped up into my mind as well. It sounds like you would like to decrease your withdrawal.
Client:	Yeah. I know that because . . . it's kind of like running away from my problems in some ways. I kind of understand that coping strategy.
Therapist:	Correct.
Client:	I mean, it helps a little bit, but it seems like it's not the best though.
Therapist:	Right. It doesn't completely help out in the long run.
Client:	Yeah. There are better things I could do.
Therapist:	And that leads to my next question. What would be a couple examples of behaviors or activities you wish you could do a little bit more of?
Client:	Being present with my girlfriend and going out with her. Whether it's bringing the dog for a walk together or going out to eat together, going out on double dates . . . stuff like that.

Therapist:	Okay.
Client:	Those just are at least a handful of activities I could do.
Therapist:	So, getting more active. Getting out there with your dog and your girl-friend, and maybe eventually your friends, as well.
Client:	Yeah.
Therapist:	So, the goal of this monitoring log and eventually scheduling is to help get you there.
Client:	Yeah.

Therapist:	What time do you typically wake up? I know it's been tough lately.
Client:	Uh . . . I was waking up closer to six thirty, but more recently it's been about eight o'clock.
Therapist:	Oh, alright so you're getting up at eight o' clock.
Client:	Yeah.
Therapist:	Are you a shower in the night or morning guy?
Client:	Morning.
Therapist:	Okay. So when you wake up at eight . . .
Client:	I'm feeling pretty rushed.
Therapist:	You're pretty rushed? How far is work from home?
Client:	It's only like a 10-minute ride.
Therapist:	Okay. So, you have a little bit of time . . .
Client:	But it's like, again, kind of like I know that I'm sleeping more . . . it's harder to get going in the morning. I'm kind of feeling like I'm like rac-ing the clock, almost.
Therapist:	Yeah. I can sense that it's frustrating.
Client:	Yeah.
Therapist:	You're getting up at eight, you shower in the morning, and you do your hygiene.
Client:	Yeah.
Therapist:	Hopefully, you're scarfing down some breakfast.
Client:	Yeah. I try to bring something.
Therapist:	Okay.
Therapist:	So at least you have something there with you at work.
Client:	Yeah.
Therapist:	So, what you're going to do here is write that you woke up . . . maybe you wake up at seven thirty, who knows.
Client:	Yeah.
Therapist:	Then you take a shower, eat breakfast, or whatever it is . . .
Client:	Yeah.
Therapist:	Of course, if you wake up earlier you can write that down.
Client:	Okay.
Therapist:	What I'm trying to emphasize here is that what would be considered mundane activities like waking up . . . "I have to write down that I woke up?"
Client:	And that I took a shower, yeah.
Therapist:	Yeah. It's still helpful to know what the pattern is.

Client: Okay.
Therapist: There may not be anything there, but it's just for us to look over next week. The more information we know, the better.
Client: Okay.

Discussion Questions 6.1

- Does this client at least seem moderately engaged and motivated to attempt monitoring his behaviors over the next week? What are the indicators that support your perspective?
- Based on what you know about this client so far (e.g., information from his assessment and this video vignette), what patterns of behavior do you think warrant follow-up in the next session while reviewing his Weekly Activity Monitoring Log?
- Would monitoring this client's accomplishment and pleasure be helpful for his treatment? In what way?

ACTIVITY 6.1: BEHAVIORAL ACTIVIATION WEEKLY ACTIVITY MONITORING LOG

Complete your own Weekly Activity Monitoring Log for at least 1 week. As described above for your clients, try to note as many tasks and activities as possible, even those that seem the most mundane. Include your ratings of pleasure and accomplishment as well. Process with your peers what this experience was like for you (processing the actual content is addressed in Activity 6.2). What did you like the most about this experience? Was there anything you did not like? What was the most challenging? How does this provide you perspective when using this technique with your clients?

Reviewing Completed Activity Monitoring Logs and Assigning Daily Activity Schedule

Reviewing your clients' completed Weekly Activity Monitoring Log should be your top agenda item for the next session. It is important to show the value of this activity and use this opportunity to begin moving toward changing maladaptive behavioral and cognitive patterns. At this time, your focus should be on identifying completed and uncompleted activities (and any patterns), associated thoughts and feelings, and facilitate the scheduling of pleasurable and accomplishment activities. How well you accurately review your clients' activity log will determine the effectiveness of your clients' activity scheduling. This process is crucial to giving your clients a "good start" to therapy as they move toward reducing distress through completing specific tasks and solving problems.

When you begin reviewing your clients' activity log, simply ask them to share their experience of filling in each day's activities. Was this an easy or a challenging task? Was this an enjoyable or an unpleasant experience? Did they learn anything about themselves? How do they feel? What is their current motivation/hope? Also, monitor your clients' nonverbal behavior when reporting their experience. Monitoring nonverbal behavior is a basic counseling skill for all therapists but can be especially important during this time because it allows you to better facilitate reinforcing positive responses and validating any moments of frustration. For example, as your clients explain how they noticed that a particular activity elicited pleasurable feelings, you may observe that they were smiling and that their body movements were more active than in the previous session. Simply verbally acknowledging this observation and reinforcing these activities can further stimulate their engagement and motivation during transition to activity scheduling. Overall, information from such questions and observations can help inform how you move forward with reviewing the actual content of the log.

Table 6.3 provides a list of questions to help you evaluate your clients' Weekly Activity Monitoring Log. Notice that these questions focus on a variety factors to consider across days and time: completed and uncompleted activities, pleasurable and unpleasant activities, activities that elicit accomplishment and those that do not, distressing and inhibiting automatic thoughts, and involvement with other people. Keep these questions in mind both when reviewing the log and while eliciting feedback from your clients. Of course, your clients' responses may stimulate additional follow-up questions. The ultimate goal here is to get as clear and detailed a picture as possible of your clients' behavioral (and to some degree cognitive) baseline.

Table 6.3.   Daily Activity Monitoring Log Evaluation Questions

What activities or daily tasks were completed or attempted?
What activities provide pleasure?
Is there any pattern of days/times when pleasure is particularly high or low?
What activities provide accomplishment?
Is there any pattern of days/times when accomplishment is particularly high or low?
Were there activities that included other people? Did these activities provide pleasure?
Were there any obstacles that prevented activities or daily tasks from being initiated
    and/or completed?
Are there any thoughts or emotions in response to these activities or tasks?
What can be done to increase pleasurable activities?
What can be done to increase accomplishment activities?
What can be done to increase social activities?
What can be done to increase daily tasks?
Are there any activities overlooked/not included in the log (i.e., activities that used to
    be completed in the past but have now stopped/reduced)?
Is the client open to including additional/new/different activities to their schedule?
Are there potential obstacles in scheduling future activities or tasks?

After obtaining a baseline of your clients' daily activities with the Weekly Activity Monitoring Log, Table 6.4 can be used to schedule activities and tasks for a specific day with attainable goals. The Daily Activity Schedule is similar to the log but does have a few distinct features: it focuses on one specific day, planned and actual activity to track follow-through, expected pleasure (before activity) and actual pleasure (after activity) along with accomplishment, and tracking associated thoughts (believability rating) and emotions (intensity rating) for each planned/actual activity.

When your client is ready to use a Daily Activity Schedule, you may find it helpful to start off with a list of potentially pleasurable and productive activities. A key point to follow is to let clients decide on the specific activities to schedule as much as possible. Clients benefit greatly learning how to schedule and follow through with activities that they value, whether it is for pleasure or practical purposes to meet basic needs. With that said, you should be an active guide during this process by providing suggestions and input based on information from your clients' Weekly Activity Monitoring Log and your activity monitoring evaluation questions. At the very least, make sure that the chosen activities are going to have therapeutic relevance to your clients and are practical, considering their presenting problems and associated energy level and motivation. During this process, clients should also include some activities that may be perceived as "small/minor." Not only do you want them to experience success and moving forward, but it is also common for clients to overlook completing basic tasks (e.g., showering, laundry, or cooking a meal) that may be just as important, cognitively and emotionally, as completing a "big/major" task. Ideally, you need to balance challenging and gently pushing your client enough to experience success and movement, but you also do not want to set up your clients by scheduling too many and/or too difficult activities too soon. Obviously, this will have a deleterious effect on your clients' therapeutic progress if they come back the following week thinking that they repeatedly "failed" throughout the week.

In terms of specifics, how many activities to schedule depends on the clients' level of distress. You also need consider other factors, such as time of day, time between tasks, complexity of tasks, and inclusion of others (e.g., friends and family). It is appropriate to make modifications in scheduling, especially for those who have low energy, difficultly concentrating, and low motivation. For example, for one client, you may be focusing on what time to wake up in the morning and take a shower. For another client, you may be scheduling multiple activities for a day, focusing on completing a work project and social activities with friends. For all clients at their own baseline, when in doubt, start off with "easier" options and then work toward those that are more challenging.

When clients are ready to schedule specific activities, review with them the planned activity and the actual activity columns. The planned activity is what clients will write in the day before (ideally). However, it is not uncommon for planned activities to not go as planned. The actual activity column provides the opportunity to either confirm the planned activity or allow for modifications. Convey to your clients that it is okay if not all activities go as planned and to do their best to be flexible when necessary.

Table 6.4. Daily Activity Schedule

DAY: _____

Time	Planned Activity	EP	Actual Activity (Time)	AP	A	Thoughts: Believability (0–10) Emotions: Intensity (0–10)

EP = expected pleasure; AP = actual pleasure; A = accomplishment (all on a 0–10 scale).

There is also space for clients to rate their expected pleasure before and after the activity. Comparing before-and-after ratings is an effective self-report approach to assess if your clients' mood improves in response to behavioral and cognitive changes. There is also space to rate their sense of accomplishment after the activity. A common scale to use for pleasure and accomplishment is 0–10, where 0 is no pleasure/accomplishment and 10 is great pleasure/accomplishment. This approach will provide additional "evidence" to your clients that they are making progress and feeling better. It should be noted here that experiencing pleasure and accomplishment is difficult for clients experiencing significant distress. Sometimes, it is helpful to reduce expectations for feeling pleasure and accomplishment until their severe distress has been reduced.

Finally, the last column allows for clients to write any thoughts or emotions they have following an activity, even if they did not initiate or complete it, as this information is just as important. They can also record their level of believability for thoughts and intensity for emotions on a 0–10 scale. Suggest to your clients that they write down their thoughts and emotions as soon after the event as possible. The more in the moment their thoughts and emotions, the greater the chance for accuracy and relevance. Also, this will be good practice for future cognitive activities, such as tracking automatic thoughts (see Chapter 7). This information will also be helpful in upcoming sessions to help assess cognitive target areas (e.g., possible negative automatic thoughts and core beliefs for cognitive restructuring).

Before your clients put their Daily Activity Schedule into action, it might be necessary to troubleshoot for potential obstacles. This is more of a preventive plan to prepare for the "unexpected" when following through with the planned activities. You do not have to plan for every single activity. Rather, picking two or three planned activities is usually enough for a general plan to ensure effective follow-through with the schedule. Simply review with your clients what they think (i.e., predict) could go wrong. Thereafter, discuss some practical options in response to these obstacles. This process also implicitly teaches your clients the importance of being proactive and planning for potential obstacles instead of being reactive after the obstacle has occurred.

Behavioral experiments can also be helpful for clients who may be skeptical that specific planned activities (or even the Daily Activity Schedule itself) will actually not produce any desired outcomes. Rather than arguing or trying to convince them that it works, you can take a purposeful passive approach by asking them to simply "give it a shot" and see what happens. You will need their assurance that they will at least "try." Even if they truly believe that a significant portion of the Daily Activity Schedule will be a failure, it is almost inevitable that at least some parts of the intervention will be helpful; this will provide information to build off of in the future. You can buffer this approach by asking them to at least predict their levels of pleasure and accomplishment before they engage in the activity and then record their actual ratings after the activity for future comparison. If there is even the slightest report of improvement during the next session, most clients will be more receptive to future activity scheduling and identifying and testing their negative automatic thoughts.

The following are two vignettes from Video Case Examples MDD-6 and MDD-7 demonstrating reviewing a completed Weekly Activity Monitoring Log and introducing a Daily Activity Schedule. Following the vignettes are discussion questions and two activities.

VIDEO VIGNETTE 6.2

MDD-6: Behavioral Activation—Reviewing Completed Weekly Activity Monitoring Log

Therapist: Let's talk about your weekly activity monitoring log. Before we get into details—and there's no right or wrong answer for this—how would you describe your overall experience? This is your first time you really did this by yourself.

Client: It was pretty tough. There were times where it was actually kind of nice to see that I was enjoying things and I was kind of accomplishing things. But even just looking at it right now, I'm kind of like . . . feeling how tough of a week it was.

Therapist: Mhm.

Client: It was an interesting experience to actually rate everything, but as you can see here. I stopped rating things after my tough Tuesday.

Therapist: So, Tuesday was a tough day.

Client: Yeah, Tuesday was a really tough day. I wasn't able to really get as much done as I had wanted to and on the back end; I stayed an extra two hours.

Therapist: This is not a bad start. Remember, we talked about how you obviously do your best to fill it out as best you can. It's perfectly natural to have a day or two, or parts, to not follow through.

Client: Yeah.

Therapist: For what it's worth, as I look at here, most days are filled out pretty well. Remember, it isn't either good or bad. It's more . . . what you get done.

Client: Yeah.

Therapist: I definitely see some stuff here we can work on.

Client: Yeah.

Client: I did some laundry on Tuesday night. That wasn't too bad. Melissa wasn't home. It was a couple big loads. <laughing> I actually folded them instead of just sitting in the basket. Instead of just picking it out and having it be super wrinkled, I folded it and actually hung it up.

Therapist: That's great.

Client: I actually did the laundry. So that wasn't too bad. I mean I did the massive pile of dishes on Thursday and that felt like I got something done. I think that's something I've said before, is that when I actually do it, I feel like I'm doing something; but it's just getting it started that's really hard for me.

Therapist: That seems to be a theme . . . initiating it.

Client: Yeah . . .

Therapist:	It sounds like once you start doing it—not always, but a lot of times—you get it done.
Client:	Yeah.
Therapist:	And you feel pretty decent about it.
Client:	Yeah.

Therapist:	Let's go into more details of your date night.
Client:	I came home and took the dog outside and got ready. As it came time to start getting ready I said, "Okay Melissa, like where are we going to go eat?" <laughing> I mean, it's so childish . . . really such a hard thing for us to make that decision. We're going back and forth, back and forth, and she's getting frustrated with me because I can't make a decision . . . and it kind of put a sour note on it because we're spending 10, 20 minutes almost . . . I wouldn't call it arguing, but we were talking past each other. She wanted one thing, I wanted another . . .
Therapist:	Okay. This is before you even got out of the house?
Client:	Before we even got out of the house.
Therapist:	Okay.
Client:	I wasn't really in too much of a rush to get ready. It didn't seem like she was either. By the time we got out the door it was already starting to get late and I was starting to worry if we are even going to be able to find a parking spot when we get there.
Therapist:	There's a lot going through your mind at once.
Client:	Yeah. I know I'm thinking about it a lot, but it was a tough kind of start to the night. We got there eventually. It took us awhile to park. I was kind of worried about that. I mean, it's kind of ridiculous to think about finding parking, but for me it's something with my truck . . . it's a little more difficult for me to parallel park . . .
Therapist:	Okay.
Client:	It's just something that I worry about a little bit. I worry about the logistics of getting to places and I think maybe that was kind of why I'm worried about getting things started. Just because I get caught up in the logistics of it.
Therapist:	You spend a lot of time thinking about what needs to get done instead of . . .
Client:	Doing it.
Therapist:	Following through and getting it done. There could be a little bit of anxiety going on there. We've discussed before about depression and anxiety. I'm not saying it's necessarily a diagnosable anxiety, but I do notice some themes of worrying or ruminating about events.
Client:	Yeah.
Therapist:	Not just before, but sometimes afterwards as well.
Client:	Yeah.
Therapist:	You finally decide where to go, but it's a little bit later than planned. Instead of maybe enjoying the moment getting out there, you're worrying about "Where I'm going to park?" "Are we going to have a seat?"
Client:	Yeah.

Client:	The night ended pretty well. Once it actually got started and as we sat down.
Therapist:	Experiencing pleasure with your girlfriend is not an issue at all.
Client:	Yeah. It's just getting there.
Therapist:	It's getting there to that point . . . working on some of those thoughts your mind gets stuck on a few things.
Therapist:	Maybe there's a little bit of jumping to conclusions about what's going to happen. Also, perhaps not directly related is . . . we talked about dichotomous thinking as well—it's either going to be a good or bad night.
Client:	Yeah.
Therapist:	You know, it doesn't have to be a perfect night. It wasn't, but there's still a lot to take from it. So much pleasure came from that experience.
Client:	Yeah.
Therapist:	This can be an area we can talk more about when scheduling activities. We'll filter through some of those thoughts as well. I'm glad you were able to have a pleasurable experience
Client:	<laughing> Yeah, me too.
Therapist:	So, it sounds like once you got in there not a big deal.
Client:	Yeah.
Therapist:	We have to work on that front end piece and it seems like there's been other dates that have had a pattern there as well.
Client:	Yeah.

VIDEO VIGNETTE 6.3

MDD-7: Behavioral Activation—Introducing Daily Activity Schedule

Therapist:	I think we're ready to talk a little bit about the daily activity schedule. I still have your weekly activity monitoring log. We'll keep this to the side because this is going to be helpful for the daily activity schedule. I know we spoke a little bit about this activity schedule before, but this is the first time we're looking at it. What I want to do is spend some time explaining to you a little bit how this works. <using daily activity schedule>
Client:	Okay.
Therapist:	If you recall with the activity monitoring log I had you track over the week as best you could.
Client:	Yeah.
Therapist:	And you did a good job with that.
Client:	Yeah.
Therapist:	What we're going to do now is pick a day or two to focus on this coming week between now and the next session.
Client:	Okay.
Therapist:	Not now, but after you leave today, think about a day or two in advance. Instead of just tracking what you're doing during the day, now you're going to plan it out.
Client:	Okay.

Therapist:	We're going to pick a day and write down the activities that you think you're going to do.
Client:	Yeah, okay.
Therapist:	Okay. Any questions so far on this?
Client:	No, it sounds like it makes sense.

Therapist:	What I would like to do is a little troubleshooting.
Client:	Okay.
Therapist:	Can you think of maybe one or two activities where it might get a little difficult?
Client:	Yeah. The first one that I'm thinking about is just waking up in the morning.
Therapist:	Okay.
Client:	Just trying to find that time . . . I've been pretty tired lately and I've been sleeping more. Just even the thought of waking up half an hour early just seems so foreign to me. I've been so used to abusing the snooze button. <laughs>
Therapist:	Mhm.
Client:	So, I think that's going to be something that's going to be challenging to kind of try and change that routine. My body's just . . . I think it's kind of used to waking up at that later time now.
Therapist:	Yeah. Those are all valid points. You may not see the change right away, but I think it's helpful to start out with this. What do you think you could do—not guarantee—but maybe improve your chances? If you decide to wake up a half hour earlier, what could you do that might help it happen?
Client:	Um . . . I don't know. Melissa, she puts her alarm clock so that she has to get up and get it.
Therapist:	That's a good thought.
Client:	Yeah.
Therapist:	So, literally get out of the bed to do that? Okay.
Client:	Then she may yell at me if I don't want to get up and get it. <laughing> I think that might be something worth trying. Perhaps even getting to bed a little bit earlier.
Therapist:	Okay.
Client:	Maybe that half an hour might be enough.
Therapist:	Yeah. It's tough to change sleep schedules almost literally overnight.
Client:	Yeah.
Therapist:	If you had said two or three hours, that's not realistic. But for thirty minutes or so . . . give it a shot.
Client:	Yeah. I think that sounds good.

Therapist: What are your overall thoughts of following through with this as we wrap this up?

Client: I don't know. I mean . . .

Therapist: I sense a little bit of hesitation.

Client: I mean, it makes sense, but just following through with it . . . I don't know if I'm defeating myself already. I can kind of see myself taking it hard if I schedule something and I don't follow through.

Therapist: Okay. You have a thought in your mind that maybe some things won't happen. And if they don't you might be a little bit hard on yourself.

Client: Yeah.

Therapist: That's kind of similar to how life's been going in general, right? Being hard on yourself when you don't follow through. Sometimes you do follow-through and you're still hard on yourself, right?

Client: Yeah, yeah.

Therapist: I think that's really good insight on your part and I think where that can be helpful is to write down your thoughts during those particular activities. Because it's okay . . . They're probably not going to go exactly as planned, right? Because life doesn't . . . work that way.

Client: Yeah.

Therapist: But I think this is one of those moments where if they don't go as planned, it's really helpful to write down those thoughts.

Client: Okay.

Therapist: You're still going to have some hits as well.

Client: Yeah.

Therapist: Don't forget to write down those positive thoughts.

Client: Okay.

Discussion Questions 6.2

- What additional questions would you ask this client about his Weekly Activity Monitoring Log to assist you in moving forward with his Daily Activity Schedule (see Table 6.2)? In other words, what additional information do you want to know?
- Based on what you know about this client so far (e.g., information from his assessment and his Weekly Activity Monitoring Log), what specific activities or tasks would you like to see on his first Daily Activity Schedule?
- How would monitoring this client's thoughts (and believability rating) and emotions (and severity rating) be helpful for future cognitive work?

ACTIVITY 6.2: BEHAVIORAL ACTIVATION—
REVIEW COMPLETED ACTIVITY MONITORING LOG

Review your previously completed Weekly Activity Monitoring Log and answer as many questions as possible in Table 6.3. What activities provided you the most and the least pleasure and accomplishment? Do you experience any particular obstacles in completing any tasks? What can be done about such obstacles in the future? What are ways you can realistically increase your experience of pleasure and accomplishment, including basic daily tasks? Are there any new/different activities that you would like to try?

ACTIVITY 6.3: BEHAVIORAL ACTIVATION—
DAILY ACTIVITY SCHEDULE

Use the information from Activity 6.2 to complete your own Daily Activity Schedule for at least 2 days over the next week. Try your best to follow your planned activities throughout the day. Also include your expected and actual pleasure and accomplishment. Finally, include any thoughts and emotions you have for each activity. Be sure to rate level of believability for each thought (0–10) and intensity for each emotion (0–10). Process with your peers what this experience was like for you (processing the actual content is addressed in Activity 6.4). What did you like the most about this experience? Was there anything you did not like? What was the most challenging? How does this provide you perspective when using this technique with your clients?

Reviewing Completed Daily Activity Schedules and Moving Forward

In many ways, reviewing your clients' completed Daily Activities schedule is similar to reviewing your clients' Weekly Activity Monitoring Log. However, you have transitioned from assessment of baseline behavior to interventions for changing behaviors, which can provide more contextual information. You are now assessing the effectiveness of your clients' Daily Activity Schedule. You and your client will probably be eager to see what "worked" and "did not work." Table 6.5 provides a list of questions to help you evaluate your clients' Daily Activity Schedule. All of this information will be helpful not only for making modifications for future activity scheduling but also for future cognitive and possible behavioral exposure interventions.

While reviewing your clients' Daily Activity Schedule, a major focus should be on recognizing and praising their efforts, even for some activities that may have not been fully completed. Be sure to also emphasize the value of clients giving themselves credit for completing tasks that may be perceived as small/minor. As stated earlier, clients may put much emphasis on completing big/major tasks, but it is the completion of the smaller/minor tasks that often provides the most salient and immediate distress relief. Overall, be sure that your clients are giving themselves credit for their

Table 6.5. Daily Activity Schedule Evaluation Questions

What activities were initiated and completed?

What activities were initiated but not completed?

What activities were not initiated?

What are the reported levels of pleasure and accomplishment for each activity?

What are the reported thoughts (and believability) and emotions (and intensity) for each activity?

Are there any negative automatic thoughts (or behaviors) that warrant monitoring or follow-up?

Are there any adaptive behaviors that should be validated and reinforced?

What are any general thoughts in responses to the overall schedule?

If behavioral experiments were used, were obstacles avoided/solved?

Were there any negative predictions that were disproven?

How will this information inform future cognitive and/or behavioral exposure interventions?

progress, instead of externalizing their success to you (the therapist), others, or luck. It is exceptionally vital that clients be able to internalize their progress in order to enhance their sense of self-efficacy. You want to start early building your clients' self-efficacy and autonomy for being in control of their own behaviors and emotions; this provides a significant boost in motivation and hope for change. You eventually want clients to be motivated to initiate (and persist in) pleasurable and productive activities own their own.

Clients can also benefit from reviewing their ratings of pleasure and accomplishment. Clients will often report being surprised that certain activities were more pleasurable and/or satisfying than initially anticipated. Even if clients report what may seem like low levels of pleasure or accomplishment (e.g., a rating of 3 or 4), this should not be downplayed. For example, there is still value in recognizing a completed task with a pleasure rating of 3 that in the recent past was not even being attempted and/or not eliciting any pleasure. Also, consider that some activities are generally not inherently pleasurable or do not produce high levels of accomplishment. This is also a good opportunity to assess their preparedness and response to any potential obstacles, including any behavioral experiments. Typically, most predictions will be found to be invalid, even if an activity was not fully completed and/or not very pleasurable or productive. For example, a common theme for some clients is that none of their friends are interested in spending time with them. Sometimes, when they get the motivation to reach out to a friend, their request is well received but is put off to another time (e.g., too busy this weekend but available next weekend). In this case, instead of focusing on the delay in seeing this friend, the focus should be on the fact that the friend was receptive and willing to do something with the client. Overall, this may be one of the first moments when clients discover that some of their predictions are inaccurate. This can not only increase motivation to increase pleasurable and productive activities but also add much confidence to the effectiveness of therapy as a whole in reducing distress and improving quality of life.

The following is a vignette from Video Case Example MDD-8 demonstrating reviewing a completed Daily Activity Schedule. Following the vignette are discussion questions and two activities.

VIDEO VIGNETTE 6.4

MDD-8: Behavioral Activation—Reviewing Completed Daily Activity Schedule

Therapist: So Mark, let's get to our big homework assignment of the day.
Client: Yeah.
Therapist: We talked about last week of maybe trying to schedule a few activities. I took a look at it earlier when you came in and it looks like you filled it out as best you could.
Client: Yeah, I did.
Therapist: Right off the bat I give you a lot of credit. How would you describe your overall experience of working on this for the first time by yourself?
Client: It wasn't that bad, actually. I think the most helpful part was actually putting down what I was feeling.
Therapist: Okay.
Client: Yeah. I think that was something that . . . to actually write down what I was thinking was helpful.
Therapist: So thoughts and feelings were really helpful.
Client: Yeah. It was a little tough to see what didn't exactly work out, but it is what it is. It still wasn't a bad day.
Therapist: Okay.

Client: Preparing dinner with Melissa still went as planned. Well, dinner itself didn't go quite as we had planned it, but the preparation was still kind of nice.
Therapist: Okay. And it looks like it was planned as dinner with friends?
Client: Yeah.
Therapist: It didn't play out that way?
Client: Yeah. Melissa and I were going to have some friends over; my buddy George and Allison over.
Therapist: Okay.
Client: But, unfortunately, they weren't able to make it, kind of like last minute, as we were getting dinner ready. They just gave us a call . . .
Therapist: Oh, okay. Okay. So, you did plan that ahead. You called ahead and they said, "Yes," for coming.
Client: Yeah.
Therapist: But something happened on their end . . .
Client: Yeah.
Therapist: Okay.
Client: Yeah.
Therapist: Do you think you can explore your thoughts related to that as well? How that planned out.

Client:	Yeah, I mean that . . . that was kind of tough when I got the call.
Therapist:	Okay.
Therapist:	That didn't feel good getting that call? Kind of . . .
Client:	Yeah. The thing is I made the call to confirm with them about this earlier in the week—"Oh, yeah, we'll be there Mark, we'll be there."
Therapist:	Mhm.
Client:	And then Friday . . . at least they had the decency to call me instead of just shooting a text.
Therapist:	Okay.
Client:	So that was nice.
Therapist:	Okay. You at least appreciated the phone call.
Client:	Yeah.

Therapist:	Tell me a little bit more—they called you, which is good. You said that you were "upset" that your friends were not coming. Describe a little bit more what upset means to you.
Client:	I got the call right around six o'clock. I kind of had that feeling of do they even like . . . want to be friends with me? I had called the first time to invite them and then I called again to confirm . . . and then . . . something came up. They didn't tell me what it was, but there's that inkling of do they really, value me? Do they value this relationship?
Therapist:	Mhm.
Client:	They live 15 minutes away. I guess I could find out what happened. I didn't really press him.
Therapist:	It sounds like there's a little bit of automatic thought going on there. And, you phrased it as a question—"Do they want to be friends with me?" "Do they value me?"
Client:	Yeah . . . yeah.
Therapist:	We talked a little about core beliefs earlier. Maybe feeling a little bit unlikeable?
Client:	Yeah.
Therapist:	Because that seems to be coming up a lot. If I remember, was it also George you tried to contact?
Client:	Yeah, it was.
Therapist:	He didn't give you much of an explanation, at least initially . . .
Client:	Yeah.
Therapist:	There's a lot of ways we could look at this for automatic thoughts. Maybe jumping to conclusions a little bit? At the same time, maybe a little bit of personalization . . . internalizing it and making some assumptions about what's happened. Did they give you a reason why they couldn't make it?
Client:	It was just kind of like, "Oh, well we have family stuff going on." So, it wasn't . . .
Therapist:	So something came up with the family.
Client:	Yeah, and I have no idea what that was.
Therapist:	So, again, the ambiguity.

Client: Yeah. I'm kind of filling in the holes

Therapist: Filling in the holes, right? And, to be fair to them, they did kind of give you a reason, but your mind's still . . .

Client: It's still not . . . it's still not good enough.

Therapist: It wasn't good enough, right?

Client: Yeah.

Therapist: Unless it's really concrete and specific.

Client: Yeah.

Therapist: This is something we're working on. Your mind fills in those blanks to come to your own conclusions. Right?

Client: Yeah.

Therapist: When you called them up a day or two before, how did they respond when you said, "Hey, come over, we want to cook you dinner?"

Client: Well, they were excited.

Therapist: They were excited.

Client: Yeah.

Therapist: So, the chances are they probably did want to come over. Do you think they would say "yes" to you to come over if they didn't like you or didn't want to be friends with you and Melissa?

Client: I guess not.

Therapist: Just something to think about.

Client: Yeah.

Therapist: Usually if people don't want to be friends and hang out they wouldn't be excited and say "yes." I think this is something we're definitely going to talk about sooner than later.

Client: Yeah.

Therapist: Do you see where I'm going with that?

Client: Yeah, I do.

Therapist: I understand a lot of people would feel disappointed when you have a plan that doesn't play out.

Client: Yeah.

Therapist: You sometimes take it to a whole other level where you start saying, "Okay, they can't make it. This feels icky."

Client: Right.

Therapist: You notice how you just wrote down upset, but when we filtered through that a little bit it comes down to "they don't value me" or "they don't want to be my friends."

Client: Right. Yeah.

Therapist: And then it comes down to maybe not feeling likeable, when in fact there's a little bit of evidence that maybe points in the other direction. You see how this can be helpful?

Client: Yeah . . . yeah.

Therapist: It feels kind of "blah" talking about it, but it also provides a little bit of insight.

Client: Yeah.

Discussion Questions 6.3

- What additional questions would you ask this client about his Daily Activity Schedule to assist you in moving forward with additional Daily Activity Schedules and future techniques with his negative automatic thoughts and maladaptive behaviors (see Table 6.5)? In other words, what additional information do you want to know?
- Based on what you know about this client so far (e.g., information from his assessment, including his Weekly Activity Monitoring Log and Daily Activity Schedule), what specific activities or tasks would you like to see on his next Daily Activity Schedule?
- What automatic thoughts (or core beliefs) do you think warrant further attention moving forward with more cognitive techniques?

ACTIVITY 6.4: BEHAVIORAL ACTIVATION— REVIEW COMPLETED DAILY ACTIVITY SCHEDULE

Review your previously completed Daily Activity Schedule and answer as many questions as possible in Table 6.5. Especially focus on what activities were initiated and those that were not (or those initiated but not completed). Can you think of any reasons why certain activities were not initiated and/ or not completed? Review any possible changes in pleasure before and after each activity and levels of accomplishment. Were there particular activities that were more/less pleasurable than expected? Review your thoughts and emotions after each activity. Did you notice any themes of negative automatic thoughts or maladaptive behaviors? Did you notice any adaptive thoughts or behaviors? Are there any activities that you would like to continue? Are there any activities that you did not do but would like to do in the future?

ACTIVITY 6.5: BEHAVIORAL ACTIVATION— INTRODUCING AND REVIEWING WEEKLY ACTIVITY MONITORING LOG AND DAILY ACTIVITY SCHEDULE

Now that you have practiced completing both a Weekly Activity Monitoring Log and a Daily Activity Schedule on yourself, practice introducing and reviewing both of these activities with a peer. (You can either use your peers' previously completed activities or make up a generic version.) Were there any particular parts of either technique that were challenging to introduce or explain? Similarly, were there any particular parts of either technique that were challenging to review? How was reviewing the Weekly Activity Monitoring Log helpful for informing your approach to introducing the Daily Activity Schedule? After reviewing the Daily Activity Schedule, were you able to notice themes of negative automatic thoughts or maladaptive behaviors that might warrant attention or monitoring?

GRADED TASK ASSIGNMENTS

At times, there may be some tasks that are "bigger" and that can often be overwhelming for some clients. These big tasks may be a part of the Daily Activity Schedule or a separate task that is part of a specific intervention that is crucial to learn new skills and relieve symptom distress. In these cases, a graded task assignment (GTA) may be a viable option to help make these overwhelming tasks more manageable by breaking them down into smaller tasks. These smaller tasks often make it less psychologically overwhelming for your clients and provide more opportunities for accomplishment and, sometimes, pleasure. GTAs can also be used for clients who are not ready or motivated to follow through with a full Daily Activity Schedule.

When using GTAs for activity scheduling, much value can come from helping clients who have fallen behind on a particular type of task (e.g., chores). It is also not uncommon for some clients to complete many tasks on their Daily Activity Schedules, but still have a few difficult or overwhelming tasks that are repeatedly ignored or overlooked, including those that may have deadlines for completion or specific self-assigned goals. On the surface, this may come off as procrastination, but when you assess your clients' associated thoughts for not completing the tasks, it almost always comes down to being overwhelmed by the magnitude of the task (e.g., "It is just too big."). Other related factors include that the steps for the particular tasks were not broken down enough, the task was too complicated, or the task required more energy/motivation than anticipated. Sometimes with big tasks, clients can experience high levels of anxiety and self-defeating thoughts because they focus too much on the overall task rather than breaking it down into smaller parts in order to eventually reach the larger, desired goal. This may seem like an obvious process to engage in when confronted with a large task, but it is important to remember than many of these clients are already experiencing significant distress. Breaking a big task into smaller tasks affords the opportunity to reduce distress, move forward even if low in energy, and make small strides in building self-efficacy. This process might also aid in identifying particular sources of distress or difficulty with a smaller task. In other words, is there one particular part of the larger task that is especially challenging? There should also be a cognizant effort to make sure that these smaller tasks not only reduce complexity but also match your clients' level of motivation and energy. Similar to the importance of completing the smaller/mundane tasks with activity scheduling, completing these small tasks will help increase pleasure and accomplishment. The added bonus of using a GTA for a large task is that your clients may also experience some personal satisfaction and growth once they are able to look back and recognize the size of the task they were able to complete.

If you find that clients are especially stuck or frustrated with a particular big task, you can use Figure 6.2 as a visual aid as you walk them through the activity. Note that this is similar to the Daily Activity Schedule with regard to tracking thoughts, emotions, and ratings of pleasure and accomplishment. The difference here is breaking down the larger task into smaller tasks and a logical sequence with

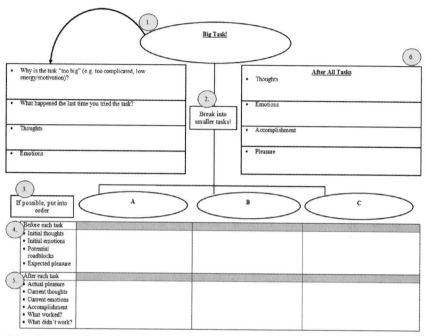

Figure 6.2. Graded Task Assignment Worksheet

room to report any thoughts and emotions specific to each task (rather than just for the overall, larger task). When initiating a GTA, simply ask what are some reasons that they think the task is "too big." Contextual information can also be obtained by asking what happened the last time they tried the task. Thereafter, ask them what are some immediate thoughts and emotions that come to mind. You may notice that even though your focus at this point in therapy is on increasing pleasurable and productive behaviors, particular negative automatic thoughts may be inhibiting their behavioral follow-through. For example, are such cognitive distortions as catastrophic or dichotomous thinking making it difficult to complete certain big tasks? In some ways, considering your clients' initial baseline, they may have some validity to their perceived inability to follow through with certain large tasks. Rather than gently cognitively challenging them on the task as a whole, it may be more beneficial to have them assist you in breaking the larger task into small parts that they think are more attainable.

When breaking the big task into small tasks, have your clients list the tasks in a logical and attainable order for completion. There are often many ways to complete a larger task; thus, it is helpful to discuss alternative approaches before developing a specific action plan. Additionally, be sure to keep in mind that each task is within the cognitive and emotional capacity of the client. As stated above for activity scheduling, it is better to have a task that is a little too easy to complete than too difficult. There is space to list thoughts, emotions, and expected pleasure before attempting each smaller task. If necessary, clients can also anticipate potential roadblocks and possible responses. After the task, clients can again share their thoughts, emotions, actual pleasure, and accomplishments. Additionally, clients can report what worked and did not work for each task. Some of this content may be too advanced for some of your clients, depending on their current therapeutic progress. Thus, use your clinical judgment for the best way to assess your clients' thoughts and emotions for this activity.

At this point, most clients should at least be able to rate their pleasure and accomplishment, as this is a part of the Weekly Activity Monitoring Log and Daily Activity Schedule. An individual rating for each smaller task makes the process more enjoyable and increases the chances for reported accomplishment. Even if clients return the following session stating that they were not able to complete all of the small tasks, you will still have the successes of the other completed (and initiated) smaller tasks to build off of. The completed smaller tasks will provide opportunities to praise their efforts and focus on any reported increase in ratings of pleasure and accomplishment. Also, it can be reinforcing and motivating to point out that although the bigger task has yet to be completed, they have made multiple successful steps (i.e., they are more much closer now than they were before). The increased motivation often observed during GTAs can go a long way toward building self-efficacy, challenging negative automatic thoughts, and increasing hope for change for completing not only this one specific task but also future tasks with increasing difficulty and complexity.

The following is a vignette from Video Case Example MDD-8 demonstrating introducing a GTA. Following the vignette are discussion questions and an activity.

VIDEO VIGNETTE 6.5

MDD-8: Behavioral Activation—Graded Task Assignment

Client:	I mean, sometimes wonder is it me or is it the company? Why aren't the people taking these jobs? Is it something that I'm not doing right? Is it something that the company's not offering?
Therapist:	Mhm.
Client:	I really don't know. I just know that recruitment is now a big part of my job, but it's something that I'm finding myself thinking a lot about.
Therapist:	So it seems like, feeling a little bit overwhelmed?
Client:	Yeah.
Therapist:	Sounds like a touch of personalization there as well?
Client:	Yeah.
Therapist:	What I have here is called a graded task assignment. We'll do a part of this now and you can do this for homework as well. <using graded task assignment worksheet>
Client:	Okay.
Therapist:	The way this particular assignment works is we've got to break it down into different parts or pieces. I get the sense here is that you're feeling overwhelmed about this.
Client:	Yeah.

Therapist:	There's a lot of stuff here to explain . . . some of this I'm going to explain in more detail right now.
Client:	Okay.
Therapist:	The big task here is what we would we call is "recruitment."
Client:	Yeah, recruitment.
Therapist:	So this is the big task here . . . we write in "recruitment," and then you notice how it gets broken into smaller parts.
Client:	Yeah.
Therapist:	We'll get to that in a second.
Client:	Okay.
Therapist:	There are also some parts here . . . where we talk about our thoughts and feelings . . . before and after each particular smaller event. I'll make a few comments about that later.
Client:	Okay.
Therapist:	There are a few questions here. You don't have to answer all of them every time, so I'm just going to highlight the ones that I think are relevant. Why do you think this task is too big? Or, to use your word, overwhelming?
Client:	It's just the nature of the beast. There are a lot of positions that are open. There's a lot of pressure from a above and sometimes I don't have quite enough time to get to it and . . . I don't know, it's just kind of overwhelming. It's just something about it I'm dreading now.
Therapist:	So, overwhelming, dreading. I think part of it that doesn't help is there's pressure from management.
Client:	Yeah.
Therapist:	Not only are you putting pressure on yourself, but the powers above are also putting a lot of pressure on you. So, I can understand. I can sense some of the overwhelmed feelings here.

Therapist:	How would you describe your thoughts when I say "recruitment"? What comes to mind right now?
Client:	One of the things is "am I doing a good enough job?"
Therapist:	Okay. "Not doing a good enough job." Could you explain that a little bit more?
Client:	I'm in charge of recruitment. I've done a good job before . . . I'm not sure if it's something with the company or if it's something with my job postings . . . or when I'm talking to a potential recruit. I don't know if I'm doing a good enough job of putting us out there as a company. And when I'm actually engaging with a person I wonder if I'm doing a good enough job.
Therapist:	So what did you say earlier—maybe you're internalizing this a little bit in the sense of self-blame?
Client:	Yeah.
Therapist:	Because it sounds like you're blaming yourself a little bit for it.

Client:	Because I mean . . . they don't pay the best for some of these positions. But at the end of the day when I make that offer and someone turns it down I take that as a reflection on myself.
Therapist:	Okay. I wrote down a few things that you just mentioned there— reflection on yourself and "am I doing a . . . a good enough job?"
Client:	Yeah.
Therapist:	It sounds like some of the themes of automatic thoughts about personalizing as well.
Client:	Yeah.
Therapist:	You do have some insight there. You externalized a little bit, but you always seem to come back to yourself.
Client:	Yeah.
Therapist:	You know, maybe it's not an either or; it's a balance.
Client:	Yeah.
Therapist:	But you're putting a lot of weight . . .
Client:	. . . on myself.
Therapist:	Yes, on the internalizing to yourself. What would be some emotions that pop up into your mind when I mention recruitment?
Client:	I said it earlier—dread.
Therapist:	Yes, that's what you said earlier.
Client:	I don't know if it's necessarily an emotion, but I mean I get this almost sick feeling . . . kind of like anxiety and I just don't want to do this.
Therapist:	Mhm.
Client:	I'm almost afraid to do this in some ways, because I don't know if I'm going to do it well enough. If it's something that I can even finish. Because sometimes I don't even have enough time in the day and I think, "Okay, well I'll put this off" and then I don't get to it at all.
Therapist:	Well, you said it yourself: regardless of whether we'll call that an emotion or not, I think that is a pretty good word.
Client:	Yeah.
Therapist:	I think dread's a good word because it does have a negative connotation.
Client:	Yup.
Therapist:	It has that kind of "blahness" to it, but it also has a future orientation of anxiety as well.
Client:	Yeah.
Therapist:	And it doesn't feel good while you're thinking about it. It fits into the other theme of how sometimes you ruminate about things and your mind gets kind of stuck. You keep thinking about it and then it makes it difficult to concentrate. I think that's some good insight on your part there.
Client:	Yeah.
Therapist:	What I would like to do then is we have three spots here where we can break recruitment into smaller parts.
Client:	Okay.
Therapist:	Does that make sense?
Client:	Yeah.
Therapist:	Tell me what would be the first part that you would identify for this task?
Client:	The first part is making the job posting.

Therapist: Okay.

Client: Writing it up and then putting it on all the different job boards.

Therapist: Okay. It's writing and posting.

Client: Putting it out there. Yeah.

Therapist: Should that be two or just one task?

Client: Put it as one because after I write it I just have to then upload it.

Therapist: It all fits into one task.

Client: Yeah.

Therapist: Okay. What would be the second task that goes with those?

Client: Actually looking at peoples' resumes.

Therapist: Okay.

Client: Looking at all the applicants that we get coming in.

Therapist: So, there is a little bit of a time lag.

Client: Yeah.

Therapist: Maybe you get something that day or two, but it can take a while.

Client: Yeah, couple weeks.

Therapist: I noticed here this is the part that you get hung up on a little bit.

Client: Yeah.

Therapist: I think this fits a theme that . . . maybe a stretch here, but if you recall the date night?

Client: Yeah.

Therapist: You don't get that concrete, specific information.

Client: Yeah.

Therapist: So you have to wait.

Client: Yeah.

Therapist: Ambiguity. What do you with ambiguity?

Client: I fill in the holes.

Therapist: Fill in the holes. And you don't fill them in with too many positive thoughts or even more realistic thoughts; they are negative. It seems like this is where the trip-up happens here.

Client: Yeah, right.

Therapist: You're thinking, "Well, who's going to respond? Who am I going to get?"

Client: Yeah.

Therapist: And you don't get that immediate behavioral indicator. It takes time to get it.

Client: Yeah.

Discussion Questions 6.4

- Based on what you know about this client so far (e.g., information from his assessment, including his Weekly Activity Monitoring Log and Daily Activity Schedule), what other big tasks could he use for a GTA?
- What would be your initial focus (e.g., thoughts, emotions, pleasure, accomplishment, obstacles, or what did/did not work) when you review his completed GTA?

ACTIVITY 6.6: BEHAVIORAL ACTIVATION— GRADED TASK ASSIGNMENT

Complete a GTA for a big task you have to complete over the next week. If you cannot think of a task that you have a concern about completing, pick a task that will at least have three small tasks. Be sure to complete the pre- and post-task content (e.g., thoughts, emotions, pleasure, accomplishment, obstacles, and what did/did not work) in as much detail as possible. Compare your responses for each part of the smaller tasks. Was any particular task more challenging than another? Did you notice any change in your thoughts, emotions, or pleasure? How would you describe your overall experience completing this activity? You can also process with your peers what this experience was like for you. What did you like the most? Was there anything you did not like? What was the most challenging? How does this provide you perspective when using this activity with your clients?

COMMON CHALLENGES FOR BEHAVIORAL ACTIVATION

Table 6.6 provides some common examples of challenges that can be experienced with CBT behavioral activation. The two most common themes for challenges tends to be clients' motivation and ability to initiate/complete activity monitoring and scheduling and therapists knowing how to utilize the information gained from such activities.

Table 6.6. Common Challenges for Behavioral Activation

Challenge	Possible Considerations
Client low motivation to initiate activity monitoring and scheduling	Do you have a good collaborative relationship with your client?
	Was your psychoeducation of the benefits of activity monitoring understood, including relationship to their current distress?
	Consider alternative methods to reduce client distress and/ or increase energy level and hope for change before moving forward.
Client struggles to complete Weekly Activity Monitoring Log or Daily Activity Schedule	Did the client understand the instructions?
	Was the client overwhelmed with the activity?
	Did working on the activity increase levels of distress?
	Remember that there is still much information to be gained for activities that were initiated and not completed (or even not initiated); good opportunity to explore related thoughts and feelings and potential obstacles.
	Some behavioral patterns are difficult to change. It may take time to see change—focus on and build off of the small steps.
	If the client has completed activities in the past, were they reviewed the following session (i.e., was there value placed on the assignment)?

Challenge	Possible Considerations
Difficulty knowing what areas to focus on in the Weekly Activity Monitoring Log to inform moving forward with the Daily Activity Schedule	Ask the client what tasks were most difficult to complete and/or resulted in the most distress.
	Ask the client what he or she thinks would be the most beneficial tasks to engage in.
	Review Table 6.2: look for patterns of behaviors, including high/low levels of pleasure/accomplishment and potential obstacles.
	When reasonable, focus on integrating activities related to your client's strengths.
Difficulty moving forward after activity monitoring and scheduling	Sometimes, clients experience much relief after completing behavioral activation activities. Depending on the client, this may or may not generalize to other areas of distress. When appropriate, consider how therapeutic gains from these activities can be applied to other presenting problems.
	Explicitly demonstrate relationship between thoughts/emotions and recent behavioral change.
	Use current distress relief and increased motivation as a springboard for implementing more challenging interventions.
	Consider how the information gained from these activities informs your CBT case formulation and future treatment goals and interventions.

REFERENCES

Beck, A. T., Shaw, B. E., Rush, A. J., & Emery, G. (1979). *Cognitive therapy of depression.* New York: Guilford Press.

Cuijpers, P., van Straten, A., & Warmerdam, L. (2007). Behavioral activation treatments of depression: A meta-analysis. *Clinical Psychology Review, 27,* 318–326.

Ferster, C. B. (1973). A functional analysis of depression. *American Psychologist, 28,* 857–870.

Lewinsohn, P. M., & Graf, M. (1973). Pleasant activities and depression. *Journal of Consulting and Clinical Psychology, 41,* 261–268.

Lewinsohn, P. M., & Libet, J. (1972). Pleasant events, activity schedules, and depressions. *Journal of Abnormal Psychology, 79,* 291–295.

Martell, C. R., Dimidjian, S., Herman-Dunn, R., & Lewinsohn, P. (2010). *Behavioral activation for depression: A clinician's guide.* New York: Guilford Press.

Mazzucchelli, T., Kane, R., & Rees, C. (2009). Behavioral activation treatments for depression in adults: A meta-analysis and review. *Clinical Psychology: Science and Practice, 16,* 383–411.

7

Automatic Thoughts

Eliciting, Identifying, Evaluating, and Modifying Maladaptive Thought Patterns

At the heart of long-term change for CBT is being able to change clients' maladaptive thinking patterns. The challenge is to first identify these thoughts and then evaluate them to see if they are negative automatic thoughts that warrant modification. As discussed in Chapter 1, one of the key tenets of CBT is that clients suffering significant distress due to their psychological distress experience distinct patterns of negative automatic thoughts. Additionally, following the cognitive model, situations do not "cause" our automatic thoughts, emotions, physiological responses, and behaviors. Rather, it is how the situation is perceived and interpreted that sets these series of responses in motion. In fact, clients experiencing psychological distress often perceive and interpret neutral and positive situations as negative. Therefore, logic dictates that efforts to modify these maladaptive thinking patterns (i.e., perceptions) can eventually lead to reduced psychological distress. Thus, it only makes sense that CBT therapists dedicate a significant portion of their treatment time to working on their clients' automatic thoughts.

Before modifying your clients' negative automatic thoughts, you will first need to identify and evaluate their relevance and validity. This is a not an easy task. Assisting clients with developing more adaptive thought patterns and being able to independently identify and modify their own negative automatic thoughts is a long process. The identification and modification phases of negative automatic thoughts are not two wholly separate processes. However, for the purpose of developing solid clinical development in specific therapeutic techniques, this chapter is divided up into many parts: (a) understanding automatic thoughts, (b) psychoeducation of automatic thoughts, (c) eliciting and identifying automatic thoughts, (d) evaluating and modifying negative automatic thoughts, and (e) working with valid negative automatic thoughts. As expected with effective CBT, you will find yourself using many of these techniques at once and across different points in therapy.

WHAT ARE AUTOMATIC THOUGHTS?

Before moving forward with identifying and modifying negative automatic thoughts, there needs to be a clear a conceptual understanding of automatic thoughts and their function. In many ways, our automatic thoughts are "pre-surface thinking" with additional underlying intricate and intertwined thoughts (A. T. Beck, 1964; A. T. Beck, Shaw, Rush, & Emery, 1979). All of us experience our own idiosyncratic automatic thoughts in response to specific situations; it is a normal part of our day-to-day experiences. However, most of the time, we often lack awareness of these thoughts. This is typically not of significant concern until people experience negative automatic thoughts that start to contribute to distress and inhibit daily function. Even still, some people are able to naturally reality test and modify these automatic thoughts on their own. However, this skill is often lacking in people who are in distress. The good news is that some basic knowledge of how automatic thoughts work can help heighten awareness of this form of thinking. Awareness is a vital step in being able to identify and modify negative automatic thoughts and reduce distress. Finally, as a related side note, the more therapists are self-aware and responsive to their own automatic thoughts, the more effective they can be in treating their clients.

Key Elements of Automatic Thoughts

In addition to the fact that we all experience automatic thoughts, there are six key elements to consider when working with clients (see J. S. Beck, 2011). First, automatic thoughts appear in "shorthand" form, often composed of a short phrase (e.g., "She thinks I'm bad at my job"). Automatic thoughts can also be a brief visual image (or both).

Second, automatic thoughts are like a "cognitive reflex." A key reason why we are often not aware of automatic thoughts is because they are experienced as spontaneous and last for only a brief period of time.

Third, automatic thoughts are experienced as emotions. Soon after we experience automatic thoughts, we experience emotions, sometimes very strong if they are negative. Thus, after a quick series of events, we are generally much more aware of the emotions than the thoughts. Although the emotions experienced are related to the content of our automatic thoughts, we often attribute it to the preceding event due to minimal to no self-reflection or evaluation of the automatic thought itself.

Fourth, automatic thoughts are almost always believed to be valid, even if in the face of contradictory evidence. There may be other events that show that the automatic thought is not valid, but this gets overlooked. An outside observer may view such thinking and corresponding emotional reaction as illogical. However, the intense emotional experience is very real if the thought is believed to be valid.

Fifth, automatic thoughts are persistent and self-perpetuating. In other words, because automatic thoughts are reflexive and perceived as valid, they are hard to stop and change. Furthermore, one automatic thought can stimulate other automatic

Table 7.1.   Key Elements of Automatic Thoughts

Element	Brief Description
Appear in shorthand form	Short phrase or brief visual image.
Cognitive reflex	Experienced as spontaneous and lasts for only a brief period of time.
Experienced as emotions	Thoughts precede emotions, but because the experience happens so fast, there is more awareness of the emotions.
Believed to be valid	Contradictory evidence is overlooked, but emotions can be intense and very real.
Persistent and self-perpetuating	Hard to stop and change and can stimulate other automatic thoughts that are part of a larger theme (i.e., core beliefs).
Based on past experiences	Historical events and significant others can shape our views of self, others, and the world.

thoughts in a chain reaction fashion. Relatedly, this is often because these automatic thoughts are connected as part of a larger theme and may have some grain of validity (i.e., core beliefs).

Sixth, automatic thoughts are learned based on past experiences. For example, historical events and significant others can shape our views of self, others, and the world (see Chapter 8). Of course, something that has been learned can also be unlearned. Table 7.1 provides a brief summary of the key elements of automatic thoughts that can be helpful for quick recall and to share with your clients during psychoeducation.

Validity and Utility of Negative Automatic Thoughts

J. S. Beck (2011) states that negative automatic thoughts generally fall into three categories based on their *validity* and *utility*. First, there is the automatic thought that has no validity and no utility. This automatic thought is not accurate even though there is objective evidence that contradicts the distortion. The therapeutic focus here will obviously be on the actual distorted automatic thought (i.e., focus on validity). Second, there is the automatic thought that is valid with misdirected and maladaptive utility. This automatic thought is accurate, but the conclusion or meaning derived from the thought is distorted. In this case, the therapeutic focus is less on the automatic thought and more on problem-focused coping and developing possible alternative conclusions or meanings (i.e., focus on utility). Finally, there is the automatic thought that is valid with no utility. This automatic thought is accurate, and the conclusion or meaning drawn from the thought is also accurate. At first, it may seem like there is nothing that can be therapeutically done for this thought. However, continuing to ruminate on this thought is maladaptive and distressful. Thus, there can still be a therapeutic focus on the utility by way of both emotion-focused coping and acceptance. Actual techniques on how to modify these automatic thoughts are discussed later in this chapter. Table 7.2 provides a summary of the three different categories of negative automatic thoughts and response strategies.

Table 7.2. Validity and Utility of Negative Automatic Thoughts

Validity of Automatic Thought	Client Conclusion	Strategy
Not true	Distorted/not true	Modify automatic thought using CBT skills.
True	Distorted	Evaluate utility and teach problem-focused coping skills while developing possible alternative conclusions.
True	Accurate	Teach emotion-focused coping skills and acceptance.

PSYCHOEDUCATION OF AUTOMATIC THOUGHTS

It his helpful to explain to your clients in the early phase of therapy (within the first few sessions) the basic components of automatic thoughts discussed in the previous section. This can be a natural transition after already discussing the basic CBT model components while providing psychoeducation about CBT. Of course, there will be continuous psychoeducation of the CBT model and the role of automatic thoughts throughout therapy, but it is important to introduce the components and mechanisms of automatic thoughts in a manner that is relatively easily comprehensible for your clients, as this information is interrelated for almost every intervention used in CBT.

When possible, there is the potential for a more natural and impactful learning moment if you can catch your clients verbalizing a series of negative automatic thoughts and associated strong emotions. As will be discussed in the next section, "Eliciting and Identifying Automatic Thoughts," when clients show strong distressing emotions, it is usually a sign of a recent negative automatic thought. You most likely do not have to be concerned if your clients will have one of these negative automatic thoughts–strong emotion moments, as it is almost always inevitable with distressed clients. It is an invaluable skill for therapists to be able to recognize client mood shifts and associated negative automatic thoughts.

If you are able to catch your clients' own negative automatic thoughts, then you can use their own events as examples to explain (or review) this key concept of the CBT model. This will typically happen when discussing a recent distressing event and/or problem. Using clients' "in-the-moment" emotions related to real-life examples can enhance attention, motivation, and learning because it has immediate relevance to their distress. It is highly recommended that you refer to Table 7.1 and visually display the CBT model and role of automatic thoughts by writing down the following points on paper or a whiteboard. When first discussing automatic thoughts, be sure to normalize the experience; all people have them. Then identify the basic elements of their spontaneity and brevity (i.e., "cognitive reflex"). You want to convey a theme that initially it seems like people may not have much control over them. Additionally, highlight the fact that people are often not aware of such thoughts and probably tend to focus on the emotions. At this point, make the transition from all people experience automatic thoughts (even negative automatic thoughts) to some people experience distress when they are not aware and/or are unable to change their negative automatic thoughts. You can also remind clients of your previous review of the CBT model, including how the perception of events affect emotions. In this case, their perceptions are distorted in some fashion (i.e., validity and/or utility) via negative automatic thoughts. If you have noticed multiple negative automatic thoughts, you can also include in your discussion how this can become ingrained and develop into a chain reaction of a larger theme. This is where you can integrate one or more of your working hypotheses of their problems based on your CBT case formulation. (This will be more effective if you have already reviewed your case formulation with your clients.) Also, highlight that such thinking is typically learned based on past experiences as a segue to future discussions of core beliefs. However, do not forget to include some optimism by emphasizing that what has been learned can also be unlearned. Clients will soon learn how to identify, evaluate, and modify their negative automatic thoughts. Relatedly, if your clients are ready, you can ask them to imagine how their emotions might change if they learned that their automatic thought was not true. Finally, throughout the process, occasionally check in with your clients to see if they have any questions. It can also be helpful to ask them to summarize to be sure that they have at least a basic understanding of automatic thoughts. At this point, your introduction of automatic thoughts should naturally flow into a more detailed discussion about how to identify automatic thoughts.

The following is a vignette from Video Case Example MDD-9 demonstrating psychoeducation of automatic thoughts. Following the vignette are discussion questions.

VIDEO VIGNETTE 7.1

MDD-9: Automatic Thoughts—Psychoeducation

Therapist: Mark, I want to talk about automatic thoughts. We've spoken a little bit about how these thoughts kind of pop into our head. I want to spend a little bit more time highlighting some of the components of automatic thoughts. I think this will be helpful for us when we start exploring, identifying, and challenging some of these thoughts. Does that sound okay?

Client: Yes, that makes sense.

Therapist: One thing that's important to know is that all of us experience thoughts, right?

Client: Yeah.

Therapist: The other thing is we all experience automatic thoughts. Part of the reason why we call it automatic is that we lack awareness of those thoughts. Many times when we talk about what happened or what's going on, we talk about our emotions, but we sometimes neglect to mention our thoughts.

Client: Okay.

Therapist: One of the components is that they appear mentally in our mind in "shorthand form."

Client: Okay.

Therapist:	What this means is it's usually a short phrase or image. It's usually not just one word. A lot of times if it's just one word, not always, but generally it's an emotion. When it's shorthand form it's something like, "I'm never going to get this done." "George doesn't like me."
Client:	Or, "I'm a failure."
Therapist:	You know, sometimes "I'm a failure" might come a little bit closer to a core belief. That's a good point. We'll talk more about those later. The core beliefs are more of a generalized term.
Client:	Okay.
Therapist:	So we could, for example, say, "I'm a failure," and could apply to almost anything, right?
Client:	Yeah.
Therapist:	Whereas if I say, "George doesn't want to be my friend," or "They don't want to hang out with me." You can see how that's tied to a specific event.
Client:	Okay.
Therapist:	But you seem to have a good understanding of this. The other thing that we've talked about a few times is automatic thoughts are almost like a cognitive reflex.
Client:	Okay.
Therapist:	If you think of a reflex . . . someone throws a ball at me, I quickly catch it.
Client:	Yeah.
Therapist:	It's really fast. It's spontaneous, but it's also brief, too. So, it's not only really fast, but it doesn't stick around.
Client:	Okay.
Therapist:	It just kind of . . .
Client:	. . . goes out of your mind.
Therapist:	Yes. So, again, we're left with the emotions that are hanging there, but they're often very strong.
Client:	Okay.

Therapist:	Any questions?
Client:	I mean, it seems like it kind of makes sense. I've gotten a little bit better at identifying automatic thoughts.
Therapist:	Yes, you've already been doing a good job with that.
Client:	I don't quite know too much about changing them just yet . . . how long that'll take. But it seems like it shouldn't be that bad.
Therapist:	No, and you've done a good job already beginning to start to identify some of them with your activity tracking. We're going to obviously revisit some of these components and one area of potential is that . . . even though it may not seem like it now . . . these thoughts, and sometimes these core beliefs, can definitely be changed
Client:	Yeah.
Therapist:	It is just going to take some time to practice with each other, and then practicing on your own.
Client:	Okay.

Discussion Questions 7.1

- Does the client appear to have at least a general understanding of automatic thoughts? What are the indicators that support your perspective?
- Of the key elements of automatic thoughts, do you notice any particular elements that are (or will be) especially challenging for this client?
- Do you have any concerns that the client may be confused about the difference between automatic thoughts and core beliefs? In what ways could you follow up to ensure that the distinction is clear?

ELICITING AND IDENTIFYING AUTOMATIC THOUGHTS

Although there may be times when clients explicitly state their automatic thoughts with minimal to no prompting from you, two vital skills that all therapists need to develop are being able to elicit automatic thoughts when warranted and also knowing how to identify them when they do occur. These skills are a required prerequisite in order to effectively modify your clients' negative automatic thoughts. While your explicit focus will be on automatic thoughts, note the implicit integral role of emotions. Guided discovery is a broad and the most common approach to eliciting and identifying automatic thoughts. Other techniques discussed include guided imagery, role play, differentiating thoughts from emotions, and tracking automatic thoughts.

Guided Discovery: Using Emotions to Elicit Automatic Thoughts

When there are emotions, there are thoughts. The power of using emotions to identify key automatic thoughts and core beliefs is highlighted by Aaron Beck's poignant statement that "emotion is the royal road to cognition" (as cited in J. S. Beck, 2011). Probably the most used strategy for eliciting and identifying automatic thoughts is guided discovery. This is a broad term that can include a variety of therapeutic techniques ranging from arousing emotional reactions and asking questions to understanding the context and associated factors related to negative automatic thoughts.

Initially, Focus Primarily on Emotions

Individuals seeking therapy are most likely experiencing negative emotions at a high level of frequency and intensity. This not only is an emotionally painful experience but also most likely inhibits their ability to clearly process information, behave effectively, solve basic problems, and experience pleasure in daily activities. From the perspective of an outside observer, the dysfunctional nature of the individual experiencing such distress may be bewildering. However, a closer look at their automatic thoughts (and core beliefs) will reveal that their emotions and behaviors are logical, at least from their perspective. It is actually often the automatic thoughts that are inaccurate and illogical. This is why it is vital that you validate your clients' emotions and do not engage in challenging and modifying them. Your goal is to focus on the specific negative automatic thoughts that are the source of their intense negative emotions.

It is not practical to address every situation when clients experience emotional distress. In part, your CBT case conceptualization will assist you in deciding what emotions, in specific contexts, to respond to. Furthermore, when you notice a shift to a negative emotion, this is a strong indicator of a negative automatic thought. Similarly, an increase in the intensity of a negative emotion is also most likely associated with a negative automatic thought. Strong mood shifts tend to be the most powerful in eliciting automatic thoughts because they represent a here-and-now moment (at least emotionally and cognitively) that most likely has significant relevance to the client. Automatic thoughts and images that are associated with these strong emotions are often called "hot cognitions." Even though your clients will be reflecting on a past event, if they experienced strong emotions at that time, there is a greater chance for recall. Of course, using recent events has a greater chance to be more accurately remembered, associated with more "raw" emotion, and have more heightened relevance than events that have occurred in the distant past (i.e., multiple weeks to months). Furthermore, when clients experience these strong emotions during a session, this can actually enhance their memory for associated events. Even if your clients' memory of the event is partially inaccurate, their emotions will provide a context where there is more immediacy and motivation to address the associated automatic thought.

Observe and Respond to Mood Shifts

In order to notice your clients' mood shifts, you should be astutely observing both verbal and nonverbal cues. Verbal cues include not only what is said but also how it is said: volume, intonation, inflection, pace, and cracking. Nonverbal cues can sometimes communicate more than what is actually said: facial expression (especially eye contact), change in posture, gestures (often hands), body movement, and muscle tensioning. When you notice these strong mood shifts, J. S. Beck (2011) recommends directly asking, "What was (just) going through your mind?" Your goal here is to immediately tap into your clients' hot cognitions to home in to their relevant negative automatic thoughts and images. For automatic thoughts, you want the actual words that are said (or seen) in their mind. For images, the greater the detail of what is actually seen in their mind, the better. Specificity for details of automatic thoughts and images is necessary for accurate evaluation (discussed in next section, "Evaluating and Modifying Automatic Thoughts").

Consider Point in Time

In relation to the triggering event, be sure to also take note of the point in time when your clients are experiencing their highest level of distress in relation to their negative automatic thought: before, during, or after. If it is before, then the focus may be more on anticipation of what could happen before the event (e.g., "She will probably be disappointed in me."). If during the situation, then the focus may be more in-the-moment, while it is happening (e.g., "I'm not going to be able to complete this test on time."). If it is after, then the focus may be on reflecting/ruminating after the event (e.g., "Once again, I screwed up.").

Follow Up on Initial Automatic Thoughts

There may be times when it is appropriate to follow up with additional questions (e.g., "What else are you thinking?") after identifying your clients' initial automatic thoughts for additional clarity and specificity. Even those who are able to provide a substantive response will most likely require some prompting for particular details. There may be a chain reaction of additional automatic thoughts that are a part of a larger theme and at the center of their distress. This information can also be helpful in developing and modifying your CBT case formulation, including hypotheses about core beliefs. Clients can also sometimes have additional automatic thoughts about their reaction to the situation rather than the actual situation (e.g., "What are your thoughts about how you responded to that situation?"). In other words, they may have a negative reaction to their responding emotions and/or behaviors (e.g., "It shows that I'm weak to let him make me so angry." "Hiding in my bedroom when I heard that noise just shows that I'm a coward."). However, although initially these negative automatic thoughts may seem separate from the actual situation, many times these thoughts are interrelated to larger themes or core beliefs. Overall, following up on initial automatic thoughts can potentially provide a clearer perspective into the mechanisms of your clients' internal dialogue.

Strategies When Clients Struggle to Identify Automatic Thoughts

There may also be times when clients struggle with pinpointing and stating their automatic thoughts and will require alternative approaches and questions. Sometimes, simply shifting the wording of the question or focusing on a particular aspect related to the event can be helpful. For example, focus on your clients' physiological arousal instead of focusing primarily on their emotions. Many times, simply asking them where they felt their emotion in their body can be a strong trigger, and they might start to experience similar sensations while in session (albeit to a lesser degree), which in turn can heighten their emotions as well. Another variation is asking the client to focus on the meaning of the event. This approach has a more cognitive slant while also attempting to personalize the event. Additionally, ask clients to "guess" at what they were thinking, or you can hypothesize a possible thought (e.g., "I wonder if you thought she doesn't think you would be a fun date after she called to cancel?") to act as a cue to identifying any possible thoughts. In this case, there is concern for accuracy or leading, but you may also

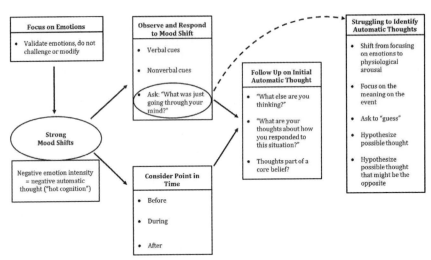

Figure 7.1. Guided Discovery: Using Emotions to Elicit Automatic Thoughts

have a starting point to move forward with more substance. Relatedly, J. S. Beck (2011) also suggests hypothesizing a possible thought that is actually the opposite of what they might have been thinking (e.g., "It probably didn't bother you that much when she canceled the date last minute.") Because your "incorrect thought" is so wrong, it may stimulate your clients' emotions and prompt their memories, resulting in a response to correct you with a more accurate automatic thought. Figure 7.1 is a flowchart of the previously mentioned common techniques used during guided discovery. This provides a visual conceptualization from focusing on emotions to identifying specific automatic thoughts.

The following is a vignette from Video Case Example MDD-10 demonstrating eliciting and identifying automatic thoughts. Following the vignette are discussion questions. An activity including eliciting and identifying automatic thoughts will follow Video Vignette 7.3 (evaluating automatic thoughts).

VIDEO VIGNETTE 7.2

MDD-10: Automatic Thoughts—Eliciting and Identifying

Client: Today was pretty tough. These last couple weeks really haven't been actually going too bad, but today was actually a lot harder than I actually expected. I tried reaching out to one of my coworkers, Jeff, to try and see if he wanted to go out for lunch . . . and . . . I don't know, he just kind of brushed me off. He didn't even really give me any answer besides "no." I don't know, I guess I've been kind of taking that pretty hard since then.

Therapist: So, this just happened today?

Client: Yeah.

Therapist: So, it's kind of fresh?

Client:	Yeah, it is.
Therapist:	I can see in your face that it seems like you're hurt.
Client:	Yeah.
Therapist:	Let me just ask you: what was going through your mind just now when you were . . . ?
Client:	I mean, again, kind of hurt. Just like this feeling of kind of rejection. I don't know, something like that. I mean, just feeling unwanted . . . kind of like worthless.
Therapist:	You do have some thoughts there. You've got the emotions down.
Client:	Yeah.
Therapist:	In terms of your thoughts for that event . . . you're doing a good job here. Do you remember now what you were thinking?
Client:	I mean, just that he didn't want to be with me.
Therapist:	Okay.
Client:	Or that he didn't want to spend the time with me.
Therapist:	Okay. I see a little bit of a pattern here.
Client:	Yeah.
Therapist:	And I can definitely see why that would hurt. When you have those thoughts it causes a lot of pain when you think someone doesn't want to be with you. I've noticed this a couple times with another friend or two, and other family. We call this a cognitive distortion. This seems like a version of personalization. It could be a little bit of mind reading—thinking what they're thinking—but here it seems like you're internalizing what's going on here. I want to explore this thought a little bit more.
Client:	Okay.

Client:	Sometimes the thought is kind of there before, but it's a lot worse after.
Therapist:	Okay. So there is a little bit of anticipation initially?
Client:	Yeah, I don't know if it's like a suspicion or just kind of like an inkling that something bad is going to happen or I'm not going to get the response that I wanted.
Therapist:	In these types of scenarios, there's a part of you that's like, "Yeah, I don't know if they're going to want to hang out with me." And then, when it does happen, it feels like the thoughts are validated.
Client:	Yeah. It's just even worse.
Therapist:	Do you spend a lot of time thinking about it afterwards?
Client:	Yeah.
Therapist:	Did you spend time thinking about it even driving here to my office after the event?
Client:	Yeah. It happened just a couple hours ago. I've hung out with Jeff before. We've gone out to lunch a bunch of times. Granted since this whole depressive episode started, I just really haven't had the time to go out with him. But I figured, hey, we've been trying to do more social activities, so why not? We used to go out all the time and I just figured, "Hey, do you want to go grab a couple subs?" And he didn't even look up from the computer.

Discussion Questions 7.2

- What did you observe as indicators that the client had experienced a strong mood shift (e.g., emotion expressed, verbal cues, or nonverbal cues)?
- What was the client's negative automatic thought? Was it associated with other thoughts?
- Based on what you know about the client so far, do you think his automatic thought is representative of a pattern of thinking (e.g., from a core belief) that should be further addressed in therapy?

Guided Imagery: Using Images to Elicit Automatic Thoughts

There will be times when some of your clients have difficulty elaborating on their negative automatic thoughts. This approach can also be helpful for clients who are reporting primarily images but need help with clarity and details. In these cases, it can be helpful to have clients visualize the distressing event. One way to look at this technique is helping clients "see" their thoughts by guiding them through reliving particular events in their mind. The use of images can greatly aide in stimulating emotions and thoughts related to the target event. You can also enhance physiological arousal, as discussed in the previous section "Guided Discovery."

Before engaging in this activity, you should explain in advance what you would like to do, as it will seem awkward to some clients without any prior prompting or permission. You want your general disposition throughout the process (e.g., tone of voice and body posture) to convey that this is a safe activity and you will be there to support them throughout the process. One of the more effective ways to start guided imagery is to have your clients try to think/imagine what was going on right before the event of interest (e.g., "What was happening before the event?" "What was going on in your mind leading up to the event?" "What were you feeling before the event?"). Thereafter, you can follow up with additional questions to help your clients recall the actual event by focusing on relevant details (e.g., "Where are you?" "Describe your surroundings?" "What are you doing?" "Do you recall any sounds or smells?" "What are you wearing?" "Who else is there?" "What do these people look like?" "What are these people saying?" "Is there anything else you can see or hear?"). As you ask these questions, astutely watch how your clients react. You are trying to notice if any questions are a strong enough hit where there is an emotional reaction/mood shift. From there, you can integrate similar questions/techniques addressed in guided discovery while also focusing on details of the event. Your goal is to make the image as clear as possible with emotion (and physiological response), which can ultimately lead to remembering distinct negative automatic thoughts.

Role Play: Re-Creating Interactions to Elicit Automatic Thoughts

If your clients are struggling to recall details of the distressing event and it was interpersonal, then you can consider doing a role play. Although this role play will obviously not be the same as the actual event, sometimes acting out a recent event can assist memory recall. Typically, when you start with a role play, you take the role of a person who interacted with your clients while the clients play themselves. Your ultimate goal is to simulate the original interaction to stimulate recall of particular details, which can in turn heighten emotions and physiological arousal. Gathering any information about the event and the person who interacted with the client can help your accuracy in providing a realistic interaction. Try to start the role play a few moments before the event and then work your way toward the moment you think your clients experienced heightened emotional arousal. You may even notice that your clients experience a strong mood shift during the role play. If appropriate, you can naturally integrate the mood shift question (i.e., "What was just going through your mind?"). Similar to guided imagery, once clients begin to gain clarity of the event, you can begin integrating the questions used for guided discovery. When necessary, you can also reverse the roles where the clients play the other person and you play the clients. In this case, you can serve as a model for your clients to observe and learn how to respond (e.g., thought processes, social skills, and behavioral responses) in these situations.

Differentiating Thoughts from Emotions

There will be moments when your clients struggle to differentiate between their thoughts and emotions. Sometimes, clients briefly confuse the two when discussing an event, and it may not even need to be addressed (e.g., it naturally resolves or they misspoke). Other times, there is some confusion that warrants its being addressed subtly with brief redirection or prompting. However, there will be some clients who are truly confused about the difference between the two. Keep in mind that some clients may conceptually understand the difference between thoughts and emotions when reviewing the CBT model but struggle with actual application when asked to review a specific, personal event. In fact, this may be indicative, at least in part, of some the distress they are experiencing (i.e., difficulty processing the source of distress).

Clients commonly mistake emotions (e.g., hurt) for thoughts (e.g., "I know my boss gave me an extra shift over the weekend on purpose because he does not like me."). If clients are still struggling with the difference after reviewing the CBT model, you can provide a few examples by writing out some thoughts in one column and associated emotions in the next column. Then ask them to see if they notice anything different between how the two columns look. Without even looking at the content of each column, it can easily be observed that thoughts are longer. More specifically, thoughts are full sentences (or phrases), while emotions are one word. You can have your clients remember the statement, "Full sentence = thought. Single word = emotion." Ultimately, it is the content of the thoughts (i.e., full sentences) that influences emotions (i.e., a single word). You can also remind your clients that in the near future, they will learn how to modify their thoughts in order to have different, less distressing emotions. Emotions are not modified, as this would be a futile task because, in many ways, their emotions are understandable based on their thoughts. It would also not be validating to try to change their emotions. The focus will be on the source of the distressing emotions (e.g., negative automatic thoughts).

Having a good understanding of your clients' CBT case conceptualization can provide some assistance in recognizing if there are any inconsistences between how the event connects with their emotions and automatic thoughts. If clients report emotions that appear to not connect with their automatic thoughts and the context of the event, you should follow up for clarification. This discrepancy may be due to your not having a full understanding of the presenting problems or clients having difficulty in identifying their emotions and/or the source of their emotions. If the former, you can ask additional clarification questions and make the necessary adjustments, particularly in your understanding of the event and the automatic thought. If the latter, your focus can range from psychoeducation on labeling emotions to reviewing CBT model basics with an emphasis on how thoughts precede emotions.

Whether clients have a poor vocabulary for emotions or struggle labeling their own personal emotions, the following approaches can be helpful. One effective technique that is simple and basic is providing a list of negative emotions followed by a brief discussion. Table 7.3 provides a sample list of common negative emotions often

Table 7.3. Negative Emotions and Negative Automatic Thoughts Worksheet

Emotions	Client-Specific Negative Automatic Thoughts
Anxious, worried, scared, fearful, dread	
Sad, unhappy, lonely, empty, hopeless, unloved	
Angry, mad, annoyed, frustrated, rage, irritated	
Hurt, wounded, rejected, unworthy	
Confused, disconnected, uncertain	
Disappointed, disheartened, discouraged	
Suspicious, distrustful, skeptical	
Envious, jealous, greedy	
Insecure, inadequate, intimidated, vulnerable	
Resentment, revengeful, bitter	
Disgusted, revolted	
Guilty, remorseful	
Humiliated, ashamed, embarrassed	

associated with negative automatic thoughts in the first column. The second column is blank to allow you to enter any client-specific negative automatic thoughts. You can tailor this list to best fit the needs and presenting problems of your clients. Your clients can keep this list with them in their therapy notes to use as a quick reference. Visually seeing these words along with a brief example of their own negative automatic thoughts may be enough psychoeducation to improve emotion awareness and emotion communication skills.

If there is more of a concern for psychoeducation on the relationship between events and emotions, you can have clients develop a list of negative emotions (use Table 7.3 if necessary) and examples of distressing events. Table 7.4 is an example template that can be used to list separate negative emotions across the columns and associated events across the rows. The goal here is simply to visually connect their common negative emotions with specific events. Also review with your clients that many events can have different emotional reactions depending on the individual (e.g., date canceling at the last minute could be sad for some and angry for others). Again, clients can keep this template with their therapy notes to use as a resource when they experience strong negative emotions. If you keep a few columns or rows blank (or an additional blank sheet), it can also be used as part of a homework assignment for practice between sessions.

Table 7.4. Negative Emotions and Associated Events Worksheet

Sad	Anxious	Angry	_____
1. Date cancels at the last minute.	1. Having to give a public presentation for work.	1. While driving on the highway, you get cut off by an aggressive driver.	
2. Received a failing grade on your psychology exam.	2. Finding out that your pet requires a major operation.	2. Submit a work project late because your colleagues did not do their parts.	
3. Cannot find a friend to hang out with over the weekend.	3. Realizing you might not have enough money to pay next month's bills.	3. Friend accidentally breaks an expensive piece of furniture in your house.	
4.			
5.			
6.			

Tracking Negative Automatic Thoughts

A further step in writing down emotions and events is writing down negative automatic thoughts as soon as possible when then occur. At this point, the use of this technique assumes that the client has a solid grasp of understanding the difference between thoughts and emotions. Actively engaging in this technique heightens awareness to relevant thoughts as they occur throughout the day. This process helps clients develop their own version of self-assessment in identifying their own automatic thoughts and sets the stage for eventual evaluation and modification of negative automatic thoughts. In other words, often the act of writing down negative automatic thoughts and visually seeing the words can stimulate their own evaluation process of their thinking patterns (e.g., "Why did I think that? It makes no sense."). In some ways, clients may start to make modifications to such thoughts own their own. If this occurs, this provides you a great opportunity to naturally guide these clients to specific techniques and interventions to change their negative automatic thoughts. Table 7.5 is a tracker that can be used as a template to track specific negative automatic thoughts throughout the day or week. Note that its content is similar to Tables 7.3 and 7.4 but now includes room to identify events, negative automatic thoughts, emotions, and body sensations. Again, like the other related techniques, this should first be done in session and then assigned as homework. In the next section, this figure expands even further to include identifying and labeling specific cognitive distortions, associated behaviors, consequences, and ways to dispute and develop alternative thoughts. You are essentially scaffolding your client to eventual use of a negative automatic thought record (discussed in the next section "Evaluating and Modifying Automatic Thoughts").

Table 7.5.   Negative Automatic Thoughts Tracker

Event	Negative Automatic Thoughts	Emotions	Body Sensations
1.			
2.			
3.			
4.			
5.			
6.			
7.			

Remember: Use Your CBT Case Formulation

Do not forget to use your CBT case formulation for shaping the direction of your questions to elicit emotions related to relevant automatic thoughts. Although your CBT case formulation is still evolving, you should still have enough information to at least hypothesize on what sources of distress to focus on for your questions. For example, what you know about precipitating and maintaining factors, presenting problems, and background history can make your assessment of automatic thoughts more efficient and concise. Additionally, the information gained from these questions can help further develop your CBT case formulation, including possible core beliefs. This point reiterates that assessment and interventions are a continuous process where information in one domain informs the other.

EVALUATING AND MODIFYING AUTOMATIC THOUGHTS

After going through the process of eliciting and identifying automatic thoughts and images, the next step is not to immediately jump into modifying these thoughts. You will need to first evaluate these thoughts to see if they have practical and therapeutic relevance and if it is appropriate for modification. In other words, not all negative emotions and negative automatic thoughts are worth discussing. It is helpful to look at evaluation as a form of "emotion and thought assessment" and modification as a form of "emotion and thought intervention." Utilizing the following evaluating and modifying techniques for automatic thoughts is not a one-time event. Rather, these are skills that will be continuously used until the final session. Ideally, your clients will be able to naturally integrate these techniques into their daily lives as therapy progresses.

The Evaluation Process: Focusing on Relevant Automatic Thoughts

Rating Emotion Intensity

Once negative emotions with associated automatic thoughts have been identified, clients should be asked to rate their degree of intensity for their emotions. Assessing the intensity of an emotion will help you determine if the automatic thought merits further examination. You will find that sometimes your clients will express negative emotions and associated automatic thoughts, but these emotions might not be very intense. If this is the case, these automatic thoughts are probably not as relevant to your clients' distress and identified problems as other thoughts with more intense emotions. You will have only so much time each session for modifying your clients' thoughts; thus, you will need to focus on other automatic thoughts that have greater potential for therapeutic value.

You can provide a brief explanation to your clients that emotions can vary by degree (e.g., slightly angry, somewhat angry, or extremely angry). Even though many clients may intellectually understand this concept, it can be a little more challenging to apply this concept to their own emotions. A simple but effective way to have

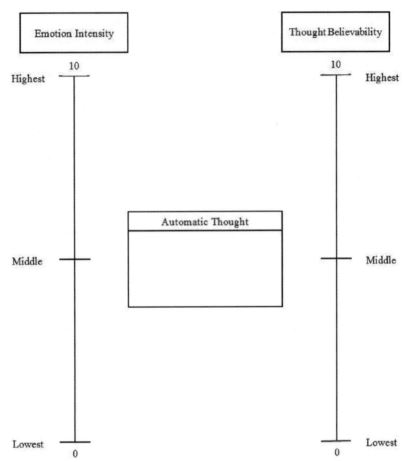

Figure 7.2. Emotion Intensity and Negative Automatic Thought Believability Scale

clients rate their intensity of emotions is to have them use a 0–10 scale, with 0 being essentially no intensity and 10 being the most intensity (e.g., "If 10 is the saddest you've ever felt or you could imagine feeling and 0 is not feeling sad at all, how sad did you feel when you found out that you did not get the job?"). If necessary, you can use Figure 7.2 as a visual scale to compare both emotion intensity and thought believability (discussed next) at once.

Although this assessment of emotions is subjective, this is not a concern because what is important is how clients perceive their own emotions. This also provides clients another opportunity to be more self-aware of their emotions, including other stimulating events and negative automatic thoughts. Furthermore, clients will use this skill when they later use negative automatic thought records. In sum, rating clients' emotion intensity provides you an opportunity to determine if it is therapeutically appropriate to follow through with the associated negative automatic thought. This information can also be used to assess the effectiveness of modifying clients' automatic thoughts by having them rate their emotions later in therapy (i.e., pre- and post-assessment of specific emotions).

Rating Thought Believability

Once you determine that your clients' negative emotions are strong enough to move forward, you will need to assess how much they actually believe the negative automatic thought or image. In other words, you want to determine the likelihood of your clients to have this negative automatic thought again and if they will experience emotional distress in the future. For example, sometimes clients will report that they no longer believe the automatic thought because they were able to resolve the problem on their own or they have a plan to respond if the problem occurs again. This information will help you determine if this is an automatic thought that warrants modification.

Having clients rate how much they believe their thoughts is essentially the same process as rating the intensity their emotions. You can have them rate how much they believe their thoughts using the same 0–10 scale for their emotions, with 0 being no longer believe the automatic thought and 10 being fully believe the automatic thought (e.g., "If 10 is you fully believe your thought and 0 is no longer believe your thought, how much do you believe your thought, 'I turned them off with my personality during the interview'?"). Just like rating emotional intensity, you can use Figure 7.2 as a visual scale to compare both emotion intensity and thought believability at once.

Focus on Event

If you and your clients are confident that there is a negative automatic thought that is strongly believed and contributing significant emotional distress, then also take the time to focus on the context of the event for further clarification. For example, you will want to clarify details about the actual event that occurred to "trigger" the automatic thought. Additionally, determine where (e.g., work or school) and when (e.g., weekend morning or weekday evening) the event happened. Also ascertain if any other individuals were associated with the event. This is also a good time to follow up on any other additional emotions and physiological arousal. Correspondingly, follow through with any other possible distressing thoughts or images associated with the events. Finally, determine the specific behaviors that followed this event–emotion–thought process, including the outcome/consequences. Overall, the more detail you know about the actual preceding event and other related thoughts, the better for both your CBT case formulation development (i.e., automatic thought patterns and core beliefs) and upcoming modification strategies.

The following is a vignette from Video Case Example MDD-10 demonstrating evaluating automatic thoughts. Following the vignette are discussion questions and an activity that also includes eliciting and identifying automatic thoughts.

VIDEO VIGNETTE 7.3

MDD-10: Automatic Thoughts—Evaluating

Therapist: Let's use your word "hurt." You've used that word a lot.

Client: Yeah, yeah.

Therapist: On a scale of 0 to 10, where would you put that emotion?

Client: Right now?

Therapist: Yeah, while you're talking about this scenario.

Client: Right now, I mean maybe like a 6.

Therapist: Okay.

Client: It's there, when I'm thinking about when it actually happened I mean, probably an 8 or a 9.

Therapist: Okay. So, in the moment it was 8 or 9.

Client: Yeah.

Therapist: I think 6 is still high enough to check into it.

Client: Yeah.

Therapist: How much do you believe the thought that Jeff doesn't want to spend time with you right now?

Client: I think that's a little higher. That's a 7 or 8. Because again, it's kind of a common pattern.

Therapist: Right.

Client: I mean, not necessarily with Jeff, but I've been trying these things and the results that I'm getting aren't what I want.

Therapist: I think it is something worth exploring a little bit more. Are you okay with that?

Client: Yes.

Client: Then I went over and popped into his office and I was figuring I'll just strike up a quick conversation, but then when I actually asked him, "Do you want to go out for lunch?" he was just laser-focused on his computer.

Therapist: Okay.

Client: I was like, "Okay, do you want to go for lunch?" and he's like "I don't really have time for that, Mark. Maybe another time." I mean when I walked in there, he wasn't even really even doing anything.

Therapist: Right.

Client: He was just kind of typing around on this computer. He didn't seem that busy. We've gone out to lunch before. It was Friday, typically a lot of people in our office like to get out of the office and go for lunch. There are a couple great sub shops that are in the area that we've been to before.

Therapist: Okay.

Client: I would've even bought lunch for us. I didn't say that, but I just figured . . . I don't know. I guess I thought that it would've been a sure bet . . . that Jeff would be like, "hey, let's go." Not "I'm just typing away." It just kind of seemed like I wasn't that important when I was talking to him.

Therapist:	Even though you thought it was a sure bet there's still a part of you that thought you might be rejected?
Client:	Yeah.

Client:	It seemed like he wasn't that busy. Yeah, he might've been typing up an e-mail or something, but it's not a busy time of year for him. I didn't think he would be that stressed or that he would be that busy on a day like that.
Therapist:	It appears that you're making some assumptions in the sense of what you think could be going on.
Client:	Yeah.
Therapist:	Whereas, who the heck knows what could be going through his mind?
Client:	Yeah.
Therapist:	But from what you know from his routine you try to fill in the holes.
Client:	Yeah. It seems like it.
Therapist:	But we don't know what else could have been going on.
Client:	Yeah.
Therapist:	Could be right, could be wrong, we don't know.
Client:	Yeah.

Client:	I want to be around people and I'm trying. But sometimes I get down on myself. If one person doesn't want to be around me, maybe I should just go and get my lunch and just eat it by myself.
Therapist:	And let me guess, when you were sitting there eating by yourself, were you thinking about just what happened earlier?
Client:	Yeah. And I think that was when I felt the most hurt. Just thinking and processing it . . . kind of filling in the holes with all those kind of assumptions . . .
Therapist:	Yeah.
Client:	I kind of almost started laughing when you said it because it almost seems silly because it's the truth. I'm filling in a lot of the holes that I don't really have all the information for.
Therapist:	Right. But you find ways to fill in those holes. You notice that the longer you ruminate it's almost infinite . . .
Client:	Yeah.
Therapist:	There's different ways we can fill in the holes.
Client:	Yeah.
Therapist:	When we're alone it's easier to ruminate. It sounds like it did hurt you in the moment when he said "no," but the real pain seemed to kick in when you're sitting there eating alone. You're not just thinking anymore about Jeff not wanting to eat with you, but now you're maybe generalizing it: "Well, other people don't want to have anything to do with me either."

Client: Yeah. The feeling isn't as strong right now, but I'm still thinking about it. At least now that the feeling's not as strong I think it's a little bit easier to try and . . . I don't need to fill in all those holes for Jeff because I don't know.

Therapist: Yes.

Client: You make a great point—how can I know what's going on in his life? It could just be like me.

Therapist: Right.

Discussion Questions 7.3

- By evaluating this negative automatic thought, what else did you learn about the client's thinking pattern?
- What is significant about the event associated with the negative automatic thought?
- Is there any other information about the negative automatic thought and/or event that you would like to know?
- Based on what you know about the client so far, do you think his negative automatic thought warrants modification?

ACTIVITY 7.1: AUTOMATIC THOUGHTS— ELICITING, IDENTIFYING, AND EVALUATING

Practice eliciting, identifying, and evaluating negative automatic thoughts with a peer. Have one of you play the role of the "client" by describing an event and then show a mood shift. While the other plays the "therapist," respond to this mood shift ("What was just going through your mind?") to elicit a negative automatic thought. You can also ask follow-up questions to assess when the thought occurs relative to the event (i.e., before, during, or after) or if it is related to a core belief. You can also challenge yourselves by having the client struggle to initially identify a negative automatic thought, requiring the therapist to shift the approach (e.g., focus on physiological arousal instead of emotions or hypothesize a thought that might be the opposite). Thereafter, follow up with rating the intensity of the emotion and believability of the negative automatic thought. Conclude with obtaining additional details about the event related to the thought (e.g., other individuals involved or resulting behaviors/consequences). Was it difficult to notice the mood shift and respond with a follow-up question to identify the automatic thought? Does it become more challenging when an automatic thought is not provided immediately after your initial questions? Were you comfortable deciding to explore the negative automatic thought further based on rating the emotion intensity and thought believability?

Socratic Techniques: Evaluating to Modifying Automatic Thoughts

Socratic questioning is a common term used in CBT that refers to asking clients direct questions about their negative automatic thoughts to help them "get to the truth" own their own. In other words, you do not want to "tell" your clients what to think; rather, you want to help "show" them so they can see it for themselves. Here, the term "Socratic techniques" is used because this approach does not exclusively involve continuous questions to reach a desired outcome. Rather, there are a variety of techniques that go beyond questions that you can use to help clients eventually modify their negative automatic thoughts and regulate their emotions autonomously. Overall, you want a natural transition from evaluation to modification that is collaborative.

The following are some of the most common and effective Socratic techniques for evaluating and modifying negative automatic thoughts. It is important to note here that not all of these Socratic techniques will be used for every automatic thought; it depends on the context for each thought. Some of the following techniques may not be appropriate for some thoughts, while in other cases it may not be pragmatic to use every technique. Furthermore, these techniques can enhance the collaborative nature of the therapeutic relationship, foster engagement and motivation, and supplement further understanding of the CBT model. Thereafter, other effective techniques for evaluating and modifying thoughts are also discussed, many of which are extensions from Socratic techniques that promote awareness, responsiveness, and eventually prevention of future negative automatic thoughts. Table 7.6 provides a list of each Socratic technique and associated questions to be used as a quick reference while in session, especially when learning each approach.

1. Examine the Evidence: Determine if the Negative Automatic Thought Is Invalid

If you and your client are confident that there is a negative automatic thought that is strongly believed and associated with high emotional intensity, you must first establish its validity by examining the evidence, as this will determine your next approach. If the negative automatic thought is initially determined to be largely invalid, then you will most likely continue with modification techniques, whereas if it is largely valid (i.e., for the most part true), then you will have to shift your approach because the focus will be more on how to cope with such thoughts (see the section "Working with Valid Negative Automatic Thoughts").

When a negative automatic thought is determined to be initially largely invalid, you still need to be careful not to immediately attempt to modify the negative automatic thought. J. S. Beck (2011) provides three reasons for such caution: (a) you do not know how much a negative automatic thought is truly distorted (i.e., a portion may still be valid), (b) immediately modifying a thought may be invalidating to the client, and (c) modifying a thought without the client's involvement does not adhere the CBT principle of collaborative empiricism. Generally, all CBT therapists should

Table 7.6. Socratic Techniques and Common Questions for Automatic Thoughts

Socratic Technique	Questions
Examine the evidence	"What is the evidence that supports your thought?" "What is the evidence against your thought?"
Decatastrophize perceived negative outcomes	"What is the worst that could happen?" "Even if it does happen, what effect would this have on you? What can you do to cope with this?" "What is the best thing that could happen?" "What is the most realistic thing that could happen?" "What is the probability of the worst-case scenario actually happening on a 0%–100% scale?" "What is the probability of the best-case scenario actually happening on a 0%–100% scale?" "What is the probability of the most realistic scenario actually happening on a 0%–100% scale?"
Explore possible alternative explanations	"Is there another explanation for what happened other than . . . ?"
Assess the impact of believing the negative automatic thought	"What is the outcome of believing that [negative thought]?" "What could be the outcome of changing your thought?" "What could be the outcome of thinking that [negative thought is not as bad as initially thought]?"
Separate self from negative automatic thought	"What would you tell your [family member/friend] if they had a similar thought as you?" "I wonder if what you would tell your [family member/friend] could also apply to you. What do you think?"
Shift attributional biases	"Are there other people or related factors that could have influenced the outcome of this event, even if a small amount?"

be cognizant of the fact that most automatic thoughts have some level of validity (i.e., not 100% erroneous). Even if you still decide to move forward with modifying a negative automatic thought, many times it is appropriate to acknowledge what may be true about the thought. This acknowledgment can be validating for many clients, which can result in increased motivation and engagement to work collaboratively.

First, ask clients for any evidence that supports the validity of their thought (e.g., "What is the evidence that supports your thought?"). Thereafter, ask clients for any evidence that contradicts the validity of their thought (e.g., "What is the evidence against your thought?"). These are basic but important questions that will often provide you with enough information to assess the actual validity of the thought. Remember, most automatic thoughts have some validity. What is important is for you to assess if this thought is invalid and relevant enough to warrant further exploration and eventual modification.

This approach is often most helpful for clients when using Table 7.7, a two-column worksheet for writing down both the evidence for and the evidence against the negative automatic thought. Sometimes, visually seeing the written comments can

Table 7.7.   Examining the Evidence Worksheet—Automatic Thoughts

Negative Automatic Thought:	
Evidence for Thought	**Evidence Against Thought**
Is the Thought Valid?	
Yes	**No**
Socratic techniques not necessary	**Possible Socratic Techniques**

Validity of Conclusion?		Decatastrophization, alternative explanations, impact of believing thought, separating self from thought, shift attributional biases
Accurate	**Distorted**	
Consider acceptance and emotion-focused coping skills	Evaluate utility and consider problem-focused coping skills	**Possible Cognitive Distortions**

help clients process the validity of the thought. Thereafter, you can assist your clients in deciding on the validity of the thought and how to move forward if necessary. Typically, it is more convincing for your clients to "see" how much particular thoughts are invalid by objectively acknowledging that some part of the thought also has some credence. Furthermore, this information can be used by clients in their therapy notes as a reference guide and supplement future homework assignments.

2. Decatastrophize Perceived Negative Outcomes

It is not uncommon for some clients to associate the worst-case scenario or worst fear with their negative automatic thoughts. This is called "catastrophic predictions of the future." Unsurprisingly, your clients' worst-case predictions are often unrealistic due to overestimation; the probability of its occurrence is minimal to none. (If the worst-case prediction is valid, then you will not focus on its unrealistic/low probability nature. Rather, a more appropriate approach can focus on coping skills in response to the possible outcome.) Your goal here is to assist your clients in their ability to consider more realistic outcomes. Rather than trying to tell your clients that their worst-case prediction will probably not happen, ask them to first speculate what is the worst that could happen if their automatic thought were true (e.g., "What if what you say is true [to some degree]? What is the worst thing that could happen?"). This is sometimes referred to as the "what if?" or "so what?" approach. Then follow up by asking clients what would be the consequence if the worst thing happened and what they could do to cope with it (e.g., "Even if X does happen, what effect would this have on you? What can you do to cope with this?"). There are two goals here: first, to show clients that even if the worst-case prediction occurs, it would probably "not be that bad," and, second, to also assist clients in recognizing that they have the ability to cope if it does happen. In other words, even it does happen, they will live through it both emotionally and physically. If necessary, you may have to review with your clients possible ways to handle such scenarios through developing a coping plan (e.g., what has worked, what has not worked, what could work, and barriers to coping).

In addition to showing your clients that even if the worst-case scenario happens the outcome is manageable, you can also help them develop more realistic outcomes. After asking your clients what is the worst thing to happen, ask them what could be the best-case scenario (e.g., "What is the best thing that could happen?"). Soon after, ask them what is the most realistic scenario (e.g., "What is the most realistic thing that could happen?"). More often than not, clients will come to recognize that their worst-case prediction is inaccurate and that the most likely outcome from their negative automatic thought is somewhere in between "the worst" and "the best."

If necessary, you can also include probability testing. Here, you can ask clients to compare the chances of the worst-case scenario, best-case scenario, and the most realistic scenario as a 0–100 percentage. First, start with asking the probability of the worst-case scenario (e.g., "What is the probability of the worst-case scenario actually happening on a 0%–100% scale?"). If deemed to be appropriate, you can also ask if the worst-case scenario has ever happened before. This approach is most effective if you know it has not happened (i.e., there is negative thinking for a scenario that has never happened). Thereafter, follow up with the same question for the best-case scenario (e.g., "What is the probability of the best-case scenario actually happening on a 0%–100% scale?") and the most realistic scenario (e.g., "What is the probability of the most realistic scenario actually happening on a 0%–100% scale?"). In most cases, comparing these probabilities will show that the most realistic scenario has a higher probability than the worst-case scenario. Thereafter, you can ask your clients if they have an alternative automatic thought that better reflects the more realistic scenario. Overall, these techniques help clients recognize that worst-case scenarios rarely happen and that, if they do, it is often not that bad and that they have the skills to cope. You can use Table 7.8 to take notes for all categories of information. Again, although this process may be basic enough to verbally process, having a visual for each written scenario and its probability can provide clients with greater clarity. There is also space to include any relevant information to develop a coping plan, if necessary.

3. Explore Possible Alternative Explanations

Many times, there are different explanations for the event associated with your clients' negative automatic thoughts and emotions. Simply ask if there is an alternative explanation for what happened (e.g., "Is there another explanation for what happened

Table 7.8. Decatastrophizing Worksheet

Negative Automatic Thought:

Scenario	Worst	Realistic	Best
Probability (0%–100%)			
How to Cope?	What has not worked? What has worked? What could work? (worth trying?) Barriers and response to coping plan?	**Alternative Thought:**	

Table 7.9. Possible Alternatives Worksheet

Event:	
Negative Automatic Thought:	
Emotion:	
Behavior/Consequence:	
Current Explanation	**Alternative Explanations**
	1. 2. 3.
Consider Your Most Likely Alternative Explanation	
Alternative Thought:	
Alternative Emotion:	
Alternative Behavior/Consequence:	

other than . . . ?"). During this process, your clients might begin to recognize that their alternative explanation is actually more valid than their initial perception and negative automatic thought. If this occurs, your clients are already learning experientially that there are alternative ways to perceive events. Thereafter, ask them to consider possible alternative thoughts and corresponding emotions in response to the most likely alternative explanation. If appropriate, you can also ask them to consider an alternative behavioral response/consequence with this alternative explanation. The effectiveness of modifying clients' thoughts has the potential to be more powerful if they are generating their own thoughts to alternative explanations rather than being told what to think. You can use Table 7.9 to help you identify your clients' current explanation and consider alternative explanations in response to a specific event. There is also space to evaluate if your clients' thoughts, emotions, and behaviors would change in response to their most likely alternative explanation.

4. Assess the Impact of Believing the Negative Automatic Thought

Another helpful approach is to assess your clients' distress and consequences for believing and not believing certain negative automatic thoughts. This technique is relatively simplistic but can be effective with clients who may be especially motivated and receptive to your CBT interventions up to this point. Simply ask your clients the outcome of believing a specific negative automatic thought (e.g., "What is the outcome of believing that you will fail your exam next week?"). Clients will almost always respond with associated negative feelings and distress. Then immediately follow up by asking your clients the outcome of not believing the specific negative automatic thought and replacing it with another. You can ask this question in general form (e.g., "What could be the outcome of changing your thought?") or with a specific direction (e.g., "What could be the outcome of thinking that you might not get a perfect score on your exam but will probably get a solid passing grade?"). If necessary, sometimes coming up with a hypothetical alternative thought can be enough to provide clients perspective in how thinking differently results in different emotions and behaviors.

5. Separate Self From Negative Automatic Thought

Sometimes, having clients separate themselves from their thoughts helps them observe the context of a situation more objectively. A common method employed is to ask clients to consider what they would tell a family member or friend if they had a similar thought (or were in a similar situation) (e.g., "What would you tell your mother if she had a similar thought as you?"). If your clients have some experience with CBT skills at this point, there is a good chance that they will be able to provide some version of an alternative interpretation. Even though the approach of this technique is obvious, many clients are able to at least temporarily separate themselves from the associated (strong) negative emotions by taking the perspective of someone else. In turn, this allows them to more objectively assess the event and thought and provide an alternative interpretation. If the alternative interpretation appears to be more adaptive and relevant to your clients' needs, then you can ask if this can also apply to them (e.g., "I wonder if what you would tell your mother could also apply to you. What do you think?"). This can be impactful because you are using your clients' own words to consider for modifying their own thoughts.

6. Shift Attributional Biases

The meanings that people assign to everyday events throughout their lives are called attributions. There are generally considered to be three different types of attributions: (a) personal internal/external, (b) permanent stable/unstable, and (c) pervasive general/specific (Abrahamson, Seligman, & Teasdale, 1978). Personal attribution refers to how much a person attributes events internally (themselves) or externally (the environment). Permanent attribution refers to how much a person attributes events as stable (it will always be this way) or unstable (it can change). Pervasive attribution refers to how much a person attributes events as global (it happens everywhere/always) or specific (it was unique/atypical). These attributional styles were initially developed to explain the learned helplessness model, which is often associated with depression. However, variations of attributional styles can be helpful in understanding your clients' distress beyond depression. Of course, people do not fall into just one category of each type; they fall within a spectrum. However, people who are experiencing significant distress tend to view negative events as

My Attributional Style	
Internal	External
Stable	Unstable
Global	Specific

X = Negative Events

O = Positive Events

Event: Negative Automatic Thought:	
Internal	External
Stable	Unstable
Global	Specific

X = Right Now

O = More Adaptive (less distressing)

Figure 7.3. Attributional Style Worksheet

internal/stable/global and positive events as external/unstable/specific. You can first explain attributional biases in a way that your client will best understand by using a diagram or drawing out on paper/whiteboard the dimensions of each attribution. You can also use Figure 7.3 to ask your clients to mark where they think they fall on the dimension for each attribution. Note that it is important to differentiate their perceived attributions by negative and positive events in order to identify potential patterns. This can help you assess their self-awareness by comparing where your clients put themselves on the dimension and your own impression of their attributional biases. If you do notice a discrepancy, it may be appropriate to gently point out how your perspective compares with your clients' and initiate a discussion. Keep in mind that not all clients will fall consistently on the dimension for each attribution type. For example, you could have a client for negative events who strongly internalizes but can view some events as unstable and specific. You can also use Figure 7.3 to review a recent event and negative automatic thought to "test the validity" of each attribution. First, ask clients to mark where they fall on the attribution dimension right now. Next, ask clients to mark on the attribution dimension where they think it would be more adaptive or less distressing. There will almost always be discrepancies between the two markings, which can stimulate a discussion about the dimensional nature of attribution styles and how even making slight shifts in attributions can influence thinking patterns, emotions, and behaviors. This information can also be saved as part of your clients' therapy notes and used as a resource for homework and future sessions to track any changes in attribution style.

Another helpful technique related to attribution, shown in Figure 7.4, is the commonly used responsibility pie. This is especially helpful for clients who have a strong proclivity to internally attribute negative events. First, have your clients identify an event with an associated negative automatic thought and emotions. Before even getting into how much responsibility to assign, ask your clients to think of anyone or something that is responsible for the negative event. There is no ideal number, but you typically want at least four or more. Because clients have a strong tendency to focus on their own flaws, you want to ask questions that get them thinking from alter-

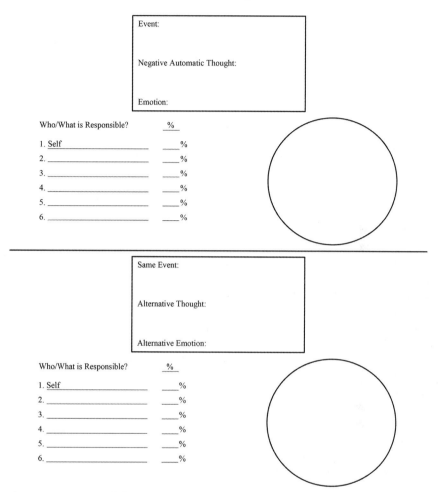

Figure 7.4. Responsibility Attribution Pie

native perspectives beyond themselves (e.g., "Are there other people or related factors that could have influenced the outcome of this event, even if a small amount?"). After completing the list of who/what is responsible, you can begin to assign a percentage of responsibility to each of the identified people and factors. Then use the percentages to complete the responsibility attribution pie. Once the pie is complete, this is a good opportunity to process your clients' reaction to the visual presentation of responsibility and assist them with shifting toward external responsibility for certain negative events. You can ask your clients to explain why the other people and/or related factors also share some of the responsibility. Many times, this prompts clients to lower their own share of the responsibility as they come to realize that their initial perception was not accurate. Also, use some of the other Socratic techniques discussed earlier to see if they can make any slight modifications to their initial negative automatic thoughts.

Thereafter, once an alternative automatic thought has been identified, have your clients use the same list of who/what is responsible (there might be an addition or two) and reassign the percentages of responsibility. After creating another responsibility pie, have your clients reflect on the difference between the two, including alternative thoughts and emotions. Your goal here is not to have your clients reduce their portion of responsibility to almost nothing. Rather, you want them to translate their shifts in their attributional styles to other sources of distress.

The following is a vignette from Video Case Example MDD-11 demonstrating modifying automatic thoughts. Following the vignette are discussion questions and two activities.

VIDEO VIGNETTE 7.4

MDD-11: Automatic Thoughts—Modifying

Therapist: Mark, let's examine the evidence here . . . check out the validity of this thought.

Client: Okay.

Therapist: I find it's helpful with the evidence to write it down. <using the examine the evidence worksheet>

Client: Okay.

Therapist: I like the way you framed this automatic thought the best. You said, "Jeff doesn't want to spend time with me."

Client: Yes.

Therapist: We're agreeable with that?

Client: Yeah.

Therapist: What I want to do here is look at the evidence for and the evidence against the thought.

Client: Okay.

Therapist: I'll always start with evidence for. "Jeff doesn't want to spend time with me." What would be some examples that you could say this is evidence that he doesn't want to be with you?

Client: The fact that he wouldn't even look at me.

Therapist: Okay, I'm going to write "not look at me" and I will emphasize no eye contact.

Client: Okay.

Therapist: Anything else?

Client: He was just like "I don't have time for this."

Therapist: Okay.

Client: So, he doesn't have time for me I guess?

Therapist: I'm putting down in quotes "I don't have time for this"

Client: Okay.

Therapist: So, to be fair to you, in terms of where you're coming from with this thought, your evidence is he doesn't even look at you (no eye contact)— nonverbal. And then, verbally, he even said "I don't have time for this."

Client: Yeah.

Therapist:	Can you think of any other evidence?
Client:	No.
Therapist:	What about evidence against the thought that he doesn't want to spend time with you?
Client:	He was legitimately busy. I've been legitimately busy the past couple weeks and I'm sure if the shoe was on the other foot . . . I don't know what I would have said if Jeff had come and asked me.
Therapist:	Okay. I'll put down "busy" with a question mark.
Client:	Okay.
Therapist:	Maybe, maybe not.
Client:	Yeah.
Therapist:	What else could we point to you for evidence?
Client:	I mean, I know he was busy.
Therapist:	Have you guys ever gone out before?
Client:	Yeah. We have gone out before. That's kind of . . . kind of an obvious one. <laughing>
Therapist:	<laughing> Yeah, right, sometimes the obvious ones . . .
Client:	Kind of get overlooked.
Therapist:	So, you have gone out before?
Client:	Yeah.
Therapist:	I'm writing "have gone out to eat before." Multiple times?
Client:	Yeah, oh yeah, a bunch of times. I would even say maybe like 10, 15 times.
Therapist:	Okay.

Therapist:	I think that's some pretty good evidence against the negative automatic thought.
Client:	Yeah.
Therapist:	Do you feel that this thought is more invalid than valid? In other words, do you think this negative automatic thought is valid?
Client:	I'm kind of leaning toward "no."
Therapist:	Okay. That's good. It doesn't have to be a hundred percent.
Client:	Yeah . . .
Therapist:	It's not that easy, right? But you're leaning more toward maybe this thought isn't very accurate.
Client:	Yeah.
Therapist:	I think this is a good exercise for you to use for homework, too.

Therapist:	For alternative explanations, what would be another way to interpret what's going on with Jeff?
Client:	He's really busy and he probably has some kind of deadlines to get done or get work done. It's not necessarily that he doesn't have time for me, but maybe he doesn't have time to go out to eat, because he needs to eat a quick lunch in the office.
Therapist:	Maybe it's not about you, it's about something else that's going on.

Client:	The work he was to do.
Therapist:	Right. Now, let me just have some fun challenging you a little bit because you said before, "Well, I know what he has to do. He should do this and do that."
Client:	Yeah.
Therapist:	Let's pretend someone was making that argument with you. How would you respond if I said, "Well Mark, what do you mean? You're supposed to x, y, and z why don't you have time for me?"
Client:	I guess now that I have to think about it, just because someone has to do x, y, and z doesn't mean they're getting x, y, and z done at specific times.
Therapist:	Yes, good. Another consideration . . . Didn't you tell me sometimes your supervisor annoys you when she comes in and just says, "Hey Mark," and plops some papers on your desk?
Client:	Yeah.
Therapist:	And says, "Do this for me now?"
Client:	Yeah. That could've happened to him.
Therapist:	Right. We may not know exactly why, but maybe he had other stuff to do that had nothing to do with you.
Client:	Yeah.

Therapist:	I think it might be worth giving it a shot for you to try separating the self from the thought.
Client:	Okay.
Therapist:	When we talk about a thought that's really personal to us it's sometimes hard to really be objective with all the emotions that are going through our mind even though we know what we're doing with the task.
Client:	Okay.
Therapist:	What would be an example of a friend that we could use? It may be Melissa or another friend that you can think of.
Client:	Melissa.
Therapist:	So, let's just pretend Melissa had a similar scenario with her job. I'm sure sometimes you come home and talk to her about how your day went. What if she comes home from work and looks kind of distressed, distraught, and blah? You say, "How was your day?" and she says, "Well, I asked one of my friends that I usually go out to eat with for lunch and she didn't want to have anything to do with me" and she gave similar details like yours?
Client:	Well, the thing is that I would be saying a lot of the things I just said. Maybe they don't have the money to go out.
Therapist:	That's a good one.
Client:	Maybe they don't have the time. Maybe they already ate. Maybe they were busy. Maybe they're . . . lactose intolerant. <laughs>
Therapist:	Yeah. <laughs>

Client: I mean, there's all sorts of different things. I just think that it's kind of silly . . . It's so easy to think of what I would say it to Melissa, but when it comes time to say it to myself, it's almost impossible.

Therapist: Alright. Did you just notice something doing this particular activity? In a sense it almost seemed easier for you to come up with alternative explanations for Melissa than it was for yourself.

Client: Yeah

Therapist: And you did a really good job coming up with alternative explanations.

Client: Yeah.

Therapist: I think you rattled off . . .

Client: Like, four or five right there?

Therapist: Yeah, at least four or five. Right? Real quick.

Client: Yeah.

Therapist: It's funny how when we just look at it from a different lens that's not related to us personally it becomes easier. I have a feeling you could have gone on listing even more.

Client: Yeah.

Therapist: You see how they're kind of similar when we're looking at alternative explanations, along with what would we tell someone else?

Client: Yeah.

Therapist: The whole purpose of this particular exercise is to consider other reasons why someone may be thinking or behaving a certain way that's negatively affecting them, or at least we perceive it that way. That's the goal. It works well with a lot of your automatic thoughts. When it comes to friends and feeling rejected and they don't want to have anything to do with you, you immediately internalize it . . . personalize it . . . and then after the fact you sit there and stew over it for a while.

Client: Yeah, that makes sense.

Discussion Questions 7.4

- After examining the evidence, do you think the client's negative automatic is invalid? In other words, is it worthwhile to move forward with modifying his negative automatic thought?
- Did the client provide some realistic possible alternative explanations? How would this information be helpful in modifying his own negative automatic thought?
- The client was able separate himself from his negative automatic thought relatively easily. What made this particular technique especially helpful for this client?
- Is there another Socratic technique that might be effective in modifying the client's negative automatic thought?

ACTIVITY 7.2: AUTOMATIC THOUGHTS—MODIFYING

Practice modifying negative automatic thoughts with a peer. Have one of you play the role of the "client" by stating a negative automatic thought (assume that it has high emotional intensity and high believability and that it is invalid). While the other plays the "therapist," start with assessing its validity by examining the evidence. Thereafter, follow up with at least two more Socratic techniques to modify the negative automatic thought. Remember, the Socratic techniques you choose to use will depend on the negative automatic thought and its context (not all techniques are equally effective). Do you think the client was able to largely independently recognize that the negative automatic thought was invalid rather than being told? What Socratic technique was most effective? Did you find any of your Socratic techniques to be ineffective? If so, why do you think this was the case? Discuss why you chose to not engage in other Socratic techniques.

ACTIVITY 7.3: AUTOMATIC THOUGHTS—MODIFYING 2

Practice using a responsibility attribution pie on yourself with a negative automatic thought in relation to a specific event. Identify individuals or other factors that contributed to the outcome and assign percentages of responsibility. While viewing the visual of the responsibility pie, consider options for shifting yourself toward external responsibility. Consider why other people or related factors also contribute a portion of the responsibility. Also use any other appropriate Socratic technique to develop an alternative automatic thought. Now reassign responsibility and create another responsibility pie. Do you see any differences in external responsibility between the two pies (i.e., less responsibility attributed to yourself)? What shift in responsibility surprised you the most? Does the visual comparison help you recognize the change from your initial negative automatic thought to your alternative automatic thought? You can also try this Socratic technique with a peer as a role play.

Identifying Cognitive Distortions: Modifying Specific Thought Patterns

The title of this section may include the word "identifying," but the content fits best here because the focus is to label certain patterns of thinking in order to aid interventions focusing on evaluating and modifying negative automatic thoughts. Clients' identification of specific cognitive distortions is a skill that develops over time and has more therapeutic value once they have practiced other identifying, evaluating, and modifying techniques. You will also feel more comfortable labeling your clients' negative automatic thoughts once you have had enough time to assess their thinking patterns and integrate into your CBT case formulation. Furthermore, clarification on possible distorted thinking patterns can also inform future/concurrent assessment and interventions for core beliefs (see Chapter 8).

A. T. Beck (1976; A. T. Beck et al., 1979) coined the term "cognitive distortions" during his early work with people experiencing "emotional disorders," especially those with depression. Beck noticed that many of his distressed clients had certain consistent patterns in thinking that were noticeably illogical to him but not to them. Additionally, Beck noticed these patterns of negative biases in thinking not only within but also between his clients. In other words, even though his clients varied in the source and type of their distress, they still displayed similar thinking patterns (i.e., different in content but similar in process). Many different types of cognitive distortions have been proposed since Beck introduced this concept. Table 7.10 provides a list of some of the more common types of cognitive distortions and examples (see A. T. Beck, 1976; A. T. Beck et al., 1979; J. S. Beck, 2011; Burns, 1980).

The primary purpose of using cognitive distortion labels is to help clients recognize their own patterns of maladaptive thinking. This can heighten clients' self-awareness of their own automatic thoughts, which can aid in making the necessary modifications when they do occur. This cognitive awareness is sometimes referred to as "thinking about thinking," or metacognition. Eventually, some clients will be able to "prevent" and respond to such thoughts from occurring when they are able to recognize certain patterns of thinking before they spiral out of control.

Clients will learn how to recognize their own cognitive distortions through psychoeducation and your own modeling in session when you recognize and point out patterns in their maladaptive thinking. As noted earlier, this is a technique that is generally implemented when clients have already developed at least a basic understanding of automatic thoughts and have engaged in a few Socratic techniques. Thus, it should not be surprising or off-putting to clients when you introduce the topic and purpose of identifying specific cognitive distortions. You can also provide your clients a list of cognitive distortions, such as those in Table 7.10, if you think they will be receptive to it.

You will probably notice that identifying and labeling negative automatic thoughts can be very challenging for some clients. There are many cognitive distortions and corresponding definitions, and there can also be overlap of multiple cognitive distortions. Many of these thinking errors have been repeated (and in some ways at least partially reinforced) for many years and are now ingrained as part of their information processing system. To help buffer potential frustration and reduction in motivation, you may need to explain to clients that this is a skill that takes time to develop with continued practice. (Initially, this practice will come from repeated therapist exposure by using this technique in session and eventual use between sessions as part of their everyday lives.) You can also convey to your clients to not get caught up with having to correctly identify all cognitive distortions for every automatic thought. What is important for your clients to understand is the broader theme of being able to more consistently and accurately recognize their own maladaptive thought pat-

Table 7.10. Cognitive Distortions and Examples

Cognitive Distortion	Example
Dichotomous thinking (all-or-nothing thinking)—When you view yourself, others, or events in two categories (e.g., hated or loved, all bad or all good) instead of on a continuum.	"She does not love me, so she hates me."
Personalization—Perception that others' negative experiences or negative external events are because of you with little or no evidence; alternative explanations are not considered.	"My boss did not look at me when he walked by. He is mad at me."
Catastrophizing (fortune-telling)— Predicting worst-case outcomes with little to no evidence (or history) while ignoring evidence for more plausible outcomes.	"I know that I will mess up my class presentation and everybody will laugh at me."
Magnification/minimization—When you view yourself, others, or events by either magnifying the negative or minimizing the positive.	"I received a 'C' on my midterm. This proves I'm a pathetic student." "I received a standing ovation for my piano performance, but I know I'm not competent."
Overgeneralization—You make a conclusion about a single or a few events and then extend it across multiple events.	"I felt really uncomfortable at the last party I went to. I'm not going to any more parties because they are bad experiences and I probably won't make any friends."
Selective abstraction (mental filter)—You focus only on the minor negative information while ignoring the larger body of evidence of positive information.	"One of my friends cancelled my dinner invitation tonight (four others will be attending). This means people don't want to be around me."
Mind reading—You assume what other people are thinking about you with minimal to no evidence while not considering other information and possibilities.	"She just got up from her seat soon after I sat down. She must think I'm a loser and is embarrassed to be next to me."
"Shoulds and musts"—You have a very specific view of how you, others, or events must function, and you believe that it would be horrible if these expectations were not met.	"I must always meet every deadline. It would be horrible if I don't turn this project in on time."

terns in order to think more adaptively and reduce distress by effectively responding to life stressors and problems.

As you continue to integrate/model automatic thought identification through cognitive distortion labels, it should soon become a habit for clients to pick up on such thinking (e.g., "There I go again. . . . My initial thought was dichotomous in nature. I need to recognize that it is still okay if things do not go as planned."). Thus, if you believe that cognitive distortion identification can benefit your clients, you will need to make sure that you are consistent in identifying and addressing these distortions while also integrating Socratic techniques. It takes time and much practice to effectively integrate metacognition skills into one's everyday life. A great supplemental intervention for cognitive distortions, especially as a homework assignment, is using thought records.

Negative Automatic Thought Record

A great intervention to integrate into identifying, evaluating, and modifying negative automatic thoughts is the use of thought records. Additionally, effective use of thought records facilitates distress regulation, changes maladaptive behavioral patterns, and helps assess outcomes. Thought records also provide a great opportunity to track and log therapeutic progress over time. There have been a variety of versions of thought records since A. T. Beck et al. (1979) introduced the "Daily Record of Dysfunctional Thoughts" as a therapeutic worksheet to assist clients with monitoring their negative automatic thoughts when distressed. J. S. Beck (2011) has introduced a more contemporary thought record to better reflect the evolution of CBT. Table 7.11 is another version of a thought record, the Negative Automatic Thought Record (NATR), that best matches the CBT content and skills presented in this book, especially the Socratic techniques and integration of cognitive distortions. The use of the NATR is not necessary for all clients, especially if they are responding well to the Socratic questions alone. However, you will find that most of your clients will receive some benefit to integrating at least some form of the NATR into your treatment plan; at the very least, the NATR helps consolidate and organize relevant CBT concepts.

There is a lot of information in a NATR, and it can be overwhelming to some clients. At this point, you should already be using some of the previously mentioned Socratic techniques. When you use the NATR the first couple of times, it can be helpful to walk through each step while writing in the information provided by the client. Other options include using a whiteboard and eventually having clients complete it themselves while you verbally guide them. By the time you start using the NATR, you have most likely already at least elicited strong emotions and an associated negative automatic thought. If you have not already done so, be sure to also be clear on what was the triggering event. You now already have information that can go into the first three columns for the top row under "Before": "Day/Time Event," "Negative Automatic Thought(s)," and "Emotion(s) (Body Sensations[s])"). When

Table 7.11. Negative Automatic Thought Record

BEFORE:

Directions: When you notice that you are experiencing strong emotions (or body sensations), immediately record any thoughts or images that comes to mind in the "Negative Automatic Thought(s)" column and then finish the rest of the columns.

Date/Time Event	Negative Automatic Thought(s)	Emotion(s) (Body Sensation[s])	Behavioral Response	Outcome
What was the event or image that is associated with your current distress?	(a) What are the specific thoughts and/or mental images? (b) Rate the believability of each thought (0–10). (c) What cognitive distortions did you make?	(a) What are the emotions or body sensations? (b) Rate the intensity of each emotion or body sensation (0–10).	What were your behaviors in response to your thoughts and emotions?	(a) What was the outcome of your behavior? (b) What are your thoughts and emotions about this outcome?

AFTER:

Date/Time Event (Same as Above)	Alternative Thought(s)	Alternative Emotion(s) (Body Sensation[s])	Alternative Behavioral Response	Alternative Outcome
What was the event or image that is associated with your current distress?	(a) Respond to any Socratic technique appropriate for your negative automatic thought. (b) How much do you believe each response (0–10)? (c) What is your alternative thought? (d) Rate the believability of this thought (0–10).	(a) What emotions or body sensations do you feel now? (b) Rate the intensity of each emotion or body sensation (0–10).	What will be (or are) your alternative behaviors in response to your thoughts and emotions?	(a) What would be an (or was the) alternative outcome of your behavior? (b) How much do you believe your original negative automatic thought and your alternative thought?

Socratic Techniques: (a) What is the evidence that supports your thought? What is the evidence that contradicts your thought? (b) What is the worst/best/realistic scenario that could happen? What is the probability of each scenario? If the worst scenario happened, how could you cope? (c) Is there another explanation for what happened? (d) What is the outcome of believing your thought? What could be the outcome of changing your thought? (e) What would you tell friends or family members if they had a similar thought as you? (f) Are there other people or related factors that could have influenced the outcome of this event, even if a small amount?

reviewing automatic thoughts, also rate the believability of each thought and identify corresponding cognitive distortions if appropriate. Similarly, also rate the intensity for emotions and body sensations.

The next column, "Behavioral Response," might be new to your client depending on what has been covered up to this point. Here, you can simply ask your clients to report anything they did after (or while) experiencing their thoughts/emotions. Some clients might say "nothing" when they did do something, but it was noneventful (e.g., took a nap, watched television, or washed dishes). Thus, be sure to walk them through and use behavioral descriptions of any actions taken.

The last column, "Outcome," focuses on any possible outcomes resulting from their behaviors (e.g., behavior—took a nap; outcome—missed class). As your clients develop a greater understanding of their thoughts, you can ask them if they experienced any thoughts (e.g., "I screwed up again") or emotions (e.g., frustration) in response to the outcome. Your goal here is to see if your clients engage in certain maladaptive behavioral patterns, possibly reinforcing their negative automatic thoughts. Some clients may not immediately think there is any outcome to their behavior. Thus, the behavioral response and outcome columns provide a good therapeutic opportunity for clients to recognize the relationship between their behaviors and how it influences other aspects of their life. You can even take this a step further by eventually including their initial negative automatic thoughts and emotion/body sensations. You can do this by summarizing and processing your clients' reactions by starting at the event and working your way across from left to right. The key theme here is for clients to "see" the interrelationships among their thoughts, emotions, and behaviors. Recognizing how certain negative automatic thoughts contribute to their current distress can provide additional motivation for modification techniques.

Once your clients have a good awareness of their negative automatic thoughts and have been exposed to multiple Socratic techniques, you can review with them the columns on the bottom row under "After." This is essentially the modification portion of the NATR. You should walk through each of these steps at least a couple of times before having your clients attempt it on their own. The event remains the same as above, while the focus is on alternative thoughts, emotions, and behavioral responses. The "Alternative Thought(s)" column is extensive because it focuses on using a variety of Socratic techniques for modifying their original negative automatic thought. Noted above the "After" columns is a summary of the Socratic techniques. Remember that not all Socratic techniques are appropriate for all negative automatic thoughts. If you think it can be helpful, ask your clients to rate how much they believe their responses to each Socratic technique. Thereafter, ask them to develop an alternative thought based on reviewing the above "Before" section and completing some Socratic techniques. It is also helpful to rate the believability of this alternative thought. Do not expect your clients to rate their alternative thought believability at 70% or higher most of the time. Even a believability rating of 50% is a good start. If their rating is much lower than 50% (e.g., 35%), you can review their Socratic techniques or wait to reassess once the other alternative columns are completed.

Once your clients have developed a somewhat believable alternative thought, have them complete their alternative emotions/body sensations (and intensity) and behavioral responses. In many cases, this is a hypothetical estimate of emotions and behaviors based on having a new thought to the original event. Thus, it is okay for clients to speculate on different emotions or behaviors now that they have modified their original negative automatic thought. (Later, there may be times when clients are completing the "After" section right after they have developed an alternative thought and acted on it. In this case, they would be reporting on actual rather than hypothetical emotions and behaviors.) At this point, it is a good time for clients to compare their alternative emotions and behavioral responses to their original/actual emotions and behavioral responses in the above "Before" section. Simply ask your clients to reflect on these differences and if their alternative thought has the potential to be less distressing than their original negative automatic thought.

Finally, completing the "Alternative Outcome" column has the potential to show clients how an alternative thought can result in different life consequences that they have at least some control over. Similar to the "Before" section, you want your clients to recognize the interrelationships among their thoughts, emotions, behaviors, and outcomes. Clients often feel empowered because this process instills a greater sense of control and autonomy in being able to recognize and modify their negative automatic thoughts. Of course, clients are also able experience reduced levels of distress. A nice capstone to this exercise is to ask clients to rate their believability of the original negative automatic thought and compare it to their current believability of the alternative thought. If completing the NATR was at least somewhat successful, you should see a higher rating of believability for the alternative thought. Again, you are not looking for 100% believability. Rather, your goal is to see progressive improvement in believing the validity of their alternative thoughts over their negative automatic thoughts over time.

NATRs are great to be used as a supplement or primary focus for homework assignments. Once you believe your clients are ready to complete a NATR independently, you can have them complete the columns you determine to be appropriate. Typically, it is best to have them first complete the "Before" section (or select parts) as homework. Once they have mastered this process, you can eventually consider having them complete the "After" section as homework once it has been reviewed in session. Using NATRs provides a great opportunity for clients to practice their newly learned skills between sessions, which can help build autonomy and self-efficacy in their CBT skills. Over time, you may even notice clients generalizing their adaptive thinking skills across multiple events and problems beyond areas not of primary focus in therapy. Furthermore, clients are recording their negative automatic thoughts "live" as they occur rather than trying to recall events after the fact, which can be prone to gaps in memory and reduced intensity in emotions. Even if clients get stuck in completing their NATR homework, it is okay. This is information that can be addressed in the next session by presenting these moments of getting stuck as opportunities for further learning and practice. This information can also be used to inform the direction of future interventions, including modification of other negative automatic thoughts and possibly related core beliefs. Overall, there is a wealth of information that can be used in therapy sessions for further assessment, processing, and feedback.

The following is a vignette from Video Case Example MDD-12 demonstrating completing the "Before" section of a NATR. Following the vignette are discussion questions and two activities. (Note: See Video Vignette 4.2 (MDD-13) for another example of reviewing the "Before" section of a NATR during the early session stage.)

VIDEO VIGNETTE 7.5

MDD-12: Automatic Thoughts—Negative Automatic Thought Record

Therapist: So, for the thought record, I want to use this particular automatic thought we've been discussing about Jeff. . . . We're going to practice one now, using the event we just discussed with Jeff. It's fresh and a little bit easier to go through for a practice exercise. We'll talk later about how maybe practicing one or two of these between now and next week could be helpful when we come back and review your homework. The piece down here ("After"), is eventually we're going to consider some alternative ways of thinking. We actually already did some of these; we talked about validity, alternative explanations, and what we would tell a friend, but I don't want to do too much too quickly. It's one thing to do it in session together, but I first want to have you practice this alone and then we come back and try it, okay?

Client: Okay.

Therapist: So, this part is a no brainer. We don't have to worry about the exact date, but what's today? <using the negative automatic thought record>

Client: Friday.

Therapist: Okay, sometimes days of the week play a role; sometimes time of day too. We know it was afternoon, so we'll put afternoon. What was the actual event, I know we just discussed it, but how would we describe it?

Client: Asking Jeff to lunch.

Therapist: There you go. Sometimes we do have thoughts and feelings where we are not even aware of how they started. "Triggering event" might be too strong of an expression, but there's something that started it. Granted you were feeling a little emotion before then, but the key point is this is where it started: when you asked Jeff. Okay, so you asked Jeff to lunch. Did Jeff say yes or no?

Client: No.

Therapist: Jeff said no, just to provide a little more context there. So then, what's been the specific automatic thought we've been talking about?

Client: That Jeff doesn't want to spend time with me.

Therapist: How much at the time did you believe that thought?

Client: Probably at an 8 or a 9.

Therapist: You said that earlier too, that it was in the 8-ish range, so I wrote down 8 or 9. What kind of cognitive distortion have we been calling this?

Client: Personalization.

Therapist: Sometimes the way they're labeled, they don't always follow the exact scope. There's other ways you could argue you maybe jump to conclusions, but I think for you to call it this, where you really personalize events, is a good theme for you to focus on. So, I would agree with that. As a little tip, we have reviewed cognitive distortions a little bit. If you're not sure, because you may have a different type of thought, do your best to fill it in, but don't worry if it's wrong or right. That's more for us to talk about next session. It may or may not be relevant. There was one particular emotion especially you used that stuck with me when you described it.

Client: Hurt.

Therapist: And at the time, how intense was that emotion?

Client: Again, probably an 8, maybe even closer to the 9.

Therapist: So at least an 8, maybe a 9. So, you asked Jeff to lunch, he says no ("Jeff has no time for me."). What was your response—what did you do?

Client: I still went out to lunch, not the sub shop that I wanted to go to. Then I just went and sat by myself in the park.

Therapist: You still went out to lunch to McDonald's and then you sat by yourself in the park and ate there. What was the outcome of your behavior?

Client: I guess I felt lonely. I felt isolated. And the outcome, I still got lunch but . . .

Therapist: Still got lunch, felt lonely, isolated. Just because I'm getting to know your thinking a little bit more, I might even put in rumination. The point is the outcome is not only you sitting there isolated . . .

Client: Yeah, I'm thinking . . .

Therapist: You're thinking, exactly. And then the last part, as you're sitting here even now or even afterwards when you're reflecting, how did you feel about the outcome itself?

Client: I felt bad. I kind of felt sad and maybe a little guilty that I had done this by myself and kind of just alone.

Therapist: I wrote down bad, sad, guilty. A little bit of that self-perpetuating component. Do you remember any of the thoughts you may have had? There was something that you mentioned as well. It's okay if you don't remember. It was kind of a core belief.

Client: Maybe just that I'm hard to like.

Therapist: Yes. I don't remember the exact words you said before as well, but it was something to the effect of "hard to like" or "people don't want to be with me."

Client: Yeah, "people don't want to spend that time with me."

Therapist: . . . What I would like you to do—and we'll review this later before we go to clarify the details—I want you to at least try one maybe two. I'm feeling a little ambitious with you because you did so well with the evidence.

Client: Okay.

Therapist: . . . Next week, do the best you can to fill it out. Don't worry if it's perfect. We'll review at least one, maybe two, and then we'll decide if you're ready to then use the thought record to challenge those thoughts afterwards . . .

Client: That's pretty doable.

Therapist: You ready to move forward then?

Client: Yeah.

Discussion Questions 7.5

- Was this a relevant negative automatic thought worth exploring? What additional information did you learn about the client that might help your conceptualization of his presenting problems and distress?
- Was the client able to clearly identify his behaviors in relation to the outcomes? How is the client's response to the outcome (emotionally and cognitively) helpful to understanding his distress?
- Is it worth moving forward to modify this negative automatic thought with the "After" section of the NATR? What would be effective Socratic techniques to modify his negative automatic thought?

ACTIVITY 7.4: AUTOMATIC THOUGHTS—
NEGATIVE AUTOMATIC THOUGHT RECORD—"BEFORE"

Practice completing the "Before" section of the NATR with a peer. Have one of you play the role of the "client" by sharing a negative automatic thought (assume that it has high emotional intensity and high believability and that it is invalid). While the other plays the "therapist," start with assessing the context of the negative automatic by identifying the preceding event. You can then move on to asking details about the negative automatic thought (e.g., rate believability and type of cognitive distortion). Thereafter, identify any related emotions and/or physiological arousal (rate intensity). Next, focus on identifying the behaviors in response to the negative automatic thoughts and emotions. Finally, conclude with identifying the outcome of the behaviors and associated thoughts and emotions in response to the outcome. Did you find using the NATR helpful in organizing your questions and the content of the information provided? Do you think the NATR is a helpful technique for clients to see the relationship between negative automatic thoughts and related emotions, behaviors, and outcomes? What are some possible indicators that this negative automatic thought warrants modification (i.e., the "After" section)?

ACTIVITY 7.5: AUTOMATIC THOUGHTS—
NEGATIVE AUTOMATIC THOUGHT RECORD—"AFTER"

Practice completing the "After" section of the NATR with a peer. If possible, continue with the same client–therapist roles and negative automatic thought as Activity 7.4. Begin with the "Alternative Thought(s)" column by completing one or more of the noted Socratic techniques. Remember that the Socratic techniques you choose to use will depend on the negative automatic thought and its context (not all techniques are equally effective). If you think it will be helpful, you can ask to rate the believability for the response to any of the Socratic techniques. Based on the responses to the Socratic techniques and information from the "Before" section, develop an alternative thought and rate its believability. Next, identify possible alternative emotions and/or physiological arousal (rate intensity) in response to the alternative thought. Similarly, identify any possible alternative behaviors in response to the alternative thoughts and emotions. Finally, conclude with identifying an alternative outcome and compare the believability of the original negative automatic thought to the alternative thought. Did you find using the "After" portion of the NATR helpful in selecting appropriate Socratic techniques to modify the negative automatic thought? What Socratic technique was most effective? Did you find any of your Socratic techniques to be ineffective? If so, why do you think this was the case? Discuss why you chose to not engage in other Socratic techniques. Do you think the NATR is a helpful technique for clients to see how their emotions, behaviors, and outcomes change in response to an alternative thought? Was the NATR helpful in developing a believable alternative thought?

Cognitive Rehearsal: Imaginal Cognitive Exposure

Although some of your clients may naturally integrate what they have learned into their day-to-day lives through your Socratic techniques and NATRs, others may benefit from a more formal process of "thinking before acting" through cognitive rehearsal. To some degree, many of us already rehearse our thoughts by playing out scenarios before engaging in particular behaviors. For some clients who have already developed a few CBT skills, this technique can be used to help formalize the process for particular event–thought–emotion–behavior patterns that have been difficult to effectively modify. In some ways, cognitive rehearsal is like "imaginal cognitive exposure" with problem solving and eventual live application. The following steps are helpful to effectively put cognitive rehearsal into practice: (a) identify the particular event of concern (or events with similar characteristics), (b) identify any precipitating events or triggers before the event occurs, (c) identify negative automatic thoughts with high believability (and possible cognitive distortions), (d) identify associated emotions with high intensity, (e) identify possible behavioral responses (including past behaviors to similar events), (f) modify the

Table 7.12.   Cognitive Rehearsal Steps Worksheet

Steps	Notes
1. Identify event	
2. Identify precipitating events or triggers before the event	
3. Identify negative automatic thoughts (and possible cognitive distortions)	
4. Identify emotions	
5. Identify behavioral responses	
6. Modify negative automatic thoughts using Socratic techniques	
7. Mentally rehearse alternative thoughts and behavioral responses	
8. Assess emotions and outcomes resulting from alternative behavioral responses	
9. Develop new strategy for future similar events	
10. Assess thoughts, emotions, and behaviors using the new strategy	

negative automatic thought using previously effective Socratic techniques, (g) mentally rehearse the alternative thoughts and behaviors, (h) assess emotions and possible outcomes resulting from the alternative behaviors, (i) develop a new strategy for future similar events, and (j) assess thoughts, emotions, and behaviors in response to the new strategy. What worked? What would you do differently? This is an activity where having your clients use their client therapy notes can be help assess the effectiveness of their cognitive rehearsal between sessions. Of course, you should first assist your clients in practicing these steps while in session. Table 7.12 is a quick reference guide to walk your clients through each of these steps while taking notes. This will help ensure that no steps are missed and provide you with the opportunity to "troubleshoot" for any problems at a specific step.

Behavioral Experiments

There may be times when you can develop experiments with your clients to test the validity of a specific automatic thought. Many of the previously mentioned modification techniques naturally lend themselves to behavioral experiments because you will often ask your clients to practice their new skills between sessions. Typically, such behavioral experiments fit very well when modifying negative core beliefs. However, there may be times when setting up a formal behavioral experiment for a negative automatic thought is necessary. See Chapter 8 for a detailed discussion on using behavioral experiments for negative automatic thoughts and negative core beliefs.

WORKING WITH VALID NEGATIVE AUTOMATIC THOUGHTS

As discussed earlier, a significant portion of your clients' negative automatic thoughts will be largely invalid, and the previously mentioned modification techniques discussed in this chapter will generally be effective. However, there will be times when your clients will have largely valid negative automatic thoughts but are still experiencing distress. In these situations, you will not want to target the negative automatic thoughts with any Socratic techniques. Rather, your concern is more on the consequence/utility of the thought (see Table 7.2). In some cases, the valid negative automatic thought is associated with a distorted conclusion or meaning. The focus here can be on the utility of the automatic thought by developing possible alternative conclusions and considering possible problem-focused styles of coping. In other cases, both the valid negative automatic thought and the conclusion or meaning are accurate. The focus in this case can be more on accepting the reality of the situation and more emotion-focused styles of coping. The following are some helpful strategies when working these valid negative automatic thoughts.

1. Assess the Validity of the Conclusion

Some clients may have a valid negative automatic thought, but the resulting conclusion can be inaccurate/invalid, at least in part. Instead of challenging your clients' thoughts, you can challenge their conclusions. Some of the Socratic techniques used for automatic thoughts can be applied to clients' conclusions. For example, you can assess the evidence both for and against the validity of your clients' perceived conclusion.

2. Consider Alternative Conclusions

Once your clients have made some progress in recognizing the lack of validity in some of their conclusions, you can implement basic techniques aimed at considering possible alternative conclusions. For some clients, it may be important to emphasize to them that CBT is not "positive thinking"; rather, it is more accurate thinking that is adaptive. Simply replacing negative thoughts with positive thoughts that are not realistic may initially feel good but always ultimately results in failure and compounded distress. Your goal here is to develop conclusions both that are accurate (i.e., not made-up self-positive talk) and that contribute to adaptive functioning and distress reduction. In some cases, this will include addressing the reality of the problem/situation, including genuine risks and personal flaws and limitations. Alternative conclusions will also almost always include enhancing and/or developing alternative coping strategies.

3. Problem-Focused Coping

Some clients may have an accurate/valid perception of the situation, but it may be possible to consider a few strategies to problem solve and alter the situation (at least in part). It is important to remind yourself that not all problems can be solved. In many situations, a problem can be solved only partially. Thus, although the discussion in this section differentiates problem-focused from emotion-focused coping, many times both strategies are used when confronted with a distressing situation (Lazarus & Folkman, 1984). Effective problem solving can enhance clients' self-efficacy and also reinforce the notion that they have more influence over some situations than initially perceived. Overall, this approach acknowledges that even when certain thoughts are valid and the initial assessment of the possible outcome/consequence is accurate, clients can still effect change and alter the outcome for the better.

4. Acceptance and Emotion-Focused Coping

Sometimes, there are conclusions that are accurate and do not necessarily warrant alternative conclusions. However, ruminating over these conclusions can result in significant distress. One similar Socratic technique is to ask clients to assess the impact of ruminating over their negative conclusions. This can help clients understand that although they cannot change the outcome/conclusion, they can still control how they emotionally cope. In other words, not all problems have a solution, especially for events that have occurred in the past. Sometimes, clients continue to experience distress because they have feelings of guilt and/or they have unrealistic expectations that the problem will naturally resolve over time when there is no chance of this happening. Therefore, some clients will need assistance in accepting the outcome, often through emotion-focused coping. This process can focus on other areas of your clients' lives that are positive or rewarding and possibly assist in developing new personal, adaptive meaning of the event (i.e., although the outcome cannot change, what clients make of it can). In extreme cases, such as strong feelings of guilt after a significant loss, you may need to shift your attention to specific interventions for this type of distress (e.g., trauma focused).

COMMON CHALLENGES FOR AUTOMATIC THOUGHTS

Table 7.13 provides some common examples of challenges that can be experienced working with automatic thoughts. The two most common themes for challenges tend to be identifying relevant negative automatic thoughts and choosing appropriate Socratic techniques for modification.

Table 7.13. Common Challenges for Automatic Thoughts

Challenge	Possible Considerations
Difficulty identifying relevant negative automatic thoughts	Are you eliciting negative automatic thoughts or images that are high in emotional intensity and believability? Be sure to respond to the client's mood shifts.
	Shift your focus from intense emotions to intense physiological arousal.
	Focus on recent events that appear to have the most relevance and associated distress to the client's daily life. If therapeutically appropriate, ask clients to record their emotions and thoughts "live" as close as possible to the actual event (Figure 7.4 is helpful for this).
	Consider working backward, starting with the client's behaviors and outcomes, which can sometimes stimulate strong emotions.
	Utilize other approaches beyond guided discovery: guided imagery and role playing to elicit more intense emotional and/or physiological intensity.
	Use your CBT case formulation to inform what client problem areas to focus on what questions you use.
	Ask client to "guess."
	Hypothesize a possible thought that might be the opposite.
Client struggles to understand the difference between emotions and thoughts	Review with clients the "trick" to quickly know the difference: emotions are a single word; thoughts are a phrase or sentence.
	Provide example comparisons between thoughts and emotions using the client's own words.
	Remember to use Figures 7.2 and 7.3, which focus on negative emotions and associated thoughts and events.
Difficulty selecting appropriate Socratic techniques to modify a negative automatic thought	Remember to always start with examining the evidence to determine if the negative automatic thought is invalid. Only largely invalid negative automatic thoughts warrant modification.
	Play out the scenario of modification with a specific technique in your mind and assess possible outcomes.
	If one technique does not work, simply try another.
	Sometimes, more than one technique can work (and may be necessary) to modify particular negative automatic thoughts.
	If available, review previously completed Negative Automatic Thought Records, including possible patterns of cognitive distortions, to assess previously effective modification techniques.
Difficulty working with valid negative automatic thoughts	Remember not to modify automatic thoughts that are largely valid.
	Focus on the consequence/utility of the thought.
	If the valid negative automatic thought has a distorted conclusion or meaning, focus on developing alternative conclusions and problem-focused coping.
	If the valid negative automatic thought has an accurate conclusion or meaning, focus on acceptance and emotion-focused coping.

REFERENCES

Abrahamson, L. Y., Seligman, M. E., & Teasdale, J. D. (1978). Learned helplessness in humans: Critique and reformulation. *Journal of Abnormal Psychology, 87,* 49–74.

Beck, A. T. (1964). Thinking and depression: II. Theory and therapy. *Archives of General Psychiatry, 10,* 561–571.

Beck, A. T. (1976). *Cognitive therapy and the emotional disorders.* New York: International University Press.

Beck, A. T., Shaw, B. E., Rush, A. J., & Emery, G. (1979). *Cognitive therapy of depression.* New York: Guilford Press.

Beck, J. S. (2011). *Cognitive behavior therapy: Basics and beyond* (2nd ed.). New York: Guilford Press.

Burns, D. D. (1980). *Feeling good: The new mood therapy.* New York: Signet.

Lazarus, R. S., & Folkman, S. (1984). *Stress, appraisal, and coping.* New York: Springer.

8

Core Beliefs

Identifying and Modifying the Source of Maladaptive Thought Patterns

In order to enhance long-term change for CBT, it is sometimes necessary to go beyond clients' negative automatic thoughts by exploring their negative core beliefs. As discussed in Chapter 7, it is not unusual for some clients to have concrete, specific maladaptive patterns in thinking. If their patterns of thinking are pervasive, then there is a good chance that their negative automatic thoughts may be an "external" representation of "internal" negative core beliefs. While automatic thoughts may be represented by words or images, core beliefs are ingrained and global sources from which automatic thoughts develop. Therefore, although modifying negative automatic thoughts may be enough for some clients, others will need to "dig deeper" to get at the true source (at least in part) of distress.

Similar to automatic thoughts, before modifying your clients' core beliefs, you will first need to identify and evaluate specific core beliefs. Although a challenging task, effective work with automatic thoughts will better facilitate recognizing and evaluating relevant core beliefs contributing to your clients' distress. Modifying core beliefs utilizes some similar techniques as automatic thoughts but also requires a few additional unique skills. Soon after clients begin modifying their core beliefs, you will also need to consider integrating new, more adaptive/positive core beliefs. Similar to automatic thoughts, for the purpose of developing solid clinical development in specific therapeutic techniques, this chapter is divided into many parts: (a) understanding core beliefs, (b) psychoeducation of core beliefs, (c) identifying core beliefs, and (d) evaluating and modifying core beliefs. As expected with effective CBT, you will find yourself using many of these techniques at once and across different points in therapy while also working on automatic thoughts at the same time.

WHAT ARE CORE BELIEFS?

Broadly speaking, core beliefs are the templates that provide rules for our information processing. Core beliefs are all-or-nothing statements that are typically rigid, global, and overgeneralized views about the self, others, and how the world "works." J. S. Beck (2011) notes that some authors often use the terms "core beliefs" and "schemas" interchangeably. However, A. T. Beck (1964) views schemas as cognitive structures as part of the mind, and core beliefs are the specific content that derives from these schemas. Thus, when working with clients, it is generally best to simply stick with using the expression "core beliefs." Also, for therapeutic pragmatic purposes, it is best for most therapists to conceptualize clients' distress and origination of automatic thoughts within the context of core beliefs.

Three Categories of Core Beliefs

Core beliefs are typically placed into three categories (A. T. Beck, 1999; J. S. Beck, 2005): helplessness (e.g., "ineffectiveness in getting things done, protecting oneself, achievement"), worthlessness (e.g., "bad, unworthy, dangerous to other people"), and unlovability ("defective in character so as to preclude gaining the sustained love and caring of others"; J. S. Beck, 2011, p. 232). As would be expected, sometimes clients have negative core beliefs that fall into only one category, while others have core beliefs that fall into multiple categories. In addition to these three categories, core beliefs are typically expressed through at least one of three lenses: self, other people, and the world. Table 8.1 provides examples of common core beliefs for each category (for a more extensive list, see J. S. Beck, 2011). As will be discussed in the next section, common patterns of negative automatic thoughts (i.e., cognitive distortions) are typically strong indicators that they are extensions of specific core beliefs. The more you understand your clients' core beliefs, the more you can understand their thinking and behavioral patterns contributing to their distress.

Table 8.1. Three Categories of Core Beliefs

Helplessness	Worthlessness	Unlovability
"I am helpless."	"I am worthless."	"I am unlovable."
"I fail at everything I try."	"I am disgusting."	"I am unlikable."
"I am a weakling."	"I am a disaster."	"I will always be alone."
"I am stuck."	"I am greatly flawed."	"I will eventually be rejected."
"I am defenseless."	"I shouldn't be allowed to live."	"I will never be cared for."

Key Elements of Core Beliefs

Just like automatic thoughts, there are six key elements to core beliefs (see J. S. Beck, 2011). First, core beliefs most likely developed during childhood into adolescence due to significant life events and people and biological vulnerability (can also develop during adulthood). Also, when these core beliefs developed, they may have been valid at the time and served a functional purpose but are presently invalid. On the other hand, other core beliefs may have never been valid, with little to no utility. The next section, "Core Belief Development," explains in more detail how core beliefs develop.

Second, strongly held negative core beliefs are biased. In other words, negative core beliefs develop over time across multiple events through a lens that recognizes only supportive information and disregards contrary information (or distorted contrary information to be supportive). In some cases, negative core beliefs do not necessarily contribute to significant personal distress. However, negative core beliefs can become prominent after a series of stressful life events (i.e., activated).

Third, as noted earlier, core beliefs fit into one of three categories: helplessness, worthlessness, and unlovability. It is possible to have negative core beliefs that fit into one category or all three categories.

Fourth, negative core belief are self-perpetuating. Negative core beliefs are reinforced (i.e., validated) with patterns of negative automatic thoughts (i.e., cognitive distortions), strong negative emotions, and maladaptive behaviors. This negative reinforcing pattern can be difficult to break without deliberate attempts to modify the core belief associated with the negative automatic thoughts.

Fifth, negative core beliefs can be modified and replaced by more accurate/ adaptive core beliefs. Many of the Socratic techniques used for negative automatic thoughts can be used for negative core beliefs (there are also a few different techniques). A new core belief will most likely reduce the emotional intensity and distress experienced by the associated negative automatic thoughts.

Sixth, positive core beliefs often get overlooked due to presenting distress. Sometimes, preexisting positive core beliefs can be used to modify other negative core beliefs and reinforce new positive core beliefs. Table 8.2 provides a brief summary of

Table 8.2. Key Elements of Core Beliefs

Element	Brief Description
Usually develop during childhood into adolescence	Contributing factors include significant life events and people and biological vulnerability; negative core beliefs may have served a functional purpose but are no longer valid
Negative core beliefs are biased	Negative core beliefs tend to be reinforced by supportive information while disregarding contrary information
Three categories	Helplessness, worthlessness, unlovability
Negative core beliefs are self-perpetuating	Negative core beliefs are reinforced and validated by patterns of negative automatic thoughts, negative emotions, and maladaptive behaviors
Negative core beliefs can be modified and replaced by more accurate/adaptive core beliefs	Many of the Socratic techniques used for negative automatic thoughts can be used for negative core beliefs
Positive core beliefs often get overlooked due to presenting distress	Positive core beliefs can be used to modify negative core beliefs and reinforce new accurate/adaptive core beliefs

the key elements of core beliefs, which can be helpful for quick recall and to share with your clients during psychoeducation.

Core Belief Development

Core beliefs generally develop at an early age, from childhood to adolescence (even adulthood), based on interactions with significant and influential individuals, such as parents/guardians, teachers, coaches, and peers. Significant life events, including both traumatic experiences and successes, can also contribute to core belief development. Genetics and biological vulnerability (e.g., intelligence, temperament, and specific skills or lack thereof) can also contribute to the development of core beliefs. The overall interaction of these three factors (significant others, significant events, and genetics) are reciprocal, where different mechanisms are reinforced/validated; the more so, the more concrete the core belief. J. S. Beck (2011) states that most people tend to have core beliefs that are relatively positive and realistic (e.g., "I am a generally likable person." "I tend to be competent at most things I do."). It is perfectly normal to have both positive and negative core beliefs. However, negative core beliefs become more prominent when experiencing psychological distress. Figure 8.1 provides a visual depiction of the interaction of these three factors eventually developing into negative core beliefs that surface under psychological distress. In many ways, the development of negative core beliefs follows a pattern similar to a stress-diathesis hypothesis. In other words, when there is minimal or manageable psychological distress, the predisposition and existence of negative core beliefs may not have any significant negative effects, but when there is excessive and unmanageable distress, they can become salient with profound negative impacts on thinking and behaving (Clark, Beck, & Alford, 1999).

Benefits of Changing Negative Core Beliefs

As can be seen in Figure 8.1, core beliefs provide the prototypes for how people perceive and take in information from the environment, cognitively process information, and behaviorally respond to the environment. Helping your clients with their negative core beliefs has the potential to change the way they view themselves, interact with other people, and perceive the world. Effective modification of negative core beliefs can diminish overall distress by reducing the frequency and intensity of negative automatic thoughts. Furthermore, this process can act as an "immunization" to resist future stressors due to an improved ability to independently recognize and modify negative automatic thoughts. It is important to not forget that although your clients will have profoundly negative core beliefs, they will also have some positive/adaptive core beliefs that can contribute to helpful coping. These positive core beliefs can be increasingly uncovered and strengthened while working on negative core beliefs. Additionally, positive core beliefs may be used to help modify negative core beliefs. Thus, the value of finding, improving, and utilizing positive core beliefs can be greatly beneficial both during and after therapy.

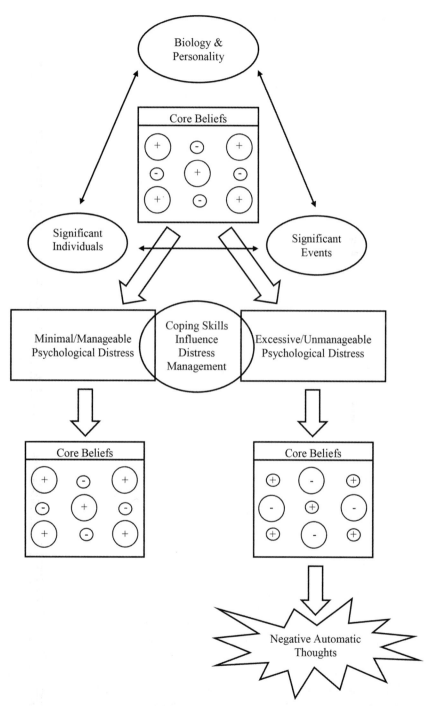

Figure 8.1. Core Belief Development

Benefit to Treatment

The more you have a comprehensive understanding of your clients' core beliefs and associated maintaining negative automatic thoughts and reinforcing behaviors, the more comprehensive your CBT case formulation and more effective your interventions can be. Even though you may not necessarily introduce the concept of core beliefs to your clients within the first few sessions, you should be internally conceptualizing your clients' core belief development and influence on their presenting distress.

It is important to note here that the CBT theoretical approach also recognizes the intermediary influence that intermediate beliefs (i.e., assumptions, attitudes, and rules) exert between automatic thoughts and core beliefs. Although this concept absolutely has theoretical value, most clients benefit from recognizing the role that the interaction between automatic thoughts and core beliefs has on views of self, others, and the world. Delving too much into theory can be cumbersome and esoteric to most clients. Thus, it is best to keep your approach to explaining the theory as simple as possible while maintaining maximum therapeutic gain. For a detailed discussion of intermediate beliefs, see J. S. Beck (2011).

PSYCHOEDUCATION OF CORE BELIEFS

Similar to automatic thoughts, as soon as therapy begins, you should be hypothesizing and listening for your clients' activated core beliefs. Over time, determine the categories and lenses of the core beliefs and related automatic thoughts, emotions, and behavioral responses. The greater clarity you have about your clients' core beliefs, the more effective you will be in introducing this topic to them in a way that can be easily understood and does not put them on the defensive. When you do present to your clients your conceptualization of their core beliefs and automatic thoughts, it is best done in a tentative manner. At this point, you should have already identified and worked on at least a few negative automatic thoughts. However, your hypothesized core beliefs can still be inaccurate and are rather personal to clients, as you may be identifying the source of potentially maladaptive thoughts, emotions, and behaviors for the first time. It is often helpful to present your hypothesized core beliefs within the context of supportive related negative automatic thoughts that they have had across multiple situations (you may have even already grouped some negative automatic thoughts as specific cognitive distortions). In fact, sometimes your clients may be ready to identify an underlying pattern on their own ("Do you notice any patterns with your negative automatic thoughts/cognitive distortions?").

Reviewing the key elements of core beliefs does not necessarily have to be as extensive as reviewing automatic thoughts. Even a general discussion of core beliefs can be difficult to understand for many clients and potentially be off-putting. However, a few themes should be touched on. First, explaining the development of core beliefs is helpful to clients because it can highlight specific significant past life events and individuals that may have shaped their development. Clients generally do well reflecting on historical information that may have influenced particular aspects of their present selves. Second, explaining the three categories of core beliefs (i.e., helplessness, worthlessness, and unlovability) can have benefits in using particular modification techniques that target persistent themes of negative automatic thoughts. Integration of core belief categories in conceptualizing clients' distress has the potential to provide broader insight and long-term growth by resolving long-standing "unfinished business." Third, explaining how negative core beliefs are self-perpetuating can be helpful for some clients if they understand this concept for negative automatic thoughts. Here, the focus is broader because you are addressing the reinforcing nature of core beliefs on negative automatic thoughts. In other words, you are going beyond simply stating that thoughts, emotions, and behaviors are related. Finally, you can provide some hope to your clients by acknowledging that core beliefs can be modified, which can result in significant distress reduction. Furthermore, recognizing positive core beliefs and noting their role in modifying negative core beliefs can also provide optimism.

The following is a vignette from Video Case Example MDD-14 demonstrating psychoeducation of core beliefs. Following the vignette are discussion questions.

VIDEO VIGNETTE 8.1

MDD-14: Core Beliefs—Psychoeducation

Therapist: Mark, we've been doing a lot of work on automatic thoughts and you've been having some insight and it sometimes come naturally. I've already thrown out the word core beliefs and explained it a little bit; and we even did a thought record a few days ago where we talked about how one of your thoughts was a core belief. We've also done a couple of diagrams. Does this sound a little familiar?

Client: Yeah, the "I'm worthless" one, right?

Therapist: Yes, that's a really good one. The two big ones for you seem to be "I'm worthless and I'm unlikable." We've been making progress. Basically, we've been identifying and modifying some of these automatic thoughts and you've been making good progress with it. I'm also noticing though there's still some lingering distress. It is perfectly natural but I want to continue making progress and I think what's going to be important for you is to really go a little deeper into where some of these automatic thoughts are coming from and those core beliefs that we've touched upon . . .

Client: Yeah, that sounds good.

Therapist: For the most part, core beliefs are due to significant life events that have happened in the past. This could be either events or people involved in those events. For example, we've talked about worthlessness and unlikable. There might have been something that has happened to you, even as a child or adolescent. A lot of times people talk about how core beliefs start off as children or adolescents but it could be events that happened not too long ago in our adulthood as well. That's something we're going to talk more about. Does sound okay to explore a little bit?

Client: Yes.

Therapist:	Now the good news is that we can modify these core beliefs, not exactly the same way but very similar to automatic thoughts. Some of the techniques that we've already been doing for automatic thoughts we can also use for core beliefs, but you'll notice they'll feel and process a little different. It's one thing to talk about one specific event and say, "Oh I can think differently about it"—and you've been doing a great job with it. Now this will feel a little different in that we're not talking about just one event, we're talking about generally . . .
Client:	. . . the big picture.
Therapist:	Yes, the big picture. Some of the techniques will be similar but the process, emotionally, might feel a little bit different and there are some techniques that are specific to core beliefs. The good thing is that we can develop some new core beliefs. They don't have to be this way. I don't like to use the word more positive. But the way I look at it is maybe we can make some of these negative core beliefs more valid, honest, accurate, logical, whatever word or language we want to use. Does that make sense?
Client:	Yeah.
Therapist:	. . . And we're not going to go through 10 or 12 core beliefs but I think there are two or three core beliefs that we can identify and clarify as we modify them. Let's see if we can make them more adaptive or more accurate.
Client:	That makes sense. If we can push the needle just a little bit, it would make me feel a little bit better and change the way I am thinking.
Therapist:	Correct. That's a good way to put it. You're already getting it. We're not going from one point to another but . . .
Client:	. . . just a little bit.
Therapist:	Yes. We're moving on a continuum. We'll go as far as we can realistically go and each core belief might be a little bit different and you're absolutely right: if we can shift those core beliefs, then maybe we'll affect those thoughts that pop into your head a little bit too often than we want to.
Client:	Cool.
Therapist:	So the next thing we're going to do then is start identifying or clarifying what core beliefs we want to focus on, okay?
Client:	Okay. Let's do it.

Discussion Questions 8.1

- Does the client appear to have at least a general understanding of core beliefs? What are the indicators that support your perspective?
- Of the key elements of core beliefs, which one(s) do you think are the most relevant to address for this client considering his background?
- Based on this client's past and current reported negative automatic thoughts, what core belief(s) deserve the most attention for modification? What information do you have that supports your decision?

IDENTIFYING CORE BELIEFS

Some of the techniques discussed here for identifying core beliefs may precede or occur concurrently with providing psychoeducation for your clients. There is no specific formula because it is not possible to predict the process of identifying core beliefs (e.g., spontaneously or purposeful) due to each client's varying level of distress and history. In general, identifying and modifying core beliefs is more challenging than automatic thoughts due to their ingrained, pervasive, and global nature. However, the degree of difficulty will be different for each client. For example, some clients may unknowingly state their core belief while expressing it as an automatic thought. In this case, it will be up to you to notice and make this distinction. Other times, clients who do not express significant emotional distress in session are less likely to state their core beliefs than those who experience high levels of in-session emotional distress. Here, it is important to recognize that, similar to automatic thoughts, core beliefs are more naturally activated where there is high emotional arousal.

Many of the techniques used for identifying automatic thoughts can also be used to uncover core beliefs. However, there are additional Socratic techniques idiosyncratic to the nature of core beliefs. What techniques you choose to use will be based on your clinical judgment, including how "deep" and pervasive the core beliefs are. While utilizing the forthcoming techniques, it can be especially helpful to hypothesize in advance possible core beliefs your clients may have. Having a good estimate of possible core beliefs can guide you in choosing the most appropriate approach to identifying the core belief. Looking for patterns in previous automatic thoughts can help develop hypotheses. In fact, at this point in therapy, you have probably noticed maladaptive thinking patterns in both content (i.e., helplessness, worthlessness, or unlovability) and style (i.e., specific categories of cognitive distortions).

Guided Discovery: From Emotions to Automatic Thoughts to Core Beliefs

These techniques were already discussed in Chapter 7 for use with eliciting and identifying automatic thoughts. The focus here is on the nature of these techniques specific to core beliefs. If there are thoughts when there are emotions, then there can also be core beliefs underneath these emotionally laden thoughts. For core beliefs, you can follow the same approach used for automatic thoughts (i.e., eliciting strong emotions, identifying the triggering event, and recognizing the relationship between thoughts, emotions, physiological arousal, and behaviors), but instead of stopping when an automatic thought(s) is identified, you can continue by summarizing any possible themes and asking further follow-up questions (e.g., "Do you think you a have rule in your mind about . . . ?" "Do you find that these types of thoughts about . . . have a pattern that come from a deeper source?" "I wonder if these thoughts about . . . come from a fundamental belief?"). If necessary, you can follow up with guided imagery, especially if clients are having a hard time verbalizing their images with clarity and important details. If you are on the right path, in most cases clients will respond with at least some insight that their automatic thoughts are based off a firmly held belief about themselves, others, or the world.

Core Beliefs Expressed as Automatic Thoughts

Sometimes, when attempting to identify an automatic thought, your clients might unknowingly state a core belief. Depending on where you are in therapy, you may choose to point out this core belief during the session or take note of the core belief and return to it in a future session when it is more therapeutically appropriate. Whenever you do choose to share this core belief with your client, it is still prudent to provide supportive evidence by way of related negative automatic thoughts. Sometimes, presenting a core belief by itself can be too much too fast and put some clients on the defensive.

Core Beliefs Embedded in Patterns of Automatic Thoughts

Initially, this technique is less about explicitly asking clients specific questions and more about paying astute attention to what they say when discussing negative automatic thoughts. Across sessions (and Negative Automatic Thought Records [NATRs] and other related activities), there is a good chance that you will notice certain patterns in the way your clients perceive themselves, others, and the world. This includes not only styles of thinking by way of cognitive distortions but also certain themes in how negative automatic thoughts cluster together across a variety of situations. These themes may be more salient with clients experiencing significant emotional distress, which may be an indicator of a strong and firmly held core belief. If you are confident in your hypothesis about a particular core belief, you can share it with your clients and ask them for their perspective on its validity. You can even directly ask your clients if they can identify a recurrent theme if you believe they may have the insight to reflect on their own thoughts. Even if this technique does not immediately result in a "discovery" of a core belief, it can set the foundation for other techniques, such as the downward-arrow technique and the core belief flowchart (discussed shortly).

Be Direct: Ask Client for the Core Belief

Sometimes, you can simply frame a question within a specific context and simply ask clients directly what is their core belief ("We have been discussing your pattern of [negative automatic thoughts/cognitive distortions]. I wonder if you can think of a core belief that represents this particular style of thinking."). This is most effective if you believe that your clients have good insight and if there has been a prior identification of core beliefs using other techniques.

Downward-Arrow Technique: Digging Deeper for Core Beliefs

The downward-arrow technique is a more concerted effort to search for a core belief by both the therapist and the client (see Burns, 1980). As the technique is named, you will guide your client in searching for a core belief by starting with a clear negative automatic thought and then follow with repeatedly asking questions to get at the "core" of the thought. When using this technique, you may already have a hypothesis of a possible negative core belief associated with the negative automatic thought (and other related negative automatic thoughts). However, rather than simply telling clients their core beliefs, it can be more effective if they are able to "discover" it on their own. In therapy, "showing" rather than "telling" has more long-term therapeutic effectiveness. Of course, before engaging in this technique, you should be sure you have a good therapeutic rapport and explain the rationale and process. You can remind your clients that collaborative empiricism during this technique is important for accurately identifying core beliefs that require modification, which will ultimately lead to reduced distress. Otherwise, it will most likely be off-putting to your clients if you simply keep repeating the same questions every time they provide an answer in response to potentially distressful thoughts. Furthermore, at this point in therapy, there should be previous therapeutic successes in modifying negative automatic thoughts. Having past "evidence" of the effectiveness of such techniques may alleviate some potential anxiety about the process and outcome. The following highlights the necessary steps for effectively implementing the downward-arrow technique.

1. Identify a Relevant Negative Automatic Thought

Be sure you are confident that the negative automatic thought you select still elicits strong emotions and is believed to be true and, for the most part, is not valid. Remember that the more relevant and distressing the negative automatic thought is, the more likely there is an underlying negative core belief. As touched on earlier, if you already have a hypothesis of what could be the core belief, there is a greater chance for clients experiencing a "successful" cognitive process, including possible added insight.

2. Ask the Client the Meaning of the Negative Automatic Thought

First, remind your clients of your rationale, including your approach to asking multiple continuous questions. Second, begin asking clients questions about what the thought means to them. Due to the potential sensitive nature of the content that may develop from your questions, having a supportive and empathic tone in your approach can put your clients at ease while maintaining their motivation to continue the process. The questioning process can be a very therapeutic experience if done in a supportive yet persistent manner. In order to at least somewhat reduce the repetitiveness, there are a variety of ways in which these questions can be posed: (a) "If that is true about you, so what?," (b) "If what you say is true, what does that mean about you?," (c) "What is so bad about . . . ," or (d) "If what you say is really bad, what is the worst part about it?" Sometimes, clients may respond with an emotion instead of a thought (e.g., "I would be very sad." "That would be the most angry I've ever been."). Unless clients continue to repeat emotions, you do not have to worry about redirecting them to thoughts. Simply validate their feelings and continue with your questions, and they will often naturally progress back to thoughts on their own.

3. Stop Asking Questions at the Core Belief

As you observe your clients while asking these questions, they often will initially appear focused with mild affect. However, you will often know when to stop asking questions when you notice a strong negative shift in their affect. Along with their shift, you may also notice a pause and have a "look of insight." Sometimes, they will also verbalize their self-awareness that it feels like they just stated a core belief. Additionally, if you and/or your clients do not initially identify the stated core belief, you will soon notice that regardless of the question asked, the core belief is simply restated in similar words. Of course, as you gain experience with this technique, you will know when you have reached a core belief when you simply hear it.

4. Process the Client's Response to the Core Belief

It is essential that you are supportive and provide empathy to clients once their core belief is uncovered. The impact of coming face-to-face with one's negative core belief can provide such feelings as sadness, hurtfulness, and/or frustration. For others, it can sometimes provide relief or satisfaction. Regardless, be sure to remind clients of the purpose of this process, including the possible necessity to modify the core belief, which can ultimately result in reducing distress and promoting long-term change and well-being. In addition to the clients' emotions, ask them to share any other thoughts they may have about the process and the recently uncovered core belief. You want to give clients the opportunity to process the experience before deciding if the core belief warrants modifying.

5. Consider Options to Modify the Core Belief

If necessary, you can use additional techniques discussed in this section to ensure that the core belief has relevance to the clients' presenting distress and that it is at least partially invalid. The point here is that not all core beliefs need to be modified. However, if you had an initial hypothesis about the core belief from the beginning, there is a good chance that if the process is successful, then it is probably necessary to move forward with modification techniques.

Figure 8.2 is a diagram of the Downward-Arrow Worksheet, which you can use to assist in identifying negative core beliefs. It provides a simple visual "flow" of the process and includes the most common questions asked to eventually reach the core belief. There also some additional questions to consider: (a) "Is this a core belief that is largely invalid?," (b) "Is this core belief relevant/believed?" (can use a 0–10 believability scale), (c) "Is this core belief causing significant distress?," (d) "Are ad-

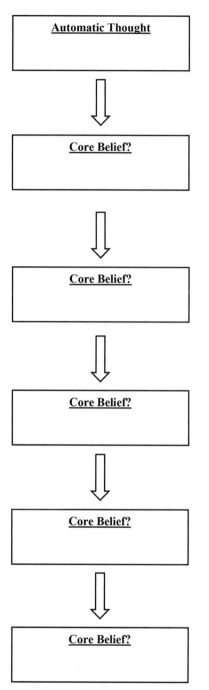

Automatic Thought

Meaning of Automatic Thought
- If that's true, so what?
- If what you say is true, what does that mean about you?
- What is so bad about…?
- If what you say is really bad, what is the worst part about it?

Core Belief?

Continue Until:
- Negative shift in affect
- "Look of insight"
- Verbally confirm belief
- Restating belief in similar words

Core Belief?

Circle Core Belief and Consider:
- Process thoughts and feelings
- Is this a core belief that is largely invalid?
- Is this core belief relevant/believed?
- Is this core belief causing significant distress?
- Are additional identification techniques necessary?
- Does core belief warrant modification? If so, what techniques?

Core Belief?

Core Belief?

Core Belief?

Figure 8.2. Downward-Arrow Worksheet

ditional identification techniques necessary?," and (e) "Does this core belief warrant modification? If so, what techniques?"

The following is a vignette from Video Case Example MDD-15 demonstrating the downward-arrow technique. Following the vignette are discussion questions and an activity.

VIDEO VIGNETTE 8.2

MDD-15: Core Beliefs—Identifying—Downward-Arrow Technique

Client: Yeah, I talked about Jeff a couple weeks ago and we had been able to go out one time for lunch, but I asked him again, "Hey Jeff, you want to go out for lunch?" and he told me that he already had plans . . . I did lunch on my own, but I saw him coming back with a couple of our coworkers and so I was kind of like, oh you already have plans with a couple of our coworkers. Why couldn't I have tagged along or why wasn't I invited or something like that? I know them, I'm friends with them . . . well not necessarily good friends, but acquaintances. I would've been able to fit around the lunch table. I was hurt. I definitely wasn't really feeling too bad when he had first told me that he already had plans.

Therapist: . . . You said, walking back into the office you felt some pain. So, of course you know what I'm going to ask you: do you recall what you were thinking at that time?

Client: Just that they didn't want me around. Yeah, that they didn't want me to be there with them.

Therapist: So, this here is called a downward arrow worksheet. What I did when you were talking is that I just wrote down in quotes, if you're okay with this one, "they don't want me around." That's your response to the event of them coming back from lunch and you weren't with them. What this technique does is I'm going to ask you some questions in a few moments . . .

Client: Okay.

Therapist: What I want to do, in a gentle way, is challenge you a little bit on this thought. And then see what else you think after I ask that question. The goal here is to find where this potential thought is coming from. In other words, is there a core belief it's stemming from this negative automatic thought? I have some ideas and, obviously, you might too, but I want to see how it plays out. And the reason why I wanted you to use this example is because I think it's a good example of something that comes up a lot in therapy and in your life. I think it is worthwhile to explore it. So, are you okay if I challenge you a little bit with some of these questions?

Client: Yeah.

Therapist: We'll start off: "they don't want me around." Again you can take your time on this as well. What if I said to you, "If that's true, so what?" I said, "Mark, what's the big deal?"

Client: I just still feel really hurt by it, I just feel kind of like unwanted . . . like I'm not really valuable or anything. I do a lot of work with these people, and to me, kind of being left around and not included in things is just really painful.

Therapist: Okay, that's a good one. You said, "feel hurt" and that's an emotion but you kept talking. There was something else I may have missed at the end, but I think you said something like not being valued?

Client: Yeah, I don't know if I'm not worth anything to them—that might be kind of that worthlessness thing—just that I'm not as valued by them.

Therapist: Okay, not valued. I'll put that down here. If you're not valued, if they don't want you around, "What does that mean about you then as a person?"

Client: I don't know if it means I'm not a good person. I put a lot of emphasis on being liked by people by having people like being around me. To have these people not include me on things is really tough for me . . .

Client: . . . I think kind of in the heart of hearts I know people like me, but there's still that inkling of doubt that people don't like me. So, if I really had to choose with how I'm feeling right now, I would say that people don't like me, but there's still that part of me that knows in some way . . . that some people do.

Therapist: That some people do. First of all, you did a good job. I know it's not easy. I give you a lot of credit going through this. The way you explain it makes sense to me as well. Part of it is that you've been doing a lot of good work and this is where the therapy is paying off. The other part that you said is that cognitively, intellectually, you're a thinker but sometimes that backfires because thinkers sometimes ruminate too much: "Intellectually, I know Melissa likes me, I know Melissa loves me, and I know I have some friends like George and Jeff and others," but emotionally you don't feel it all the time. And in the moment, you're feeling, at least when we're doing this, "I'm unlikable."

Client: Yeah, that makes sense.

Therapist: Now, this core belief, "unlikable," how strongly is it believed on a 0–10 scale?

Client: It kind of depends on the day and what holes I fill in, but some days it could be a 7 or 8 that I'm really feeling strongly about it.

Therapist: And it seems like in the moment at least it was on the higher end versus the lower end. You can correct me if I'm wrong on that, but I think that's pretty self-evident. What I also have here are some questions to consider saying there other techniques I can use. These are reminders for the therapist and client to go through. For example, is this core belief largely invalid? I think we want to test this a little bit. I think we kind of know, but I want to go through some steps to really test it and get at it in a different way as we work toward modifying.

Client: And I think I'm pushing that needle. There's that part of me that knows intellectually that people like me, but it's still in the moment when I'm stuck with the thought that people don't like me, I'm completely thrown off.

Therapist: . . . So, you can see maybe if we can tweak that core belief a little bit, make it a little bit more realistic or accurate, it might change those thoughts. What I want to do next with you—even in CBT we do a little bit of history, we don't belabor on it—I think it might be helpful to talk about where this particular core belief came from, because that will help us then for the next step when we start working on some more specific modification techniques. And while we're doing that, maybe we can change it to a more new or adaptive core belief. You want to do that?

Client: Sure.

Discussion Questions 8.2

- Was the downward-arrow technique effective in leading to the client's core belief based on his negative automatic thought and considering his background?
- What other questions could have been asked to identity this client's core belief?
- Based on the client's core belief and what you know about his negative automatic thoughts, what modification technique(s) would be the most appropriate?

ACTIVITY 8.1: CORE BELIEFS—IDENTIFYING— DOWNWARD-ARROW TECHNIQUE

Practice using the downward-arrow technique with a peer. Have one of you play the role of the "client" by stating a negative automatic thought (be sure to come up with a few more thoughts before stating your core belief). While the other plays the "therapist," start with asking questions to assess the meaning of the negative automatic thought (e.g., "If that's true, so what?" "If what you say is really bad, what is the worst part about it?"). Try your best to notice when a core belief is identified (e.g., negative shift in affect or restating belief in similar words). Do you think you were efficient in identifying the core belief (i.e., many questions and repeated client statements or just a few questions)? Did you feel comfortable asking multiple questions to transition from the negative automatic thought to the core belief? Were you able to ask the questions in a way that was sensitive to the painful nature of the core belief (i.e., your delivery)? How were you able to recognize the core belief once you heard it? How would you know if this core belief warrants being modified? Based on the core belief, what modifications would be the most appropriate?

Formal Core Belief Assessments

There may be occasions when using the previously mentioned techniques do not provide enough clarity identifying specific core beliefs. Previously identified negative automatic thoughts and other related sources (e.g., NATR) can provide insight into possible patterns of thinking linked to specific core beliefs. There may also be times when you need clarity identifying specific styles and content of core beliefs. There are a few formal assessments available to help with this process. Sometimes, seeing a list of core beliefs can stimulate clients in recognizing particular maladaptive thinking patterns (or adaptive thinking patterns). Even if the previously mentioned techniques have been helpful identifying particular core beliefs, these assessments can also aid in tracking core belief patterns over time. Furthermore, there is always the possibility that additional particular negative and positive core beliefs can be identified and used to further enhance your case formulation and treatment plan.

Assessments specifically designed for core beliefs include the Dysfunctional Attitude Scale (Weissman & Beck, 1978), the Personality Belief Questionnaire (A. T. Beck & Beck, 1991), and the Young Schema Questionnaire—Short Form (Young, 2005). Also available is the Automatic Thoughts Questionnaire (Hollon & Kendall, 1980), which, contrary to its title, assesses mainly core beliefs. Reviewing each item that has a strong endorsement can reinforce previously known core beliefs and highlight "new" negative and positive core beliefs. This is also an opportunity for clients to process their reactions to completing these assessments, which can provide additional information about the development and maintaining factors of their core beliefs. Remember that these assessments are rarely used independently. Rather, they can be a great supplement to the previously mentioned identification techniques, including formative monitoring of overall therapeutic progress.

Core Belief Flowchart—Part A: Historical Events and Present Patterns

It is sometimes helpful to explore the key historical individuals, events, and contextual factors that may have led to the development of certain core beliefs. This process is not necessary for all core beliefs but can be helpful for negative core beliefs that are especially ingrained and pervasive across multiple life domains. This is where introducing the Core Belief Flowchart—Part A (CBF-A), shown in Figure 8.3, can help explain this concept because it allows you to focus on a client-specific personal example. A key purpose for using the CBF-A at this stage is to review the historical nature of relevant core beliefs. The second half of the CBF-A looks similar to the NATR by providing a visual depiction of common negative automatic thoughts that result from the specific core belief. Additionally, there is also space to record associated emotions and behaviors. The information in the CBF-A related to the NATR can be helpful to provide a visual depiction of how patterns of thinking, feeling, and behaving stem from a specific negative core belief. Finally, identifying positive formative influences that may have promoted particular positive core beliefs also has therapeutic utility, especially when developing adaptive thoughts and behaviors.

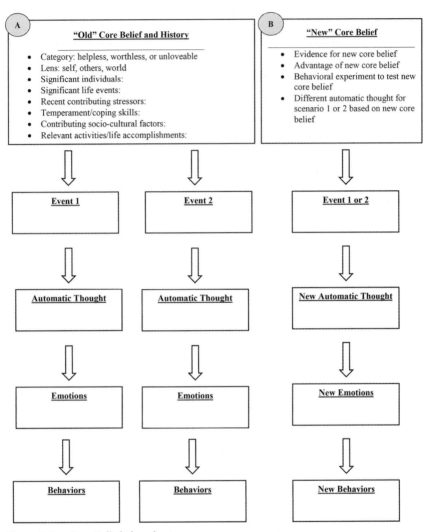

Figure 8.3.   Core Belief Flowchart

(CBF-B, also shown in Figure 8.3, is introduced in the next section, where the focus is on modifying the negative core belief after relevant historical information has been gathered and related thinking patterns have been identified.)

In addition to the previously mentioned techniques for identifying core beliefs (especially information from the downward-arrow technique), the following highlights the key domains for relevant information and helpful questions to ask for the "Core Belief and History" section of the CBF-A. Table 8.3 provides a list of each domain to assess and associated questions, including space to record relevant client information.

Table 8.3. Core Belief Flowchart Domain Questions Worksheet

Domain Questions	Notes
Category Helpless, worthless, unlovable Lens Self, others, world	
Significant Individuals "Which people have influenced your life the most?" "Which family members have influenced the way you think?" "Besides family members, who has influenced the way you think?" "Has anyone ever given you great support or inspiration?" "Has anyone ever caused you harm or belittled you?"	
Significant Life Events "Have you experienced any (positive or negative) life events that you believe shaped/influenced/transformed who you are today?" "Did you learn anything about yourself during/after this experience?" "Is it possible that you experienced an event that changed/transformed your view of how the world/others work?" "What negative messages did you get about yourself from all of the arguments with your family?" "Can you think of any attitudes or beliefs that you have that may be a result of that experience?"	
Recent Contributing Stressors "Has anything recently happened in your life that has been especially stressful?" "Has anything recently been on your mind that you can't stop thinking about?"	
Temperament and Coping Skills "What quality about yourself do you like (dislike) about yourself the most?" "How would others describe you as a person?" "Is there any characteristic/quality about yourself that could probably never be changed (or you don't want to change)?" "How do you cope with day-to-day stressors?" "How do you handle situations that are out of your control?"	

(*continued*)

Table 8.3. *Continued*

Domain Questions	Notes
Contributing Sociocultural Factors "How does your sociocultural background (or race/ethnicity, gender, sexual orientation, age, socioeconomic status, or immigration status) influence how you view and interact with the world?" "How does your sociocultural background influence your self-concept?" "Have you ever been treated differently (for better or worse) by others because of your sociocultural background?" Is there anything about your sociocultural background (or how others respond) that is currently contributing to your current distress?"	
Relevant Activities or Life Accomplishments "What personal accomplishments are you most proud of?" "How do your interests/abilities reflect who you are as a person?" "Is there any activity or life accomplishment that best defines how you see yourself?" "How has your job (or schooling or education) influenced your view of the world and yourself?" "Have you had any 'life learning' events or opportunities that have changed the way you approach life?"	

1. Category and Lens

To start, simply identify the category (i.e., helpless, worthless, or unlovable) and lens (i.e., self, others, or world) of the core belief. You can process the meaning of the clients' core belief to segue to the following questions.

2. Significant Individuals

Certain individuals can have a significant impact on our lives, good or bad. In some cases, these individuals can shape our core beliefs about ourselves, others, and the world. These individuals are typically people with whom we have frequent contact, value, and/or admire (e.g., parents/caregivers, friends, teachers, spiritual leaders, or coaches). The following are some questions to elicit information about such individuals: "Which people have influenced your life the most?" "Which family members have influenced the way you think?" "Besides family members, who has influenced the way you think?" "Has anyone ever given you great support or inspiration?" "Has anyone ever caused you harm or belittled you?"

3. Significant Life Events

Similar to specific individuals, specific positive and negative life events can also shape our core beliefs. In some cases, such events can be transforming life experiences. These events can shape our core beliefs by influencing how we view the world and ourselves based on how we respond to the event (cognitively and behaviorally). (Many times, these significant life events are also associated with significant individuals.) In addition to how the core belief first developed, it is also useful to explore how it was maintained over time. The following are some questions to elicit information about such events: "Have you experienced any (positive or negative) life events that you believe shaped/influenced/transformed who you are today?" "Did you learn anything about yourself during/after this experience?" "Is it possible that you experienced an event that changed/transformed your view of how the world/others work?" "What negative messages did you get about yourself from all of the arguments with your family?" "Can you think of any attitudes or beliefs that you have that may be a result of that experience?"

4. Recent Contributing Stressors

Everybody experiences multiple stressors throughout their lives, be they relatively small day-to-day stressors or occasional major life stressors. Here, you are most interested in recent life stressors that may have precipitated (i.e., triggered) or maintained any personal distress related to the core belief. The following are some questions to elicit information about such stressors: "Has anything recently happened in your life that has been especially stressful?" "Has anything recently been on your mind that you can't stop thinking about?"

5. Temperament and Coping Skills

It can also be helpful ask questions about how clients perceive their own characteristics/personality and coping skills. This information can be most helpful when considering techniques for modifying core beliefs and developing coping plans. The following are some questions to elicit information about temperament and coping skills: "What quality about yourself do you like (dislike) about yourself the most?" "How would others describe you as a person?" "Is there any characteristic/quality about yourself that could probably never be changed (or you don't want to change)?" "How do you cope with day-to-day stressors?" "How do you handle situations that are out of your control?"

6. Contributing Sociocultural Factors

There can also be a variety of sociocultural factors contributing to your clients' current presenting distress. Some of these factors may be completely out of your clients' control. However, such factors may still have an influence on precipitating and maintaining negative core belief development, which may have relevance for conceptualizing presenting distress. There may also be other factors that are opportunities for change and influence. The following are some questions to elicit information about relevant sociocultural factors: "How does your sociocultural background (or race/ethnicity, gender, sexual orientation, age, socioeconomic status, or immigration status) influence how you view and interact with the world?" How does your sociocultural background influence your self-concept?" "Have you ever been treated differently (for better or worse) by others because of your sociocultural background?" Is there anything about your sociocultural background (or how others respond) that is currently contributing to your current distress?"

7. Relevant Activities or Life Accomplishments

What clients perceive as relevant activities and/or life accomplishment can also provide important information about self-perception and cognitive/behavioral response patterns to stressors. The following are some questions to elicit information about relevant activities and life accomplishments: "What personal accomplishments are you most proud of?" "How do your interests/abilities reflect who you are as a person?" "Is there any activity or life accomplishment that best defines how you see yourself?" "How has your job (or schooling or education) influenced your view of the world and yourself?" "Have you had any 'life learning' events or opportunities that have changed the way you approach life?"

The following is a vignette from Video Case Example MDD-16 demonstrating the CBF-A. Following the vignette are discussion questions and an activity.

VIDEO VIGNETTE 8.3

MDD-16: Core Beliefs—Identifying 2—Core Belief Flowchart—Part A

Therapist: Mark, what I want to do is explore your core beliefs a little further using the one we just discussed—unlikable.

Client: Okay.

Therapist: What I have here is a core belief flowchart that has a bunch of fancy words of questions to ask you to explore a little about your history. I'm going to ask you a few questions about the history of this core belief. You may notice here—as I write "unlikable" here—excuse me—I put "old" but technically it is not "old" yet but our intention is to make it "old." You'll notice here it says "new" and there is a separate column. We're not going to do that until a little later. We will do it a little later. <using the core belief flowchart>

Client: Okay.

Therapist: What I want to do first is just briefly touch upon these events and then ask a few questions about your core belief. The event here is relatively recent: friends had lunch without me so your thought was, "They don't want me around." . . .

Therapist: The first couple questions here might be straightforward because I think you are doing a good job with this. The first question here is for category: helpless, worthless, and unlovable. I think your unlikable statement would fall into unlovable here.

Client:	Yes.
Therapist:	We also have what we call the lens. I look at this like how we view this core belief. Do we look at this more toward yourself, others, or the world? How would you look at that when you hear yourself, others, or the world? I know we've used these terms before . . .
Client:	I mean, it is kind of like myself as unlikable or like I am seeing people as not liking me?
Therapist:	Well in some ways, the way you frame that one, it could be either/or of those because it could be both ways. Before you were saying you don't see yourself as likable but I don't want to speak for you in terms of how you think others perceive you as well.
Client:	I guess seeing myself as unlikable, more of a "self" thing. I mean sometimes I think that people don't like me but I think, here, it is more of myself that is unlikable.
Therapist:	What I did was circled "self."
Client:	Okay.
Therapist:	One thing here is we discussed earlier today about maybe there could be significant events or individuals in our lives that can contribute to this core belief of "unlikable." Are there any particular individuals that you can think about? You said during adolescence is when you started feeling depressed.
Client:	Yeah, I can think of a few at least right off the top of my head. We kind of talked already about how I wasn't the most popular kid in school, but I did have a good group of friends. One of my good friends, Dave, we had been friends almost as long as George. I am not sure what happened but when we got into high school . . . people change, people go their own ways but at least with Dave, it seemed like he was too cool for me. I think that was one of those first times when I was like, "Am I good enough? What about me is so unlikable that he doesn't want to be friends with me anymore? What's wrong with me?" Anyway, I was in high school and able to get over it to put it simply. I was able to hang out with my other friends, but I think that was one of those first times when I was like, "Oh man . . . like what's going on? What's wrong with me?"
Therapist:	So, for this particular event what grade were you in?
Client:	It was sophomore year.
Therapist:	Okay so it was 10th grade and his name was Dave. It sounds like you were good friends with him for a while?
Client:	Yeah.
Therapist:	If I were to ask if there was any particular event that you remember with him was there a specific experience?
Client:	That's the thing . . . we would always kind of . . . there is a big hockey arena where we lived and we would always go to the games, especially because he was playing in a lot of them. One time I asked to go see one of his games and he didn't even give any information about it, almost like he didn't want me there. It was almost like that situation with Jeff. Afterward I found out that our other friends were there and that I wasn't.
Therapist:	You thought he didn't want you to be at the game?
Client:	Yeah. I mean that is what I thought . . .

Therapist: . . . One of the questions I'd like to ask is just how do you handle situations that you think, or you perceive, are out of control?

Client: I kind of withdraw. That's one of the ways . . . the number one coping skill that . . . I have to just put some distance between myself and whatever is stressing me out.

Therapist: I think "distance" is a good word.

Client: I know I run away and it isn't the best but it was easier to face things when I was in high school and college. In terms of having that strength to do it, I just don't quite have that same amount . . . I mean I would talk to Melissa like years ago but just not as much anymore.

Therapist: I would argue that when you were in college, it was maybe hard to withdraw long term because you were surrounded by all these social outlets. Whereas now when you're living alone, besides Melissa, living an adult life. When you withdraw it can be as long as you want it to whereas in college . . .

Client: . . . People showed up. I mean Brian would bring people into the dorm . . .

Therapist: To switch up a little bit, what quality do you like about yourself the most?

Client: That's a pretty deep question. Ah man. What do I like about myself? Well, I used to be okay with ambiguity. I used to be able to take things on the fly and say, "Okay, I'll get to it. I'll be able to handle this." I guess that's one of the skills I liked about myself. I used to think of myself as a people person. I mean that's one of those things that is difficult for me right now is that I don't know if people like me as much as they really do.

Therapist: So you did a good job at describing what you used to really like about yourself in the past. I am glad you brought it up because it's something that we may be able to get at a little more. We're already working on that ambiguity theme that we've mentioned before. What about like right now in the moment? If it helps, think about your relationship with Melissa or your good friends. Another way I sometimes like to frame it is how would others describe what they like about you?

Client: Um . . . that I am dedicated. I might have those moments where I'm kind of doubting myself but I'm here every week. I hang out with Melissa. I'm there. I am present except when I am withdrawn, but I mean it's like I am trying and that's something people see: you care. I'm trying to make a difference.

Therapist: Would you say you are a caring person?

Client: Yeah.

Therapist: You mentioned that a few times—that people point that out that you're dedicated, caring. I was thinking in my own mind that I like your word "dedicated." I would even say persistent, too because even when you have bad days, or when things start off a little sour, you and whoever you were with would find ways to turn it around more times than not. That's a good strength that I think you have. It works well with you so that those days don't turn into complete disasters but even . . .

Client: . . . we salvaged something.

Therapist: Exactly. You make the most of it more times than not. Even with work, yes, you did withdraw and went to a different task . . .

Client: . . . but I got it done.

Therapist: You still went back and got it done.

Client: The glass is half full.

Discussion Questions 8.3

- In what way was the CBF-A effective in understanding how the client's core belief developed?
- What additional historical information could have been obtained to understand the development of the client's core belief?
- How can the historical information about the core belief be helpful for informing future modification techniques?
- Does this client's core belief appear to be appropriate for modification techniques to develop a "new" core belief?

ACTIVITY 8.2: CORE BELIEFS—IDENTIFYING 2— CORE BELIEF FLOWCHART—PART A

Practice using a CBF-A with a peer. Have one of you play the role of the "client" by having a negative core belief in mind with some relevant historical information. (Keep in mind that you can continue using this negative core belief with Activity 8.3 for evidence and advantages/disadvantages, Activity 8.4 for CBF-B, and Activity 8.5 for a behavioral experiment.) While the other plays the "therapist," start with a core belief already identified to assess the meaning of the negative automatic thoughts. If it helps provide context, you can identify the negative automatic thoughts and associated emotions and behaviors for "Event 1" and "Event 2." Try to gather as much information as possible by asking questions about each domain. It is best to first identify the category and lens of the negative core belief, but thereafter you can follow the flow of the dialogue to ask questions about the other domains. Do you think you were effective in identifying key historical information about the core belief? Were you able to "keep up" and conceptually understand all of the information related to the core belief? Is there any other information you would like to know? Do you think this core belief would be appropriate to modify? Based on what you now know about the core belief, what modification techniques would be most appropriate?

Tracking Core Beliefs

Similar to tracking negative automatic thoughts, you can also have your clients track their core beliefs, both positive and negative. Just simply have them write down any possible core beliefs that come into their mind between sessions. If they have demonstrated some prior skills/knowledge in core beliefs, you can also have them identify the category and lens of the core belief and any associated automatic thoughts (and cognitive distortions if appropriate). Table 8.4 can be used by clients to record this information between sessions. This information can then be regularly reviewed in future sessions, including the possible use of the CBF if a key negative core belief is identified. Also, as stated earlier, positive core beliefs can have relevant utility later in therapy when modifying negative core beliefs. Finally, developing awareness of core beliefs is something that needs much practice over time; thus, this activity can reinforce this skill so that it can be a more natural way of clients' assessing their thoughts.

Table 8.4. Core Beliefs Tracker

Core Belief	Category and Lens	Automatic Thoughts	Cognitive Distortions?
1.			
2.			
3.			
4.			
5.			
6.			
7.			

EVALUATING AND MODIFYING CORE BELIEFS

For some clients, in order to achieve long-term therapeutic gains, including prevention of future distress and adaptively responding to stressful life events, modification of negative core beliefs to more adaptive means of thinking is a must. At this stage of therapy, you and your clients have already put much time and effort into identifying a preliminary list of negative core beliefs. Just like identified negative automatic thoughts, you will first need to determine if they have therapeutic relevance and are appropriate for modification. Not all negative core beliefs are worth exploring. Also, keep in mind that it is not possible or practical to fully reduce the believability of a core belief to nothing. Similar to automatic thoughts, the following modification techniques are meant to be continuously used throughout therapy. Regardless of the techniques used, the ultimate goal for your clients is to be able to integrate these skills both in therapy and independently into their daily lives.

The Evaluation Process: Focusing on Relevant Core Beliefs

Similar to automatic thoughts, you will need to be therapeutically efficient by focusing on core beliefs that have the most relevance to your clients' distress. Core beliefs that elicit the strongest emotions and appear to be associated with multiple negative automatic thoughts patterns should receive the most initial attention. These qualities are indicators to move forward and determine how strongly the core belief is believed. You will also have to ascertain the validity of these core beliefs. With that said, there is a good chance that by the time you get to this point in therapy, you most likely already have a good idea of what core beliefs deserve the most attention. In other words, the techniques involved in identifying negative core beliefs (e.g., downward-arrow technique and CBF) tend to naturally provide support (or not) the necessity to move forward with modification techniques. Nevertheless, it is still important to thoroughly explore if the identified core belief warrants further exploration.

It can also be helpful to know the category and lens of the specific core beliefs of interest. Knowledge of the "deeper" meaning of a core belief will allow for a more comprehensive case formulation and purposeful modification techniques. For example, clients may say, "I'm bad." Such a thought is telling, but it is still ambiguous. Although the lens is clear (i.e., in reference to self, not others or the world), further clarification questions will be necessary to determine if they mean they are a bad person so others will not love them (unlovable category) or if they mean they are a bad person with no value or even harmful (worthless category).

A variety of techniques to modify negative core beliefs are presented in the preceding sections, many of which are similar to those used for negative automatic thoughts. There are also a few techniques that are idiosyncratic to modifying negative core beliefs. In general, modifying core beliefs is typically more challenging than modifying automatic thoughts. Remember that many of these core beliefs are deeply entrenched and have been enacted on and reinforced for many years. However, at this point in therapy, you should have already worked on modifying negative automatic thoughts, including behavioral practice/experiments. Thus, there are many transferable skills to help ease into challenging these deeply held and rigid core beliefs.

Socratic Techniques: Evaluating to Modifying Core Beliefs

As explained earlier, the primary thematic approach to Socratic techniques is to encourage a sense of inquiry where clients work toward challenging their rigid and ingrained maladaptive views of the self, others, and the world to more flexible and adaptive thinking patterns. Some of the following Socratic techniques are similar in process to what was discussed for automatic thoughts, but the content will have a different focus with core beliefs. Additionally, just like modifying negative automatic thoughts, it is typically not necessary to use all of these techniques; your approach will vary by your clients' distress and category/lens of core beliefs. Regardless of the techniques used, it is especially important that you follow your conceptualization of your clients' specific thinking patterns based on their automatic thoughts. This will ensure a clearer focus in targeting not only a relevant negative core belief but also effective modification strategies. Remember to also guide your clients to "see" the contradictions in their thought patterns by "showing" (i.e., highlighting) any cognitive and/or behavioral inconsistencies. Of course, be cautious to avoid asking leading questions. Although you want to maintain the collaborative empiricism nature of CBT, you also do not want to come off that you already know the answer. Your clients should ultimately have control of the path of their thinking and their decision to make the necessary changes to their core beliefs. Table 8.5 provides a list of each Socratic technique and associated questions to be used as a quick reference while in session, especially when learning each approach.

1. Examine the Evidence: Determine if the Negative Core Belief Is Invalid

The process for assessing the validity of negative core beliefs is very similar to what was discussed earlier for negative automatic thoughts. One significant difference from automatic thoughts is that there is a greater chance that your clients' core beliefs have at least some validity in the past and may still have some validity in the present. Additionally, many core beliefs have been part of the clients' thinking for a significant portion of their lives and reinforced by multiple negative life events and corresponding outcomes. Thus, it is not unusual if clients are able to provide substantial evidence that the core belief is true. However, this does not necessarily mean that the negative core belief should not eventually be modified if it is the source of the clients' distress. In other words, there is a good chance that a significant portion of the core belief is not valid. Remember to not get caught up in thinking in absolute terms with core beliefs; the reality is probably somewhere between the two extremes.

Similar to automatic thoughts, this approach is often most helpful for clients when using Table 8.6, which is a three-column worksheet for writing down both the evidence for ("You shared with me some personal experiences related to your core belief. What is some evidence that supports your core belief?") and the evidence against ("Can you think of any evidence that is, at least in part, against your core belief?") the core belief. Also, there is a third column for later writing down evidence for the new core belief ("Based on the modification techniques and

Table 8.5. Socratic Techniques and Common Questions for Core Beliefs

Socratic Technique	Questions
Examine the evidence	"You shared with me some personal experiences related to your core belief. What is some evidence that supports your core belief?" "Can you think of any evidence that is, at least in part, against your core belief?" "Based on the modification techniques and behavioral experiments, what evidence supports your new core belief?" "How much do you now believe your old core belief?" "How much do you now believe your new core belief?" "What do you think about the difference in believability between your old core belief and new core belief?"
List the advantages and disadvantages of the negative core belief	"How have you found this core belief helpful in your life?" "Can you think of any ways this core belief may have caused you harm/pain?" "Based on the modification techniques and behavioral experiments, how has this new core belief been helpful in your life?" "How much do you now believe your old core belief?" "How much do you now believe your new core belief?" "What do you think about the difference in believability between your old core belief and new core belief?"
Separate self from the negative core belief	"What would you tell your [family member/friend] if they had a similar core belief as you?" "I wonder if it would make a difference in your psychological distress if you thought the same way about yourself as you do your [family member/friend]? What do you think?"
View the negative core belief on a continuum	"How much does this negative core belief apply to you on a 0%–100% scale?" "Think of a few people, real or hypothetical, who have the same or similar negative core belief. How much does this negative core belief apply to them?" "How do these people think and behave that makes them so close to 100%?" "Think of a few people who do not have this core belief and fall on the other side of the scale. How much does this negative core belief apply to them?" "The people you mentioned here are not at 0%, which means they are not perfect. What are some flaws that these people have?" "Now that you have provided some examples of people who fall on both sides of the scale, where do you put yourself on the scale?" "Although you may not feel it now, where would you like to be on this scale in the future?"

Table 8.6. Examining the Evidence Worksheet—Core Beliefs

"Old" Core Belief		"New" Core Belief
Believability (0%–100%)		Believability (0%–100%)
Evidence for Core Belief	Evidence Against Core Belief	Evidence for New Core Belief

behavioral experiments, what evidence supports your new core belief?"). Probably even more so than automatic thoughts, clients will typically have an easier time identifying evidence for their core beliefs than evidence against. This is okay and to be expected. It will be especially important for clients to "see" how much their core beliefs are invalid by objectively also acknowledging that a good portion of the core belief may have been valid in the past and even some parts valid in the present. With that said, providing genuine empathy and validating their negative life events and feelings will go a long way toward clients offering evidence against such core beliefs and eventually modification. This information should be kept by your clients in their client therapy notes as a reference guide for later comparison when this core belief is eventually modified into a "new" core belief. When clients later notice that their new core belief is not the mirror opposite of their "old" core belief, they tend to be more accepting of the evidence against and embrace their new core belief. When appropriate, you can also ask them to compare the believability of their old core belief to their new core belief ("How much do you now believe your old core belief?" "How much do you now believe your new core belief?" "What do you think about the difference in believability between your old core belief and new core belief?"). Again, you are not looking for 100% believability. What is important is that, over time, the gap between believability of the new core belief and the old core belief gradually increases (discussed in more detail later in the section "Core Belief Flowchart—Part B").

2. List the Advantages and Disadvantages of the Negative Core Belief

The reason why some negative core beliefs maintain their strength (i.e., believability) over time is because there may be some benefit from their resulting thoughts and reinforcing behaviors. In other words, although there may be some significant disadvantages from the core belief, including severe psychological distress, there is still enough benefit where the disadvantages are not fully recognized. It is very common for people to have bilateral core beliefs.

Similar to examining the evidence for core beliefs, this approach is often most helpful for clients when using Table 8.7, which is a three-column worksheet for writ-

Table 8.7. Advantages and Disadvantages Worksheet

"Old" Core Belief		"New" Core Belief
Believability (0%–100%)		Believability (0%–100%)
Advantages of Core Belief	Disadvantages of Core Belief	Advantages of New Core Belief

ing down both the advantages ("How have you found this core belief helpful in your life?") and the disadvantages ("Can you think of any ways this core belief may have caused you harm/pain?") of the core belief. Also, there is a third column for later writing down advantages of the new core belief ("Based on the modification techniques and behavioral experiments, how has this new core belief been helpful in your life?"). Your goal here is to obviously minimize the advantages while still being validating and to indicate and emphasize the disadvantages. Again, similar to examining the evidence, this information should be kept by your clients in their therapy notes for later comparison when this core belief is eventually modified into a "new" core belief. The goal is for clients to naturally recognize that the new core belief can still provide the similar advantages that the old core belief provided and at the same time reduce the disadvantages resulting from the old core belief. Essentially, clients are more apt to "give up" their negative core beliefs and associated behaviors that provide them personal benefit when these advantages can also be provided by the new core belief (i.e., keep the "good" and lose the "bad"). When appropriate, just like examining the evidence, you can also ask them to compare the believability of their old core belief to their new core belief (discussed in more detail later in the section "Core Belief Flowchart—Part B").

3. Separate Self From the Negative Core Belief

This is another technique similar to what was discussed for automatic thoughts. Clients can be more objective in assessing the validity and benefits of thoughts and behaviors when they can distance themselves from their own core beliefs. The most common method is to ask clients to consider what they would tell other individuals if they had similar core beliefs. The individual can be either someone they know or hypothetical ("What would you tell your [family member/friend] if they had a similar core belief as you?"). You can even have them do a role play where they "convince" these individuals that their core belief is not valid. Ideally, if your clients are able to provide an alternative response from their own core belief, you can then suggest trying to apply it to themselves ("I wonder if it would make a difference in your psychological distress if you thought the same way about yourself as you do your [family member/friend]? What do you think?"). You primary goal here is to have your clients notice the discrepancy between what they believe about their core belief and what they believe is true for others while using their own words.

4. View the Negative Core Belief on a Continuum

As discussed earlier, most negative core beliefs are expressed in extremes and are dichotomous. Such extreme and negative thinking only sets up clients to consistently view themselves (or others or the world) with a negative lens (e.g., "I'm a failure," "I'm incompetent," or "I'm not worthy to be loved."). Viewing oneself from a negative lens and acknowledging the existence of only the ideal (opposite) lens of the continuum (e.g., "I'm a great success," "I'm fully competent," or "Everybody loves me.") essentially sets up clients for persistent distress because there is no recognition of the wide area between the two continuum end points. Stated differently, they have put themselves in an impossible position because nobody is able to obtain the ideal lens of the continuum. Thus, almost everything they do or their life events are ultimately filtered back through their lens in a distorted and negative fashion. By viewing their core beliefs on a continuum instead of two opposite poles, clients can moderate their thoughts and at least shift their core beliefs toward the middle. Any shift from the negative extreme of the continuum toward the middle will provide the client some relief.

One of the most common techniques employed for moderating negative core beliefs is to have clients consider another individual (real or hypothetical) who is at the most negative extreme of their negative core belief continuum. Figure 8.4 provides a scale, with 0% at one end and 100% at the other, to help visually track the clients' responses for this technique. For a negative core belief, the closer to 100% is how much clients believe their negative core belief applies to them (e.g., "I'm a failure."), and the closer to 0% is the opposite of the negative core belief (e.g., "I'm a great success."). First, ask them where they think they would put themselves on the scale for their negative core belief ("How much does this negative core belief apply to you on a 0%–100% scale?"). Typically, clients will place themselves in the 85%–100% range. Second, ask them if they can think of some people, real or hypothetical, who are good examples of extremes for their negative core belief—as close as possible to 100% ("Think of a few people, real or hypothetical, that have the same or similar negative core belief. How much does this negative core belief apply to them?"). You can also ask them to describe what these people look like ("How do these people think and behave that makes them so close to 100%?"). (If appropriate, you can follow up if they can think of anyone "worse" than whom they just described.) Third, ask them about anyone who could fall on the other end of the continuum—the positive core belief—as close as possible to 0% ("Think of a few people who do not have this core belief and fall on the other side of the scale. How much does this negative core belief apply to them?"). Typically, clients will respond that nobody can be perfect all the time and will place these people in the 15%–30% range. You can also follow up by asking them to identify any flaws these people may have ("The people you mentioned here are not at 0%, which means they are not perfect. What are some flaws that these people have?"). Fourth, revisit where they think they now

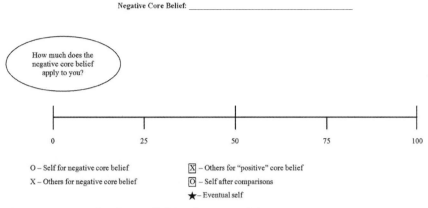

Figure 8.4. **Negative Core Belief Continuum Worksheet**

fit on the scale, considering the comparisons they just provided ("Now that you have provided some examples of people who fall on both sides of the scale, where do you put yourself on the scale?"). Clients will generally move themselves at least little more toward the middle (e.g., 65%). Finally, you can conclude by asking them where they would like to eventually view themselves ("Although you may not feel it now, where would you like to be on this scale in the future?"). Clients will also generally provide an even lower percentage (e.g., 30%). This is also a good time to point out that the core belief is no longer extreme (i.e., "I'm a failure.") but, rather, more moderate (i.e., "I sometimes make mistakes, but I generally successfully complete important tasks."). This information can be used to motivate clients to recognize that there is flexibility (or a middle ground) and that although they may have some flaws (i.e., some validity), there is room for improvement and distress relief.

The following is a vignette from Video Case Example MDD-17 demonstrating modifying core beliefs by examining the evidence and listing the advantages and disadvantages of a negative core belief. Following the vignette are discussion questions and an activity.

VIDEO VIGNETTE 8.4

MDD-17: Core Beliefs—Modifying—Evidence and Advantages and Disadvantages

Therapist: What I almost always like to do is to start out with what's called examining the evidence, and I already wrote down "unlikable." I know it says "old." It's in transition from "old" to "new." We've got evidence for the core belief. This may seem weird because we're trying to talk about changing the core belief, but I actually want you to first point out what is some evidence that shows this core belief has some truth to it? <using examing the evidence worksheet>

Client: Maybe that people blow me off? I don't know if that's filling in the holes, but I feel like people blow me off.

Therapist: You feel that way though, right? And just for sake of discussion, we don't have to write down all the names, but what would be some examples of being "blown off," both past and relatively recently?

Client: Maybe Jeff and that first incident where he didn't give me a straight answer about not wanting to go out to lunch, and then he went out to lunch with some other people after telling me that he didn't have any plans or that he did have plans but with other people. And then my old friend Dave from high school. He just decided that he was done being friends with me . . . just that people have . . . I don't know if abandoned might be a strong word, but just not a priority.

Therapist: You weren't a priority for them. And what was the name of the guy in college again?

Client: Brian.

Therapist: Brian. Would it be fair to just put that down generally? He was your roommate your first year, freshman year, he kind of faded away by the second semester?

Client: Yeah.

Therapist: And then, there was another friend of yours recently that's come up? I know you're seeing him more often now . . .

Client: George.

Therapist: George. We said at the time there was evidence for George as well.

Client: Yeah kind of the same thing. I do hang out with George, so it's kind of evidence against . . .

Therapist: That's good! That's funny; we've got George in both columns.

Client: It does go both ways. It's just how I see it I guess that day. I have more evidence against my core belief. People do like me. Jeff, we go out together for lunch. Melissa likes me . . . she might even love me. We've been together for a couple of years.

Therapist: She probably wouldn't still be hanging around.

Client: Yeah, it kind of feels a little silly now. They do like me at work. They hired me for a reason.

Therapist: I'll put down colleagues, I know you've got some friends/acquaintances as well. I think this is a good start. Do you feel comfortable with that?

Client: Yeah, we've talked about it a lot.

Therapist: So, it wasn't that bad right? It only took a few moments, especially because we've been talking about this for a while, which is helpful. That makes sense why we're doing it now here. So, evidence for core belief is the general theme of people blowing you off. . . . And then ironically, these guys pop up again for evidence for. You noticed it yourself. I didn't even have to prompt you to talk about evidence against. You right away said George, that seemed to trigger remembering Jeff.

Client: Yeah.

Therapist: You said blow off, but as we find out, it wasn't necessarily blowing you off. You do have evidence for Jeff and George where recently they are hanging out with you. . . . And then of course you mentioned Melissa, your long-term girlfriend you've been with for quite a while. In fact, it seems like she's been pretty supportive of you going through this.

Client: Yes.

Therapist: And on occasion, you've mentioned other colleagues, and maybe friends you're not as close with as George, but others that you've done group activities with as well. I think that's pretty good evidence for and against. For the believability of the new core belief, I want to tentatively put that off and revisit this. I want to keep doing this because you're doing a good job with this and I think it will be helpful for you as well. <using advantages and disadvantages worksheet>

Client: Okay.

Therapist: This is called advantages and disadvantages of core beliefs. Now this may seem a little bit odd. You could see why a therapist would ask about disadvantages, but the advantages of the core belief may seem unusual. What this is getting at is not necessarily benefits that you like. Maybe there is something that you indirectly get out of having this core belief. I don't want to say anything more because I don't want to speak for you. Everyone can really vary on what they get out of their core beliefs, even if they're negative. Take your time and think about any advantages.

Client: I guess if I'm unlikable then maybe I won't ever get close to people and get hurt by them? Because that's something that's happened before where I'll start off really well with someone, get to know them, and then when we go our separate ways. It kind of hurts me even more. That's kind of a disadvantage too, but the advantage is that if I'm not liked then I won't get close to people.

Therapist: Well, it's like when you mentioned, "If I don't get close to people it doesn't put me in a position to eventually get hurt from them, right?" You may have heard that cliché: sometimes it causes more pain to like or love someone and lose them, then it does to not at all. And that's come up before when you've talked about some friendships. . . . That's some good insight on your part. Can you think of another advantage?

Client: I don't know . . . I really feel that one. It's tough to think of the advantages.

Therapist: It's weird to try to prove or provide support for . . .

Client: I'm just going to a lot of the disadvantages. I mean, maybe if I'm not spending more time with new people, maybe I can spend time with the people who do like me?

Therapist: You've only got so much energy and time to give out to others, so at least the friends you do have, you can prioritize them. It sounds like we've covered that one. Again, this one can be a little tricky, one or two thoughts is enough. Disadvantages?

Client: Yeah, disadvantages, obviously I might be lonely in those times. . . . Melissa is obviously super supportive, but there's times when I don't want to rely so much on her. So, maybe getting that support from other people is something I lack when I'm feeling lonely because I don't even want to ask people if I'm feeling unliked. Disadvantages . . . I think one of the biggest things is it kind of just starts this negative cycle. When I feel unliked, I change the way I interact with Melissa; not even just Melissa, but people in the workplace, friends . . .

Therapist: So, feeling lonely, having to not rely on others and how it affects you, you withdraw, and changing the way you're interacting with others. Would you say the withdrawal piece has been a challenge?

Client: Yeah, definitely. It does kind of change how I interact with others, too. I just leave people alone because I don't want to bother them.

Therapist: This is helpful. I think with the information we have for evidence and advantages and disadvantages can be used to start developing a new core belief. We can think about it and talk about it. We'll do that and see how that will affect looking at how things can change if we have a new core belief. Still want to give that a shot?

Client: Yeah.

Discussion Questions 8.4

- How was examining the evidence and advantages and disadvantages techniques helpful in starting the modification process of the "unlikable" negative core belief?
- Was one technique more helpful than the other in modifying the core belief? Why was this technique more helpful?
- What information or themes obtained from both techniques will be helpful in developing a new core belief?
- What could be a possible new core belief to test with the CBF-B and a behavioral experiment?

ACTIVITY 8.3: CORE BELIEFS—MODIFYING— EVIDENCE AND ADVANTAGES AND DISADVANTAGES

Practice the examining the evidence and advantages and disadvantages techniques with a peer. Have one of you play the role of the "client" with the same negative core belief used for CBF-A. (Keep in mind that you can continue using this negative core belief with Activity 8.4 for CBF-B and Activity 8.5 for a behavioral experiment.) While the other plays the "therapist," start with examining the evidence. Always start with examining the evidence for the core belief and then continue to evidence against the core belief. Next, do advantages and disadvantages for the core belief. Again, always start with advantages for the core belief and then continue to disadvantages for the core belief. Hold off completing evidence and advantages of the new core belief until Activity 8.4 for CBF-B. Do you think you were effective in modifying (at least in part) the negative core belief using these two techniques? Was one technique more effective than the other? If so, why do you think this is the case? What information or themes were obtained from these techniques that will be helpful in developing a new core belief? What could be a possible new core belief to test with the CBF-B and a behavioral experiment?

Core Beliefs Flowchart—Part B: Modifying Old Core Beliefs and Developing New Core Beliefs

CBF-A was discussed in the previous section, where the focus is on identifying relevant historical and contributing events. Here, Figure 8.3 (same as CBF-A) focuses on synthesizing information from the previous modification techniques of the negative core belief in order to eventually develop a new, more adaptive core belief. Not all of the modification techniques have to be used, but generally the more information is available, the easier it is to begin developing a new core belief. Ideally, try to focus on more realistic (which may be more positive) new core beliefs that will reduce their distress and improve adaptive functioning. This is a great point to return to Tables 8.6 and 8.7. If you have not already done so, complete the evidence and advantages for the "'New' Core Belief" columns. Be sure to compare the believability between the old core belief and the new core belief. Remember that it is not possible (or desirable) to have a percentage for the old belief at or near 0%. Generally, you want to get at least around 25% to 30% for the old belief and 70% to 75% for the new belief. Figure 8.4 can also be helpful by referring to their most recent percentage of how much their negative core belief applies to them and where they would like to be. The primary focus should be on information that supports the new core belief (in the past or present) and reframing any "old evidence" that supports the negative core belief. The new core belief does not have to be the polar opposite of the old cold belief. Rather, as probably already done at this point with your clients using the modification techniques, an appropriate new core belief is less extreme and may acknowledge imperfections. In order to provide perspective, Table 8.8 provides some examples of old core beliefs and corresponding new core beliefs. Notice that the old core belief is extreme, while the new core belief is more adaptive but is not as extreme. Sometimes, developing a new core belief consists only of changing one or two words of the old core belief. Other times, it may require a significant shift in wording. Finally, once a new core belief has been chosen, practice at least one of the events used for the "old" core belief. However, this time, develop a possible new automatic thought that might result from the new core belief. Thereafter, consider what emotions and behaviors can develop from these new thinking patterns. The purpose here is to demonstrate if the new core belief can result in new adaptive cognitive and behavioral patterns that can reduce distress. For some clients, the cognitive processes associated these worksheets is still not quite enough evidence that the new core belief can reduce distress. In these cases, using behavioral experiments for actual life experiences is necessary (see the next section, "Behavioral Experiments"). In fact, it is okay to return to the CBF-B after completing any behavioral experiments to reassess the new core belief, which will most likely require at least some rewording.

The following is a vignette from Video Case Example MDD-17 demonstrating the CBF-B. Following the vignette are discussion questions and an activity.

Table 8.8. Old Core Beliefs Versus New Core Beliefs

"Old" Core Belief	"New" Core Belief
"I am helpless."	"Although there may be times when I don't have much control, there are many other times when I am in control."
"I fail at everything I try."	"I sometimes make mistakes, but I generally successfully complete important tasks."
"I am worthless."	"I do have value to others, and sometimes I am able to value some parts of myself."
"I am greatly flawed."	"I do have some flaws just like other people, but I also have some great strengths as well."
"I am unlikable."	"I'm a generally liked person."
"I will never be cared for."	"People have cared for me in the past, and I can be cared for in the future."

VIDEO VIGNETTE 8.5

MDD-17: Core Beliefs—Modifying—Core Belief Flowchart—Part B

Therapist: Let's go back here to the core belief flow chart. It says here evidence for new core belief and advantages of new core belief; we're going get to that in a moment. Unlikable, what would be another way to frame that differently? <using core belief flowchart>

Client: I think I hit on it a little bit earlier, but I do have some redeeming qualities. People do like me, and it's not like I have absolutely no friends by any means. I have a lot of good people in my life.

Therapist: So, you're not 100% unlikable.

Client: Yeah, maybe I'm just a good guy. Maybe I'm generally likable. Maybe not everyone likes me but some people like me. I don't know quite how to put that as a core belief but maybe somewhere in the middle like not everyone loves me but not everyone hates me.

Therapist: You said something I really like: I'm generally a likable person. The reason why I like that one is obviously you're not saying you're unlikable. We're going to use this as a continuum—that's way over here. And then over here it's everyone likes me. I don't know too many people that would think that. You said middle. Don't forget this isn't set in stone; this can be tweaked over time. But based on the way that you're wording it and the fact that without me even prompting you that much you can identify that you do have friends, you're likable, and Melissa loves you. I think this is a good start—"I'm generally a likable person." What do you think about that?

Client: I think I am generally likable. I mean there are those times that I question that and that's what's always tough for me. People do like me and people are friends with me.

Therapist: So, we do have evidence like we did earlier that you are a likable person. Let's work with that. Now you recall from this core belief flowchart, we picked two scenarios. We picked one that was relatively recent and one from the past. What we're going to try to do is see if there's a different way we may think about one of these scenarios based upon having this new core belief. Do you know which scenario you'd like to focus on?

Client: I'm thinking more of the work one. There are more people there that I'm not quite sure how much they like me. I know at the end of the day George likes me.

Therapist: I wrote Jeff and other friends have lunch without me. What perhaps could be a new automatic thought? Before you wrote they don't want to be around me or don't want me around. What would be a different?

Client: Maybe they already had plans. Maybe they didn't know if I would want to come. I'm trying to think of other ones. . . . Maybe they just didn't think to invite me. I know I don't talk to them all the time . . .

Therapist: . . . And behaviorally, what did you do last time when this happened?

Client: Withdrew.

Therapist: You said you locked yourself in your office, turned off the lights. Keeping your new automatic thoughts in mind, how might that change your behaviors?

Client: Maybe I could ask them how lunch went. Maybe ask where they went. I don't know. I don't want to invite myself out with them, but maybe if I show some interest instead of hiding in my office it might be more likely that they invite me out next time.

Therapist: So, maybe not turning off the lights in your office, not hiding in the office, and even if you don't explicitly bring up lunch when you interact with them; just a normal everyday interaction instead of being withdrawn or aloof. And of course, you can always ask how was lunch. Definitely different form being withdrawn.

Client: It would just feel better. That's the thing. I feel like I'm running away from a lot of things. Maybe I can try doing something like that—being a little bit more upfront and talking to people.

Therapist: I think that's something we can definitely do for one of your homework assignments. We've done a couple of behavioral experiments with your automatic thoughts, I want to give it a shot for your core beliefs. This is good, but it's one thing to talk about it, it's another thing to go out and apply it. Before we do that, I want to go back to examining the evidence and advantages. Your new core belief is I'm generally a likable person. What would you say is your believability of your old core belief, unlikable?

Client: The more I think about it, some days it would feel like a 50-50 thing, but the more we've been talking about, it's still there, maybe it's a 25-75. Somewhere there's more of the good core belief, the new one. We've been looking at the evidence where people like me and I have good relationships with some people. It's just some days that suspicion, that 25%, if I'm having a really tough day, really holds onto that old core belief.

Therapist: I wrote down 25% (old core beliefs) and 75% (new core beliefs). Everything you're saying made complete sense. It's not 100%. It's, "I'm generally a likable person." What would be some examples of evidence for this new core belief?

Client: That I do have friends. I do have valuable relationships with my friends, like Melissa. I do have good acquaintances at work.

_____

Therapist: Advantages for the old core belief we wrote: not get hurt by new people and spend less time with them in order to spend time with others. Now that you think you're a generally likable person, what are some advantages of having that core belief?

Client: Maybe I put myself out there a little bit more?

Therapist: I like that one.

Client: Maybe I would make some new friends. I know that maybe there would still be a little bit of doubt that one day I will drift away from them, but it might be still worth it in the end to try and make some new friends. I could get some support from them. Then, I guess, I wouldn't be as hard on myself. I think that's something, whether it's work or home or even back in school, that would pop up into the back of my head. For example, "I don't like myself right now," and it's hard to kind of sit with that and be okay with it. The more I think about I'm not a bad person, people like me . . . it feels good.

Therapist: I like that.

Discussion Questions 8.5

- Does the client's new core belief appear to be appropriate based on the original negative core belief? In other words, is it a good balance on the continuum between an extreme negative core belief and an extreme positive core belief?
- How did the new core belief influence/change the automatic thought, emotion, and behavior of the event on CBF-B?
- Based on the client's evidence and advantages for the new core belief (and CBF-B), has the negative core belief been successfully modified to facilitate adaptive thoughts, emotions, and behaviors?

ACTIVITY 8.4: CORE BELIEFS—MODIFYING 2— CORE BELIEF FLOWCHART—PART B

Practice using the CBF-B with a peer. Have one of you play the role of the "client" by using the same negative core belief used for CBF-A. (Keep in mind that you can continue using this negative core belief with Activity 8.5 for a behavioral experiment.) While the other plays the "therapist," start with CBF-B. Use the information from examining the evidence and advantages and disadvantages techniques to help develop a "new" core belief. You can

complete the "Advantages of New Core Belief" columns (including believability) now or after you complete the revised event with the CBF-B. The order
depends on what you think is the best method to identify and apply the new
core belief. Do you think you were effective in identifying a new core belief?
Was one technique (e.g., evidence for new core belief, advantages for new
core belief, alternative event for CBF-B, or a combination of two or all three)
more effective than the others? If so, why do you think this is the case? How
do you know if the new core belief will be able to have an adaptive influence
on future thoughts, emotions, and behaviors? Are there other ways to "test"
this new core belief to ensure its validity and effectiveness?

Behavioral Experiments: Testing Old Core Beliefs and Applying New Core Beliefs

Similar to automatic thoughts, you can develop experiments with your clients to
test the validity of a particular belief. Sometimes, behavioral experiments can have a
stronger influence on modifying an old core belief and reinforcing a new core belief
than verbal dialogue and cognitive techniques. In other words, these experiments
create experiences that clients can "see" and "feel" for themselves in the moment; a
change in behavior can result in a change in thinking. Most beliefs will require at
least some cognitive techniques, but how much varies on the strength of the belief.
A relatively weak belief might not require much cognitive work, and you can quickly
shift to some behavioral approaches. Of course, a relatively strong belief will probably require more initial cognitive modification techniques before a client is willing
and able to make behavioral changes. As clients begin to change their behaviors, you
will notice that their original negative core belief will continue to weaken while their
new core belief will strengthen. This can result in a continually reinforcing process
for new/adaptive cognitive and behavioral processes. Ultimately, you will want all
clients working on their core beliefs to eventually practice them "in action" outside
of session; this is where long-term change occurs.

Sample Form 8.1 is a Behavioral Experiment Worksheet, which is a helpful guide
to formally putting together a plan to test a new core belief between sessions. First,
you can list the old core belief, the new core belief, and associated believability before
the experiment. Second, clients can identify specific thoughts and behaviors that are
good indicators of the new core belief. Try to be as clear and specific as possible for
any identified thoughts and behaviors. This will minimize ambiguity and make it
easier to track. Third, with your clients, develop a plan to strengthen the new core
belief. In other words, this is the experiment to "test" your new core belief by identifying specific actions that will be taken. Fourth, have your clients identify possible
problems or obstacles that may occur with following through with experiment. Often,
past events related to the core belief can be good indicators of possible automatic
thoughts, maladaptive behaviors, or external factors. Thereafter, you can assist your
clients in developing a preemptive way to cope and problem solve for each potential

problem or obstacle. Fifth, if your clients are having some trepidation, you can ask them how likely they think they will attempt the experiment (0%–100%). If they report 80% or lower, it may be necessary to follow up on their motivation and possibly consider revising particular parts of their experiment and review their potential problems and obstacles. Sixth, before your clients engage in the experiment, you can ask them to predict the outcome. This information can provide you some insight about their expectations and self-efficacy to reinforce their new core belief. At this point, you do not have to challenge their predications. Instead, wait until the experiment is completed and compare the actual outcome to what was predicted. Seventh, when the experiment is completed, ask your clients to report on the outcome with an emphasis on their thoughts and behaviors associated with their new core belief. You can also examine any evidence for and against the new core belief. Thereafter, revisit your believability of the old core belief and new core belief. There is also space at the end for clients to share any thoughts or feelings moving forward. Finally, be sure that you review this behavioral experiment during your next session in order to assess what worked and what did not. If necessary, this information can be used for additional modification techniques and to revise the behavioral experiment for future testing. It is not unreasonable to follow up with another behavioral experiment for the same new core belief. Also, this is a good time to return to the CBF-B to apply their new core beliefs to one of the events noted in the CBF-A and reassess its believability.

The following is a vignette from Video Case Example MDD-18 demonstrating the Behavioral Experiment Worksheet. Following the vignette are discussion questions and an activity.

SAMPLE FORM 8.1

Behavioral Experiment Worksheet

"Old" Core Belief: _____
      Believability before experiment (0%–100%): _____
      Believability after experiment (0%–100%): _____

"New" Core Belief: _____
      Believability before experiment (0%–100%): _____
      Believability after experiment (0%–100%): _____

Specific Thoughts and Behaviors Associated With New Core Belief (i.e., what to look for)

1. _____
2. _____
3. _____
4. _____

Plan to Strengthen New Core Belief (i.e., what is your experiment?)

_____
_____
_____

Potential Problems/Obstacles (e.g., automatic thoughts, maladaptive behaviors, external factors)

1. _____
    Coping and problem-solving strategy _____
2. _____
    Coping and problem-solving strategy _____
3. _____
    Coping and problem-solving strategy _____

How likely is it that you will attempt the experiment? (0%–100%): _____
    Explain: _____

What is your predication for the outcome of this experiment?

_____
_____
_____

What was the outcome of this experiment? (i.e., thought or behaviors associated with new core belief)

_____

_____

_____

      Evidence for New Core Belief?

_____

_____

      Evidence Against New Core Belief?

_____

_____

Thoughts and feelings moving forward:

_____

_____

VIDEO VIGNETTE 8.6

MDD-18: Core Beliefs—Modifying 3—Behavioral Experiment

Therapist: Why don't we take a look at your behavioral experiment?

Client: We've been working on the old core belief that I'm unlikable and kind of integrating that into I'm a likable guy. As we discussed, I was going to go ask a couple of my coworkers if they wanted to go out to eat with Melissa and I with their significant others. Looking at this I can see almost how apprehensive I was about how it would go. I was thinking "are they going to have the time for me?" "Are they going value me?" I wanted to have fun with them. <using Behavior Experiment Worksheet>

Therapist: Yes.

Client: I was really excited for it, but there was still a bit of doubt if I'm going to get the exact results that I want to have.

Therapist: Right.

Therapist: What are some indicators that you're working on this new core belief . . . that shows that you're getting there? You wrote simply "spending more time with colleagues and friends."

Client: Yeah.

Therapist: And, having fun and feeling valued. We developed a plan to strengthen this new core belief based on that.

Client: Yeah.

Therapist: And, like you already said, your plan was to simply ask out a couple of your colleagues to go out with you and Melissa, kind of like a couples date . . . to see how that would go. It looks like it went well.

Client: Yeah.

Therapist: What I want to do is review the potential problems and obstacles that we hypothesized could happen.

Client: Yeah.

Therapist: The first one . . .

Client: It's pretty obvious—they could say "no." I think that's been something that I was kind of worried about. I mean, once in a while, whether it was George or Jeff, or really anyone. I was just kind of looking back on it; it kind of feels silly taking it personally if they said "no," but they obviously didn't say "no." I'm glad we made it past that pitfall.

Therapist: Yes. What was the coping strategy that you developed for this potential obstacle if they had said "no"?

Client: If they had said "no," there's no reason I still can't go out with Melissa, or give Jeff or George a call or see if one of Melissa's friends would want to go with us.

Therapist: Good. Why is that a good coping skill? How is that different from how you would've responded in the past?

Client: Because before I would kind of shut down and withdraw.

Therapist: Exactly.

Client: But here I'm still doing it and still committed to that original plan.

Therapist: Yes.

Therapist: For your prediction of the outcome you had some apprehension asking out the couples. You were 50-50% if they would say "yes" or "no."

Client: Yeah. Because we're familiar with each other, but not necessarily best friends, by any means. I know them less than I know Jeff.

Therapist: Oh, okay.

Client: We're still kind of getting to know each other. We had had dinner a couple times before, but sometime last year. So, it had been a while since we had actually done almost anything together. And, again, there was kind of that sense of doubt of whether or not they would kind of follow through or whether they'd call and cancel at the last minute.

Therapist: Okay. To some degree your apprehension was to some point valid.

Client: Yeah.

Therapist: It's understandable.

Client: Yeah.

Therapist: There's a realistic chance they could say "no."

Client: Yeah.

Therapist: One thing I like that you put down is that regardless of whether they say "no" or not, you were 90% sure that you would at least go out with Melissa.

Client: Yeah.

Therapist: Maybe your friends don't say "yes" or you didn't have time to ask out someone else, but it wouldn't have ruined the whole day.

Client: Yeah.

Therapist: Instead of withdrawing, you would've at least spent time with her.

Client: I was really happy with how this worked out. It kind of pushed me out of my comfort zone. I think maybe even a couple weeks ago I might not have been ready to ask them out. There were days that I was having trouble even asking out George or Jeff.

Therapist: Yeah, much closer friends.

Client: Yeah. Exactly. So, I just put myself out there. It was hard, but it felt good.

Therapist: I give you a lot of credit. When you first developed this plan I thought it was a good one. . . . How would you describe how the date went?

Therapist: What would be some things you could rattle off that shows evidence for your new core belief—you're a likable person?

Client: I mean, they liked me, they laughed with me, and they wanted to do it again.

Therapist: That's not bad, huh?

Client: Yeah, it really does feel good. Granted, our plans aren't set in stone, but just the fact that the doors open for us to do something again . . . it feels really good.

Therapist: And I would point out even further, is that they said "yes" to begin with. Right? Not to say if they said "no" it doesn't mean that you're not likable, but by saying, "yes," it does tell you they probably do find something likable about you and Melissa.

Client: Yeah.

Therapist: And they definitely wouldn't ask to do it again if they did not like you.

Client: Yeah

Discussion Questions 8.6

- What other thoughts and behaviors could have been good indicators of support for this client's new core belief?
- In what way was this behavioral experiment helpful in providing "evidence" for this client's new core belief?
- Is this new core belief effective enough to facilitate adaptive thoughts, emotions, and behaviors?
- What could be another behavioral experiment for this client that could potentially strengthen his new core belief?

ACTIVITY 8.5: CORE BELIEFS—
MODIFYING 3—BEHAVIORAL EXPERIMENT

Practice planning a behavioral experiment with a peer. Have one of you play the role of the "client" by using the same old core belief used for CBF-A and same new core belief used for CBF-B. While the other plays the "therapist," use the Behavioral Experiment Worksheet as a guide to develop a plan to strengthen the new core belief. Be sure to clearly identify specific thoughts and behaviors that can be associated with the new core belief. Thereafter, develop a realistic plan ("experiment") to strengthen the new core belief, including potential problems/obstacles and coping strategies. You can also assess likelihood of attempting the experiment and prediction for the outcome. If desired, you can "make up" the outcome of the experiment and provide examples of what would be good evidence to support the new core belief. Do you think this behavioral experiment has the potential to be effective? In other words, was this behavioral experiment realistic for the new core belief? Discuss the strengths and weaknesses of this behavioral experiment. Was it difficult to identify specific thoughts and behaviors to be associated with the new core belief? How is providing a prediction for the outcome of the experiment helpful in developing a new core belief?

COMMON CHALLENGES FOR CORE BELIEFS

Table 8.9 provides some common examples of challenges that can be experienced working with core beliefs. The two most common themes for challenges tend to be identifying invalid negative core beliefs and developing a new core belief that is realistic and can apply to day-to-day life.

Table 8.9. Common Challenges for Core Beliefs

Challenge	Possible Considerations
Difficulty identifying negative core beliefs	Similar to negative automatic thoughts, clients who express thoughts with high emotional intensity are more apt to state their negative core beliefs.
	Listen for clients to state the negative core belief—it can sometimes be stated when sharing a negative automatic thought.
	Hypothesize in advance possible negative core beliefs. This will help you choose the most appropriate approach for identification.
	Look for patterns in negative automatic thoughts, including content (i.e., helplessness, worthlessness, or unlovability) and style (i.e., specific categories of cognitive distortions). Reviewing Negative Automatic Thought Records can help with this process.
	Simply ask clients if they can think of any core beliefs.
	Consider almost always using the techniques in Downward Arrow Technique and Core Belief Flowchart.
	Sometimes, using formal core belief assessments can identify the specific negative core belief or stimulate related thinking patterns.
	Ask clients to record any negative core beliefs that come to mind, including its category/lens and associated negative automatic thoughts and cognitive distortions. (Core Beliefs Tracker can assist with this technique.)
	Use your CBT case formulation to review prominent thinking and behavioral patterns that tend to elicit the most distress.
Difficulty selecting appropriate Socratic techniques to modify a negative core belief	The more you know about the specific core belief (e.g., category and lens) and its related contextual contributing and maintaining factors, the more likely you will choose an appropriate Socratic technique.
	Similar to negative automatic thoughts, always start off with examining the evidence to determine if the negative core belief is invalid. Keep in mind that clients' core beliefs have at least some validity in the past and may have some validity in the present.
	Play out the scenario of modification with a specific technique in your mind and assess possible outcomes.

Challenge	Possible Considerations
	If one technique does not work, simply try another.
	More than one technique is almost always necessary in order to modify negative core beliefs.
Difficulty identifying and developing a new core belief	Remember to start with a new core belief that is not the extreme opposite (i.e., too positive) of the old negative core belief. A "slightly" positive new core belief will be more realistic when applied real-life situations and interactions. Figure 8.7 can be especially helpful with this process.
	Return to previously used modification techniques to compare the new core belief with the old negative core belief. For example, examining the evidence and advantages/disadvantages techniques have a third column for comparison, and Core Belief Flowchart— Part B allows for examining thoughts, emotions, and behaviors with the new core belief.
	Have clients practice applying their new core belief in their day-to-day lives between sessions. Figure 8.8 provides a structured format to test the new core belief and compare its believability with the old negative core belief.
	Reinforce clients' progress while also reminding them that it takes time and practice to develop new core beliefs in place of old core beliefs that may have been present for many years.
	Emphasize that clients focus on their improved emotions and decreased level of distress associated with their new core belief.

REFERENCES

Beck, A. T. (1964). Thinking and depression: II. Theory and therapy. *Archives of General Psychiatry, 10,* 561–571.

Beck, A. T. (1999). Cognitive aspects of personality disorders and their relation to syndromal disorders: A psychoevolutionary approach. In C. R. Clininger (Ed.), *Personality and psychopathology* (pp. 411–429). Washington, DC: American Psychiatric Press.

Beck, A. T., & Beck, J. S. (1991). *The personality belief questionnaire.* Bala Cynwyd, PA: Beck Institute for Cognitive Behavior Therapy.

Beck, J. S. (2005). *Cognitive therapy for challenging problems: What to do when the basics don't work.* New York: Guilford Press.

Beck, J. S. (2011). *Cognitive behavior therapy: Basics and beyond* (2nd ed.). New York: Guilford Press.

Burns, D. D. (1980). *Feeling good: The new mood therapy.* New York: Signet.

Clark, D. A., Beck, A. T., & Alford, B. A. (1999). *Scientific foundations of cognitive theory and therapy of depression.* New York: Wiley.

Hollon, S. D., & Kendall, P. C. (1980). Cognitive self-statements and depression: Development of an automatic thoughts questionnaire. *Cognitive Therapy and Research, 4,* 383–395.

Weissman, A. N., & Beck, A. T. (1978). *Development and validation of the Dysfunctional Attitude Scale: A preliminary investigation.* Paper presented at the 62nd annual meeting of the American Educational Research Association, Toronto.

Young, J. E. (2005). *Young Schema Questionnaire—Short Form 3 (YSQ-S3).* New York: Cognitive Therapy Center.

9

Behavioral Exposure

Relaxing, Testing Thoughts, and Confronting Fears and Anxieties

In Chapter 6, a variety of techniques were addressed that are initiated largely in the early phase of therapy (but are used throughout all phases) to increase the activity level of distressed clients (e.g., depression). Here, behavioral exposure techniques are typically initiated in the early or middle phase of therapy to help relieve anxiety-related distress and cope with related life stressors. These techniques continue to be used throughout therapy. In fact, it is expected that these techniques are frequently used between sessions and long after therapy ends. There is extensive research that demonstrates the effectiveness of behavioral exposure techniques for a variety of anxiety and anxiety-related disorders (e.g., agoraphobia, obsessive-compulsive disorder, panic disorder, posttraumatic stress disorder, and social phobia; Abramowitz, Deacon, & Whiteside, 2011; DiMauro, 2014; Fava et al., 2001; Gil, Carrillo, & Meca, 2001). Many of the techniques discussed in this chapter derive from learning theory, which informs behavior therapy. However, there are times when cognitive elements are appropriate to supplement the behavior techniques.

Anxiety and fear should be distinguished as two separate experiences. Anxiety is a cognitive and behavioral process that is future oriented (i.e., before the event happens). Fear is generally a physiological process that occurs in the moment (i.e., during the event) but can soon be followed by cognitive and behavioral responses. Thus, when clients are anxious, they have negative automatic thoughts (e.g., catastrophizing) and increased physiological arousal, resulting in eventually avoiding (cognitively and/or behaviorally) their source of distress because they perceive it as threatening. (This anxiety may have developed [but not always] due to previous fearful experiences.) By continuing to avoid the source of distress, they experience a reduction in anxiety and "learn" that they are safe. Slightly more technically speaking, when clients avoid/flee from their source of distress, they feel an immediate sense of emotional relief due to reduced anxiety; this is called negative reinforcement. This avoidance (i.e., negative) "works" by providing short-term relief (i.e., it is reinforced), but in the long term it can be detrimental because they do not learn the skills to cope with the source of distress. Thus, the avoidant behavior now becomes the baseline behavior, and clients will continue to experience anxiety when confronted with the same or similar sources of distress. For example, a client becomes very anxious thinking about a presentation that must be given at work tomorrow. The client then calls in sick to work the next day in order to avoid giving the presentation, resulting in an immediate feeling of relief from the anxiety and reinforcing thoughts (e.g., "I'm safe." "Now, I'm okay."). Now the client's avoidance is reinforced. The next time the client is asked to give a presentation (or perhaps other similar public speaking events), the client will most likely continue the pattern of avoidance to manage the associated anxiety. Over time, this behavioral pattern becomes essentially ingrained, including related negative automatic thoughts, resulting in marked distress.

The theoretical rationale of behavioral exposure techniques is that the very situations that are being avoided should be confronted. Stated differently, in order to break the avoidance pattern, clients need to be exposed to what makes them anxious. This is a very effective technique because exposure has the opposite effect of avoidance. Although exposing clients to previously avoided situations will initially result in increased anxiety/fear, this physiological arousal will not last forever and will eventually decrease over time after successful repeated exposures. Eventually, clients cognitively learn that the situation is no longer threatening (i.e., negative automatic thoughts are modified: "I can do this." "It's not a big deal.") while they develop associated behavioral and coping skills to manage possible future distress.

Although exposure techniques are the driving forces to break the behavioral avoidance pattern, there is sometimes a need to work on identifying associated negative automatic thoughts (e.g., catastrophic). These thoughts, sometimes in response to the intense physiological arousal associated with the source of distress, are often what initiates and reinforces the maladaptive behaviors. Thus, identifying associated negative automatic thoughts will inform the approach in implementing particular behavioral exposure techniques. Also, in turn, changing behavior patterns will modify negative automatic thoughts. Although the forthcoming techniques are used largely for those experiencing mainly some type of anxiety-related distress, many can be used for a variety of different types of distress (e.g., difficulty relaxing, poor coping/problem-solving skills, or poor social skills). Figure 9.1 provides a visual depiction of how anxiety and fear develop into maladaptive cognitive and behavioral avoidance patterns. It is important to note here that Figure 9.1 is a general model of behavioral avoidance patterns. However, anxiety avoidance can be idiosyncratic depending on the anxiety disorder (see Barlow, 2001). This chapter begins with a review of assessing anxious and fearful cognitive and behavioral patterns. Thereafter, relaxation, thought modification, and exposure techniques are discussed.

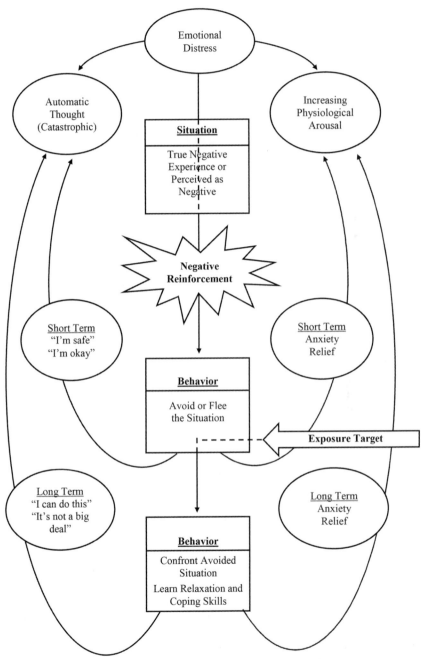

Figure 9.1. Cognitive and Behavioral Avoidance Reinforcing Anxiety

ASSESSMENT OF ANXIOUS AND FEARFUL PATTERNS

This section will seem similar to some of the content discussed in Chapters 7 and 8 with regard to assessing and modifying negative automatic thoughts and core beliefs. However, there is some variation in the targeted types of thoughts and behaviors, including physiological and emotional responses. As alluded to earlier, this type of assessment is not only for those with formal anxiety disorders. Many clients without an anxiety disorder may still be prone to anxious thoughts and behavior patterns. The following steps are in a suggested sequence to get a full contextual understanding of the clients' anxious distress, from initial precipitating factors and maintaining avoidant behaviors.

1. Triggering Events

You want to start by simply identifying any events or related factors that may have initiated the anxious/fearful experience. Such information may not be obvious to the client during the event but can be accessible soon after the experience on reflection. Sometimes, memories or images of a past or hypothetical (i.e., what might happen) event can also trigger anxiety. Also, inquire if this experience was expected (i.e., could see it coming) or unexpected (i.e., out of the blue). This information can be useful when gathering additional information related to automatic thoughts and the use of coping skills. It is helpful to get as much contextual information as possible related to the event (e.g., specific location described in detail, who was there, and what was the client doing before and after) that can be used for developing coping skills and preparing for future exposure techniques. It should be noted here that for some anxiety disorders (e.g., generalized anxiety disorder and obsessive-compulsive disorder), a single fearful event might not be the sole contributing factor in its development. However, reviewing multiple individual events has greater potential to provide substantive information in anxious patterns of thoughts and behaviors.

2. Associated Automatic Thoughts

You goal here is to identify any specific thoughts directly related your clients' presenting anxious distress. Often, there are patterns of thoughts that occur right before the anxious event. Unless there is a true threatening event, the automatic thoughts that precede the anxious response are typically distorted. Of course, there can also be thoughts during and after the anxious event/physiological response. (Chapter 7 reviews techniques for eliciting and identifying such thoughts.) Common cognitive distortions associated with anxiety focus around illogical reasoning: catastrophizing, magnification (of risk), and minimization (of own skills to cope). There also may be underlying core beliefs if there have been significant past experiences, including possible influential people, that have instilled maladaptive ways of viewing risk, danger, and means to cope with such "threatening" situations.

Identifying such negative automatic thoughts and core beliefs will be necessary for later modification interventions.

3. Physiological Response

Although physiological responses can be associated with any event or thought, the nature and intensity is generally most relevant when focused around anxious experiences. This is because anxious/fearful responses are associated with the sympathetic nervous system (i.e., fight-or-flight). In other words, there is a strong (or chronic, e.g., generalized anxiety disorder) biological response that is associated with anxiety-related disorders. There may be other associated emotions as well, but for this assessment the focus is mainly on rating the intensity of the anxiety (i.e., 0–10) and identifying specific body sensations. Physiological response information will be useful in implementing relaxation strategies (e.g., diaphragm breathing or progressive muscle relaxation) and identifying anxiety-related cues.

4. Anxiety (Behavioral) Response

This is the most important and unique step for assessing anxious distress. These are the habitual behaviors that are ultimately the response to the triggering event or memories. In other words, note specific anticipatory behaviors your clients engage in to avoid the anxious event (e.g., stay home) and/or their fearful response to the event in the moment (e.g., panic attack). You should additionally take into account the efforts that clients take to cope with the anxiety-triggering event beyond their avoidance behaviors. There can be adaptive coping skills that can be enhanced or eventually implemented (e.g., problem-solving skills, meditation, or social support). There are almost always at least a few maladaptive coping skills, including "safety behaviors." These "coping" behaviors are used to prevent, reduce, or escape/avoid perceived catastrophic events and associated distress. Safety behaviors may seem to "work" in the short term but perpetuate anxious thoughts and behaviors in the long run. Safety behaviors typically follow the mechanisms of negative reinforcement: a behavior that is strengthened (i.e., reinforced) by stopping, removing, or avoiding a negative outcome or aversive stimulus. One of the most common safety behaviors is family members or friends who help your clients cope with their anxiety. This can be a tricky pattern to break because the person providing the support has good intentions and, when done appropriately, can be helpful in reducing client anxiety. However, their help becomes a safety behavior when their support reinforces your client's avoidant behavior. Overall, these safety behaviors can significantly interfere with the effectiveness of exposure techniques and prevent distress tolerance (Blakey & Abromowitz, 2016). Table 9.1 provides some contextual examples of safety behaviors for different anxiety conditions. Knowing your clients' adaptive and maladaptive coping skills will need to be considered when implementing exposure techniques (e.g., in vivo).

Table 9.1. Examples of Safety Behaviors

An individual with agoraphobia goes out only with a trusted friend/family member.

An individual with panic disorder takes benzodiazepine when feeling early symptoms of a panic attack.

An individual with social anxiety disorder at a social gathering finds ways to avoid social interactions (e.g., hangs out near the food, makes frequent trips to the bathroom, or has to excuse oneself due to receiving a "phone call").

An individual with generalized anxiety disorder frequently seeks reassurance from a loved one to reduce excessive worry.

An individual with posttraumatic disorder due to a car accident drives a different route to work in order to avoid reminders of the trauma.

5. Outcome

The focus here is what happens after the triggering event and anxious (avoidant) behaviors. Sometimes, clients will report their anxious behavior (e.g., "I left class and went home.") as the outcome. This is accurate to point, but it can be helpful to also inquire about when time has passed after the event/experience. For example, this can include initial "relief" from not engaging in a particular threatening situation/behavior (e.g., "It felt good to get out of class and take a nap.") to later resentment toward oneself for continuing the cycle of avoidance and associated missed opportunities (e.g., "Why did I just leave class like that? I'm weak-minded." "Not only did I look like a fool to my peers, I've now fallen behind even more."). What clients do and think of themselves after the event has passed may also be a contributing factor to their anxious cycle. Table 9.2 can be used to assist in guiding your questions and tracking key information. It can also be assigned to clients to use for homework between sessions as a form of self-monitoring and as a way to track the effectiveness of current relaxation and exposure techniques, which can inform future techniques.

Table 9.2. Anxious Patterns Record

Directions: When you notice that you are experiencing a physiological arousal immediately record these sensations and any thoughts or image that comes to mind and then finish the rest of the columns.

Date/Time Triggering Event	Associated Automatic Thoughts	Physiological Response	Anxiety (Behavioral) Response	Outcome
(a) Did this event already happen, or is it hypothetical? (b) Was the triggering event expected or unexpected?	(a) What are the specific thoughts and/or mental images? (b) What cognitive distortions did you make: catastrophizing, magnification, minimization, other?	(a) Identify as many body sensations as possible. (b) Rate the intensity of your body sensations and overall anxiety (0–10)?	(a) What did you do prevent, reduce, or escape/avoid the triggering event? (b) Identify any specific safety behaviors. (c) Were there any other behaviors?	(a) What was the initial outcome of your anxious response? (b) Were there any other long-term outcomes or consequences? (c) What are your thoughts and emotions to this outcome?

The following is a vignette from Video Case Example PDA-6 demonstrating assessment of anxious patterns. Following the vignette are discussion questions and an activity. (Note: See Video Vignette 4.4 (PDA-5) for another example of assessment of anxious patterns. Also see Video Vignette 4.5 (PDA-8) for an example of tracking negative automatic thoughts and associated body sensations.)

VIDEO VIGNETTE 9.1

PDA-6: Behavioral Techniques—Assessment of Anxious Patterns

Therapist: Why don't you set it up for me? We know it happened yesterday. Where did it happen? What happened?

Client: Well, in hindsight, I feel like I was being really ambitious since our last session. My husband drove me to the grocery store and that was a really big step for me.

Therapist: Big step because you typically haven't been going to the grocery store?

Client: Well, he usually does all the shopping in general, but I wanted to make sure I didn't have a panic attack.

Therapist: Just for curiosity, you said, "really ambitious," what do you mean by that?

Client: Well, I wanted to see if I could go into the grocery store by myself.

Therapist: Okay.

Client: The drive was better than I expected and it was around 10:00 a.m. yesterday. There were a lot of people there and when I was walking down one of the aisles I could feel like my body getting warm.

Therapist: Would you describe this panic attack expected or unexpected?

Client: It was unexpected. I mean I really thought I was doing a good job. I mean, I remember you explained everything and you showed me the way things work in terms of thoughts and behaviors. I thought I had a better grip of it.

Therapist: I do think you have a good understanding of what's going on, but like you said, maybe a little ambitious at this point. I actually really appreciate and respect that—I think that's a good strength of yours—but what we might have to do is pause that a little bit and wait before you get a few more skills to give it a shot.

Client: Yeah.

Therapist: I appreciate your ambition. You could of just said, "Forget this. I'm not going to go out and do anything." So, here you are, you're in the grocery store, you thought it was going to be great, so understandably, it is unexpected.

Client: Right.

Therapist: Following the panic attack record, you rated your physiological intensity a 9.

Client: Yeah.

Therapist: That's pretty intense. That's one of the higher ones you've given in a while.

Client: Yeah.

Therapist:	Why don't you tell me some of the symptoms you experienced there.
Client:	Well, I got really, really hot and my palms were getting sweaty, and I felt like my chest getting tight, and the more I started to notice that, my heart started completely racing. It felt like it was pounding out of my chest. Then I started to notice other people could see I was struggling and I think it just made it worse and I started to feel nauseous in the pit of my stomach . . .
Therapist:	Oh, okay. I haven't heard that one in a while but I think it's because you're self-aware of or perceiving others as noticing how you were feeling.
Client:	I mean it might've been . . . I just knew I needed to get out there. I was just having those feelings of choking and then just felt like I was losing control . . .
Therapist:	Okay.
Therapist:	Help me flush out some of these thoughts. I want to get into more detail about what you were thinking both in the moment and then afterwards as well . . .
Client:	Okay. Well, with the aisle being so crowded and starting to feel those symptoms, I felt like I couldn't escape . . . what happens if I have a heart attack right there in the middle of the aisle? How am I going to get help and those people were there . . .
Therapist:	What did you do afterwards?
Client:	Well I tried to remember what you said . . . what you described in our last session, but I just had to get out. I felt like I was losing complete control and that I needed to get out. I just like ran to the parking lot and as soon as I saw my husband sitting in the car I started to feel way more relieved and ready to go home. I just needed to get away from there and back home.
Therapist:	So just to summarize, you're in the aisle having symptoms—we don't have to rehash those—I've got the form to look at. You feel like you can't escape, need some help, having a heart attack. Eventually, you just flee right out of there. You left your carriage, was it?
Client:	Yeah, I just left the carriage. And I kept telling myself, "I know I'm not having a heart attack. I know he told me . . . "
Therapist:	Okay, so you were trying to remember . . .
Client:	I tried, but my body let me know it needed to get out.
Therapist:	What you will find over therapy is that it's one thing to cognitively know it, but it's another thing to feel it. Even though intellectually you're saying, "I'm not going to have a heart attack and die" . . . at that point, in the moment, the emotions were so intense it is hard to think rationally.
Client:	Right.

| Therapist: | So, you get in the car and you feel relief. Did you go home or somewhere else? |

Client: Well, we decided not to go to the hospital. We went straight home and by the time we got home I think I was just recovering from the panic attack but the symptoms were gone.

Therapist: I'd like to talk about your thoughts after the event as well. Now you're home, you're relaxed and calm. What were your thoughts replaying the events in your mind as you sat there?

Client: I feel like I failed. I mean, I feel silly because it really should be so easy to go into a grocery store.

Therapist: Right, but it wasn't for you.

Client: Right.

Therapist: I notice you use this language sometimes—that you "failed." It seems like splitting hairs but it depends on how you look at it, right? So understandably, you're looking at the final outcome: you went to the grocery store to go shopping and you did not exit with the food purchased. You left the cart and came home?

Client: Yeah.

Therapist: Maybe it was a bit ambitious, a little bit too soon. On the other hand, the way I like to look at is the fact that you got the hope and motivation to go there. You said to me it has been a few months since you've even been to a grocery store?

Client: Yeah, that's true.

Therapist: So give yourself some credit. You at least gave it a shot. You got the cart, you pushed it around, and you got a few items in there, but didn't make it all the way.

Client: Yeah.

Discussion Questions 9.1

- Based on the context of the triggering event and physiological response, what might be an effective relaxation technique to practice?
- What would you identify as the client's primary automatic thought in response to this event? What type of cognitive distortion was her automatic thought (e.g., catastrophizing, magnification, or minimization)?
- What was the client's response to her associated automatic thoughts and physiological response? In other words, what did she do to reduce her anxiety? Did she engage in any safety behaviors?
- Consider the client's thoughts, physiological response, and behaviors. Does this pattern warrant any modification and/or exposure techniques?

ACTIVITY 9.1: BEHAVIORAL TECHNIQUES— ASSESSMENT OF ANXIOUS PATTERNS

Practice assessing an anxious pattern using the Anxious Patterns Record. Have one of you play the role of the "client" by beginning with sharing the triggering event and your physiological response. While the other plays the "therapist," start with assessing additional contextual information about the triggering event (e.g., expected or unexpected) and the physiological response. You can then move on to asking details about any associated thoughts or mental images. Thereafter, identify specific anxiety-related behaviors that were done to prevent, reduce, or escape/avoid the triggering event. Also, try to identify any specific safety behaviors. Finally, conclude with identifying the outcome of the anxious behaviors, possible long-term consequences, and associated thoughts and emotions in response to the outcome. Did you find using the Anxious Patterns Record helpful in organizing your questions and the content of the information provided? Were you able to get a clear picture of the relationship between the trigger event and the physiological response? Were you able to clearly identify an associated automatic thought? If so, what type of cognitive distortion was it? What were the anxiety-related behaviors? How were these behaviors and the outcome reinforcing of the client's thoughts and physiological response?

RELAXATION: PREVENTING AND MANAGING ANXIOUS DISTRESS

The goal of the following relaxation techniques is to help clients either cope with their anxiety "in the moment" or put themselves in a disposition where the potential for future moments of anxiety is reduced. The key mechanism for these techniques is referred to as "reciprocal inhibition," which is when high levels of emotional arousal are reduced when the client experiences a more adaptive (or positive) emotion. By having clients learn how to eventually independently induce a state of relaxation, they produce a level of cognitive and physical calmness that is incompatible with their anxious distress. Eventually, triggering events are no longer associated with negative automatic thoughts, physiological arousal, and avoidance behaviors. However, it is important to note here that for clients with high levels of anxiety, these relaxation techniques will not reduce anxiety to adaptive levels without integrating other cognitive (e.g., modification) and behavioral (e.g., exposure) techniques.

Progressive Muscle Relaxation

Progressive muscle relaxation (PMR) is a commonly used technique to induce adaptive levels of bodily awareness and calmness for anxiously distressed clients.

Tense muscles can be an indicator of stress. Many clients are not fully aware that their muscles get tense when anxious. In fact, some clients are so chronically tense that when they finally relax, what they feel is actually unnatural to them. Tensed muscles can also trigger particular negative automatic thoughts and further increase physiological arousal. PMR helps identify specific muscles and muscle groups and discriminate between feeling tensed and relaxed. This is done by teaching clients to systematically tighten specific muscles for a short period of time and then release the tension and focus on the experience. As the muscle tension is decreased, the physiological feeling of anxiety (and sometimes negative automatic thoughts) is reduced. If desired, a meditational component of calming statements and mental images can also be included. Ultimately, the primary goal here is to increase self-awareness of voluntary control over muscle groups by monitoring tension and telling oneself to relax the muscles.

PMR should first be done in session with the client while you follow a script that systematically works through all of the major muscles. The following are some basic steps for PMR (there can be many variations).

1. Explain Rationale and Method for PMR

You do not have to provide an elaborate explanation for using PMR, but the basics of the relationship between muscle tension and anxiety noted above should be explained. You want to convey that PMR can be a relatively simple but effective means of reducing anxious distress. Also, inform clients what to expect out of this experience based on the noted steps below.

2. Establish Muscle Tension Baseline and Teach Rating

Rating one's own level of muscle tension can be rather subjective. However, by having clients establish their own personal baseline, it will at least give them a "feel" for comparison. Any muscle group can be used, but using a hand is often easiest. Simply ask clients to hold our their hand in a relaxed position and give this a minimum rating of 0. Then, using the same hand, have them tighten it into a fist as hard as they can for 5 to 7 seconds and give this a maximum of 10. Then let them relax their hand and mindfully compare the difference in sensations. This process also helps reinforce for clients that they have voluntary control over the tension they feel in their muscles.

3. Guide Client Through the PMR Process

There are many variations in how one can initiate and proceed through the PMR process. Table 9.3 provides a generic but effective way to work through the key muscle groups. (There are many good-quality PMR scripts that can be found on the internet with a thoughtful search.) It is advised that you read through the script

Table 9.3. Progressive Muscle Relaxation Template

Instructions
Have clients get in a comfortable position and be sure there is minimal to no sound in the room. Also, do your best to make sure that you will not be disturbed. It is generally best to have clients begin relaxing by taking a few deep breaths or use diaphragm breathing. Below are suggested body parts and sequence for muscle groups. Use the following statement as a generic template for each body part: "Clench your hands . . . tighter and even more tighter . . . feel the tension in your hands. . . . Now relax. . . . Notice the difference when relaxed compared to tensed." Be sure to modify your words to avoid sounding monotone and match the body part (e.g., wrinkle your forehead or tighten your upper legs). You can also integrate occasional breathing techniques, relaxing images (resting on a beach), and/or relaxing statements ("let go of the tension") between muscle groups. Each muscle group should be tensed for 5 to 7 seconds and relaxed for 20 to 30 seconds. This process can be repeated or focused on specific areas of interest.

Suggested Body Parts (in Order)
Hands
Forearms
Upper arms
Shoulders
Neck
Forehead
Eyes
Mouth
Chest
Back
Stomach
Buttocks
Upper legs
Lower legs
Feet

nearly word for word (not memorized) in order to keep a good pace and not forget any muscles throughout the process. Clients can do this while lying down at home, but it is generally best done while sitting in a chair in your office. It is generally recommended that each muscle or muscle group is tensed for 5 to 7 seconds and then relaxed for 20 to 30 seconds. It is best to work the muscles top-down or down-up, not randomly throughout the body. The PMR process can be repeated or focus on specific areas of interest.

4. Integrate Breathing and Meditation Components

In order to help pace the PMR process, having clients take a few deep breaths at the start and then occasionally between muscle groups can help reach a more relaxed and self-aware state. In place of basic deep breaths, you can use diaphragmatic breathing (discussed next). Some clients may also find it helpful to include relaxing mental images (e.g., lying in bed, resting on a beach, or walking in a forest) and/or statements (e.g., "let go of the tension," "calm and rested," "relax and smooth out the muscles," or "let the tension dissolve away"). This can help clients distract themselves from anxious or wandering thoughts while also achieving a deeper, relaxed state.

5. Assign for Homework

This technique may require much practice before it reaches it full effectiveness. Also, you will want your clients to eventually use this technique independently. The use of an audio recording (your voice, their own voices, or those of a family or friend) is usually the most effective approach when done alone.

ACTIVITY 9.2: BEHAVIORAL TECHNIQUE— RELAXATION—PROGRESSIVE MUSCLE RELAXATION

Practice PMR with a peer. Take turns using a script to work through all of the muscle groups. Try to integrate breathing and meditation components as well. Be sure that you maintain good pacing (i.e., each muscle or muscle group is tensed for 5 to 7 seconds and then relaxed for 20 to 30 seconds) and use good descriptive terms for tightening each muscle part. If you use an audio recording of your own voice, you can also practice this technique independently. Even when using a script, what makes this technique challenging to facilitate? What are some variations to using PMR? Did integrating breathing or meditation components enhance the technique's effectiveness? What was the experience like using this technique on yourself?

Diaphragm Breathing

Diaphragm breathing (or breathing retraining) used to be a common technique for clients experiencing panic attacks because they often breathe too quickly, also known as hyperventilation. More recent research has shown mixed results for the effectiveness of breathing techniques for panic disorder (i.e., beneficial for some clients but can sometimes be used as an avoidance or safety behavior). Thus, some suggest that it is no longer a necessary technique for panic disorder (Craske & Barlow, 2014). However, this technique can also be used for other clients who have moments of anxious thoughts and/or irregular breathing. Chronic stress and rapid/shallow breathing associated with hyperventilation can restrict the range of movement while breathing through the chest, also known as chest breathing. Such breathing is inefficient because less oxygen gets to the blood. Ironically, more oxygen than needed is being breathed in, decreasing levels of carbon dioxide. Thus, blood vessels constrict more, and less oxygen gets to the brain and body. This experience can lead to other physiological symptoms, such as shortness of breath, light-headedness, dizziness, rapid heartbeat, and chest tightness/pain. Although these symptoms are not deadly (except in rare cases for those with a preexisting heart condition, such as heart disease), they can feel life threatening to many clients. In fact, chest breathing can trigger particular negative automatic thoughts (e.g., "I'm losing control." "I'm going to have a heart attack."), further increasing physiological arousal. The diaphragm is a large muscle located between the chest and the abdomen. Breathing through the diaphragm, or stomach, regulates breathing by being slower and deeper. Diaphragm breathing helps clients cope with thoughts of fear/anxiety in the moment, resulting in more stable breathing and less distress. If desired, a meditational component of calming statements and mental images can also be included. Ultimately, the primary goal here is to increase self-awareness of voluntary control over breathing and associated thoughts and emotions.

Diaphragm breathing should first be done in session with you physically demonstrating the technique to the client. Although the following steps may seem relatively easy, clients usually need a lot of practice to master this technique.

1. Explain Rationale and Method for Diaphragm Breathing

Providing at least some information about chest breathing/hyperventilating and its relationship to anxiety noted above can be very helpful for clients. Learning this skill will help them cope with future fearful and anxious thoughts. This technique will probably seem odd to some clients and initially cause feelings of breathlessness; thus, having some rationale should increase motivation. Also, inform clients what to expect out of this experience based on the noted steps below.

2. Guide Client Through the Diaphragm Breathing Process

There are a few variations in how to demonstrate diaphragm breathing, but the general approach to reduce the rate of breathing remains consistent. You will first demonstrate the technique and then eventually have your clients join you. Clients can do this while lying down at home, but it is generally best done while sitting in a chair in your office. It is important to follow each of the steps in the appropriate sequence while monitoring your clients once you ask them to demonstrate the skill with you and eventually by themselves. It is best to give them live feedback to correct any errors before having them do it alone for homework. The initial focus should be on making sure they are able to learn how to breathe through their stomach instead of their chest. For some clients, this will come naturally; others will initially struggle because it may seem like a brand-new way of breathing. You can begin your demonstration by putting one hand on your chest and the other on your stomach. Only the hand on your stomach should move, while the hand on your chest should have minimal movement. The next step focuses on the actual process of breathing by making sure that normal amounts of air are taken in. It does not matter whether you breathe through your nose or mouth. However, many clients find it helpful to inhale through their nose and exhale through their mouth. This is also helpful for the next component: mediation. Once clients have mastered these breathing steps, you can introduce a more explicit approach in reducing their rate of breathing. This particular step might not be introduced until future sessions. Simply have clients do the following: count (1 second), inhale (2 seconds), think of a calming word (1 second), and exhale (2 seconds). This will result in a breathing rate of 6 seconds per breath and 10 breaths per minute. The pace does not have to be perfect, as the focus is on assuring that clients are able to slow down their breathing while still using their diaphragm.

3. Integrate Meditation Components

A key supplemental technique is to have clients count every time they inhale and think of a single calming word (e.g., "relax," "release," or "peace") when they breathe out. While practicing in session, have clients count up to at least 10. The goal here is for clients to focus on their breathing and their calming words. This can be very challenging for some clients, as they will experience thoughts entering their minds. However, you can remind them that this is natural and the primary purpose of the meditative component is to filter away distracting thoughts. Remind them to not think much about the thoughts when they occur and let them pass through their minds and eventually return their attention to their breathing.

4. Assign for Homework

Because this technique takes time to get used to and can cause more distress if not implemented properly, it should be practiced at least twice a day for at least 10 minutes in a relaxing environment. It is important to emphasize to clients that they are not to use this technique during anxious/fearful situations until you tell them they are ready. If this technique is not fully developed, it can result in heightened anxiety if not used in relaxing environments.

The following is a vignette from Video Case Example PDA-7 demonstrating diaphragm breathing. Following the vignette are discussion questions and an activity.

VIDEO VIGNETTE 9.2

PDA-7: Behavioral Techniques—Relaxation—Diaphragm Breathing

Therapist: What we're going to do now is work on some relaxation techniques, and I think the first one, based upon your symptoms, is to start working on some breathing techniques. It's pretty standard for panic attacks. Many people when they have panic attacks, they overbreathe, really fast. And you've probably noticed that with yourself. In fact, a little bit of research shows that over 40% of people with panic attack or panic disorder overbreathe. I think we've already used this word a little bit, hyperventilating. . . . So, with overbreathing and panic there are two components that are going on here: initially when we start overbreathing the initial feelings start to frighten us, and then it starts to initiate some of these other panic symptoms. I noticed with you as well the thoughts then start up. But one of the first symptoms you tend to mention is the breathing and the tightness of chest. Does that sound correct to you?

Client: Yes, it does.

Therapist: . . . The one I want to focus on today is called diaphragm breathing. We already talked a little bit about when we start to hyperventilate; it's a little too much breathing in the chest and not enough in the tummy or the diaphragm muscle. What we want to do is eventually start learning to make sure that when we're taking in these breaths we're feeling it more in our diaphragm and less in our chest. The way it usually is done, and if you want you can follow me along, you can put one of your hands on your chest, right around your breastbone, and the other hand a little bit above the belly button. Without even thinking about anything else just take a deep breath in—you can use your nose or your mouth—and breathe out <both inhale and exhale>. I just noticed there that both your chest and your stomach came out a little bit there. That's okay because it's your first shot at it. The reason why we put our hands on the chest and tummy is we want this upper part here, our chest, to feel as little movement as possible. It might move a little bit, that's okay because it's impossible to have no movement, but we want to feel it mostly through our tummy. So, try again, inhale . . . and exhale <both inhale and exhale>. That's a little bit better. Try it again <both inhale and exhale>. Maybe to start off, try to purposely push your tummy out. It may feel a little unnatural, but kind of see what it feels like. So I'm going to take a breath in and then breathe out <both inhale and exhale>. There you go, keep doing it, you're doing a good job.

Client: Good.

Therapist: In a moment we'll practice counting. I'll be the one that counts out loud and you'll say it to yourself in your head. I'll kind of count for you to start. Generally speaking we want to continue up to six and do it 10 times. You'll say it to yourself, count one, then inhale for two, relax for two, and then exhale for one. What I want you to do while you're doing this is to focus as much as you can on your breathing and the words. That's kind of the purpose of meditation. . . . You want to remember that you don't have to be perfect. And anytime anybody initially tries to do a meditation technique they have thoughts that come in. It's like me saying don't think of a purple elephant, now you're going to think of a purple elephant, right? What we want to do here is if we have these thoughts that come in our mind when we're doing this—that's okay—just remember to let it flow through. If we fight it, it's going to be harder. The important thing is to not give up because what we're going to do later on is use this breathing technique when you're starting to feel very anxious.

Client: Okay, sounds good.

Therapist: You did a really good job. It's something that feels really unnatural at first. I'm guessing the reason why it was a little more challenging for you is because you really are generally a chest breather. What we're trying to do is to change the way of doing something that comes natural. With all of these panic attacks and hyperventilation, it's almost become your baseline to breathe heavily through your chest. So, we're trying to switch that up through your tummy. What I want you to do is to practice this at least twice a day for 10 minutes, two separate times. Now here's the key thing, when you practice this, you really want to make sure you're in a relaxing, quiet setting where you've got a little bit of privacy and fewer distractions. You're not ready yet to try this out when it's a really anxious situation. You first need to master this technique. I'll let you know when I think you're ready to then try this breathing technique in a real anxious situation. Any other questions on this technique?

Client: No, I think I understand.

Discussion Questions 9.2

- What makes it challenging to demonstrate a technique while also giving instructions and observing the client's actions?
- What are some behavioral indictors that the client has a good understanding of diagrammatic breathing?
- What are other possible meditation components that could be included besides counting?

ACTIVITY 9.3: BEHAVIORAL TECHNIQUES— RELAXATION—DIAPHRAGM BREATHING

Practice diaphragmatic breathing with a peer. Take turns following the instructions in step 2. This can be done lying down or sitting in a chair. First, focus on breathing through your stomach instead of your chest. Put one hand on your chest and the other on your stomach. While breathing, inhale through your nose and exhale through your mouth (the preferred method for most people). When you are ready, practice counting: count (1 second), inhale (2 seconds), think of a calming word (1 second), and exhale (2 seconds). Try to do about 10 breaths per minute. If desired, you can also try meditation using a single calming word (e.g., "relax," "release," or "peace"). What makes this technique challenging to facilitate? What parts of this technique may be challenging for clients to learn? Did integrating the meditation component enhance the technique's effectiveness? What was the experience like using this technique on yourself?

Visualization

Visualization is a meditative technique that is an effective way to relax the mind and body by picturing a relaxing scene (e.g., beach, meadow, or forest). (Imaginal exposure for mentally practicing for anxious events is discussed later.) This can include re-creating a mental sensory experience that includes not only sight but also sound, smell, touch, and taste. The primary goal for this technique is to have clients learn how to relax their minds and bodies in a grounded way. Sometimes, it is helpful to at least temporarily step outside of the present moment of anxiety. Visualization can have the opposite effect of the sympathetic nervous system (i.e., fight-or-flight) by producing a relaxed state and reducing stress. The relatively temporary moment of a relaxed state of mind can eventually be learned and reinforced to be a new baseline of adaptive functioning. This technique is also helpful in enhancing self-awareness of body sensations and breathing. It is important to note here that this technique is less about distraction and more about focusing on something else that is more pleasant/calming. The more detailed the script, including multiple senses, the more effective. Visualization is a technique that is generally accepted by clients because most find it naturally relaxing and nonthreatening.

The process for implementing this technique is rather simple compared to PMR and diaphragm breathing. Also, there is no true standardized approach, as it can vary greatly depending on the visualization scenario you use. Examples of common visualization scenarios include lying in bed, resting on a beach, watching/listening to ocean waves, walking through a forest or meadow, looking at candlelight, looking at colors in the rainbow, floating on a cloud, looking up at the stars in the night sky, and being an overall peaceful place. (There are many good-quality visualization scripts that can be found on the internet with a thoughtful search.) Before initiating a script, be sure that your clients are in a relaxed position with their eyes closed. You can also suggest that they take a few deep breaths (or use diaphragm breathing) and/or relax particular muscles (or use PMR) at the beginning to initiate a relaxed state. Throughout the process, including the conclusion of the visualization, you can gently remind clients how relaxed they feel, including particular body sensations and/or thoughts that are relevant to each client. Remember to also talk in calm tones as much as you possibly can. This is a good activity for clients to practice on their own outside of session. They may have to audio record their own preferred script because reading the script to themselves is not effective. Also remind them to practice in an environment in which they feel comfortable and that is private.

MODIFYING ANXIOUS THOUGHTS

Although the focus of this chapter is on behavioral techniques, there are particular cognitive distortions that tend to be most prevalent with anxious clients: catastrophizing, magnification (of risk), and minimization (of own skills to cope). It is sometimes appropriate to identify and initiate modification techniques before the forthcoming exposure-based techniques. For example, while engaged in behavioral exposure techniques, it might be necessary to refer clients back to their modified cognitive distortions while also actively assessing the validity of their thoughts. Thus, such modification techniques as decatastrophizing have an important role in breaking the negative reinforcement pattern between thoughts, physiological sensations, and behaviors by buffering previously learning relaxation techniques and enhancing exposure-based techniques. More specifically, reducing the impact of particular negative automatic thoughts can reduce physiological arousal and reinforce more adaptive behaviors (e.g., not avoiding) in response to anxiety. However, it is important to note that increasing evidence indicates that modifying negative automatic thoughts (or relaxation coping skills) does not yield any additional benefit to exposure alone for panic disorder and agoraphobia (Norton & Price, 2007). In fact, following the inhibitory retrieval model of extinction, some studies have shown that initial fear reduction (e.g., through modification of negative automatic thoughts) may become a safety behavior for some clients with panic disorder (Craske, Liao, Brown, & Vervliet, 2012; Craske, Treanor, Conway, Zbozinek, & Vervliet, 2014). Thus, it important to consider your clients' diagnosis and presenting distress to determine if modifying their anxious thoughts is necessary if exposure techniques are also being considered.

Decatastrophizing was addressed in Chapter 7. The focus here is to highlight these modification techniques within the context of anxious distress. You will notice that decatastrophizing not only addresses catastrophic thinking but also can be modified to include minimizing perceived risk and maximizing skills to cope. The following sections identify and explain three primary goals for using the decatastrophizing technique for anxious clients.

1. Determine a More Realistic Scenario/Outcome of the Feared Event

The purpose here is to "show" your clients that there are other possible scenarios/outcomes for their feared event. Simply ask them what is the worst, best, and most realistic thing that could happen ("What is the worst thing that could happen? What is the best thing that could happen? What is the most realistic thing that could happen?"). Use Table 7.8 (Decatastrophizing Worksheet) to write down each of the scenarios. Asking about the worst that could happen can give you information about your clients' tendency to magnify the risk. Asking about the best and most realistic provides your clients with the opportunity to consider alternative outcomes that are naturally less threatening.

2. Assess the Probability of Different Outcomes

You next want to compare the perceived chances of each scenario actually happening. Follow up with the client assessing the probability (0%–100%) that a scenario will actually happen ("What are the chances of the worst-case scenario happening? What are the chances of the best-case scenario happening? What are the chances of the most realistic scenario happening?"). If appropriate, for the worst-case scenario you can also ask if it has ever happened before. At this point, most clients will naturally recognize that there is a "better chance" that the realistic scenario will occur over the worst-case scenario. Clients will hopefully recognize that there is a continuum between worst-case and best-case scenarios. In other words, although there may be a slight chance that something very bad or very good may happen, there is a much better chance that something in between will happen. (This can be helpful for clients who also have dichotomous thinking patterns.)

3. Develop a Coping Plan for the Worst-Case Scenario

At this point, your clients should at least be a little less confident that the worst-case scenario will happen. However, clients may still be thinking, "But what if the worst scenario occurs?" You ultimately want your clients to test this for themselves through a behavioral experiment. However, it can also be reassuring for them to have a coping plan ready "just in case." You can develop a plan that can both reduce the chances of the worst-case scenario happening and outline what can be done if it does occur. Asking what has not worked and what has worked in the past is usually a good start. You can also ask if there is anything new or different that might be worth trying. Finally, it is important to also review any possible barriers to coping, and this may involve some problem solving. If you think it can be helpful, you can ask your clients to reassess the probability of the worst-case scenario after they have developed a coping plan.

The following is a vignette from Video Case Example PDA-9 demonstrating modifying anxious thoughts. Following the vignette are discussion questions and an activity.

VIDEO VIGNETTE 9.3

PDA-9: Behavioral Techniques—Modifying Anxious Thoughts

Therapist: What I want to do is decatastrophize your thoughts about failing your exam. . . . The first question I want to ask you: what is the worst thing that could happen? You walk in, you try to study, you take that exam, you get it back the next week and there it is in front of you, you failed it.

Client: I fail the class, and if I fail the class then I'm going to be out of the program. If I fail the program, I'm not going to get a job.

Therapist: I'm writing down fail class, fail program, and something about your job and your promotion. You see how they kind of self-perpetuate there? It starts off with focusing on failing the class and then it's you're going to fail the whole program and then you're not going to get that job.

Client: But I really might fail the whole program if I'm failing a class.

Therapist: Let's see how true that probably is. I won't even dispute that yet. We just did if you fail your exam, the worst-case scenario, and it is possible. I won't argue that it could definitely happen, but let's see how other scenarios work out. Now, what is the best thing that could happen when you go in and take that exam? Is there a different outcome besides failing?

Client: Passing—I could pass.

Therapist: What would be the best scenario?
Client: I get an A-plus.
Therapist: To be fair, in the past have you ever gotten A's or A-pluses on past exams?
Client: Yeah.
Therapist: So, it technically could happen. You're not thinking this one is going to happen, but it could happen.
Client: Yeah, this class is kind of hard though.
Therapist: Okay, and so what would be the most realistic?
Client: I'll pass.
Therapist: And what would be a passing grade for you?
Client: Probably a B-minus just so I can get by.
Therapist: Maybe a B-minus, maybe a B, somewhere in the B range, that's fine. We've got our worst case, our best case, and realistic. Let's go now and do probability or chance for each scenario. Just focusing right now on the class part, what's the chance that if you fail this exam that the worst-case scenario of failing the class would happen?
Client: Well, I guess when you put it like that it's probably more like 15% to 20%.
Therapist: Has this ever happened before? Have you ever failed a class before?
Client: No.
Therapist: I think that's fair to put down 15% to 20%, but at the same time, based on past evidence, you've never failed a class before. And I know right now what you're going through is a little bit different than the past. We've also talked in the past how you've been anxious as well, but you still end up doing better than what sometimes you think you would. So, I think that's fair to say 15% to 20%. What's your chances of getting an A in the class right now?
Client: I would probably say closer to 5% or 10%.
Therapist: So, not quite the same as worst case as you're still leaning more toward failing than getting an A. That's okay. The realistic one, especially based on past experience passing exams, what do you think are the chances of that?
Client: I think that's probably most realistic, so I would say 40% to 50%.
Therapist: Okay, that's good. So maybe at least almost a 50% chance of passing? That feels a little bit better than a 15% chance of failing as well. . . . We've got a box here on how to cope. Sometimes I'll ask clients questions like what has or hasn't worked before, but you've never failed an exam before so that may be hard to think about. Let's say you do fail a class, how could you possibly cope with it?
Client: I think the first thing I would do is talk to my professor. I also think that something that would have been within my control is maybe study more in advance and have better time management skills.

Discussion Questions 9.3

- Why is it generally most effective to begin with the worst-case scenario and end with the most realistic scenario?
- How could the information from this modification technique (and the process itself) be helpful for future exposure techniques?
- What other realistic possible coping options could the client utilize if the worst-case scenario did occur?
- Considering the client's response to this technique, are other techniques warranted to modify her catastrophic thought?

ACTIVITY 9.4: BEHAVIORAL TECHNIQUES— MODIFYING ANXIOUS THOUGHTS

Practice assessing modifying anxious thoughts using the Decatastrophizing Worksheet. Have one of you play the role of the "client" by beginning with a catastrophic thought that is anxiety related. While the other plays the "therapist," start with clarifying the negative automatic thought and then move on to asking about the worst-case scenario. Thereafter, move on to the best-case scenario and then the most realistic scenario. Then ask for the probability of each scenario and compare the percentages. At this point, you can ask if the client has an alternative thought in response to modifying the initial negative automatic thought. Finally, conclude with discussing coping options for the worst-case scenario, including previous ineffective and effective strategies and potential obstacles to coping. Was it helpful starting with the worst-case scenario and ending with the most realistic scenario? Did assessing the probability for each scenario provide supportive "data" to help modify the negative automatic thought? In other words, was it convincing to compare probability percentages? Did this technique provide enough "convincing" information to develop an alternative thought? How was developing coping strategies for the worst-case scenario helpful for relieving client distress?

EXPOSURE: CONFRONTING ANXIETY AND FEAR

Once clients have learned some relaxation techniques and modified any related negative automatic thoughts (if determined to be therapeutically appropriate), they are ready to begin exposing themselves to the situations that cause them anxiety and fear. For other clients, this may be their first anxiety-reducing intervention. Remember, the reason that there is so much anxiety for particular situations is because their avoidance behaviors have been reinforced (i.e., short-term relief) over time. Clients will initially experience increased anxiety (approaching the exposure) increased fear (during the exposure) and associated physiological arousal when exposed to their avoided situation. However, the fear associated with the sympathetic system (i.e., fight-or-flight) does not last forever (typically 20 to 30 minutes). When nothing harmful or threatening occurs after repeated exposures, clients learn how to adapt to and cope with the situation. Thus, the forthcoming exposure techniques are designed to stop the reinforcing pattern of avoidance by clients ultimately confronting their feared situations. Concurrently, if appropriate, they will apply their newly learned relaxation and cognitive techniques discussed earlier. Clients will first develop a hierarchy of feared situations and then engage in graded exposure, including imaginal and in vivo.

Developing a Hierarchy of Feared Situations for Graded Exposure

Developing a hierarchy for graded exposure entails identifying multiple situations that clients find fearful, providing a rating of expected anxiety for these situations, and then developing a list from least fearful to most fearful. This hierarchy of feared situations will then be followed in sequence for imaginal and in vivo exposure. It is best to focus on situations that have a related theme of anxiety. In other words, if clients have two or more different manifestations of anxiety (e.g., social phobia and fear of driving), it is best to do two separate hierarchies. This process is truly collaborative because you want your clients to be in control of identifying their feared situations, but you will still need to guide them in selecting feared situations that are therapeutically appropriate and practical. The following are the key steps in developing a hierarchy of feared situations for graded exposure.

1. Rational for Hierarchy of Feared Situations

Like any CBT technique, you should provide your clients with a clear rationale for why you want them to identify multiple fearful situations. At this point in therapy, clients will probably already have a good idea about the direction of therapy. Nevertheless, you should still be clear that this hierarchy will build off their relaxation and cognitive techniques and culminate in direct exposure of some of their most feared situations.

2. Identify Fearful Situations

You and your client probably already have a good idea of what situations are fearful to your client. Let your clients take the lead in developing their initial identification of feared situations as much as possible. There is no specific number of feared situations to identify but encourage your client to identify as many as possible. You will want to casually guide them in making sure they identify a wide range of fearful situations (i.e., not mostly very fearful or mostly mildly fearful). Once your clients have finished identifying their feared situations, you can prompt them on whether

Table 9.4. Hierarchy of Feared Situations Goals: Poor Versus Better

Poor Goals	Better Goals
Enjoy flying again	Drive to the airport and park in the garage
Stop being fearful of social activities	Spend at least 30 minutes at a social activity with familiar people before leaving
No longer be afraid of snakes	Go to the local pet store and walk down the middle of the snake aisle
Feel more comfortable in crowded places	Go to the mall early on a weekday morning and walk around for at least 15 minutes
Be relaxed when giving presentations	Practice a presentation of a well-known topic in front of a few friends in a classroom

they can think of any more, including any suggestions you may have based on past therapy sessions. At this point, you may have to combine feared situations into one if they are very similar (e.g., taking a walk at two separate but similar parks). Another very important task is to reword each feared situation like a treatment goal (i.e., specific, concrete, and measurable) when you are ready to implement your exposure technique. Table 9.4 provides some examples of poorly worded feared situations and its appropriately worded alternative. Such wording will make it clear how to move through each step of the hierarchy and assess progress in exposure techniques.

3. Rate Degree of Expected Anxiety for Each Feared Situation

Once each fearful situation has been identified and worded appropriately, ask your clients to rate how much anxiety they expect to experience using a 0–10 scale, with 0 being no anxiety and 10 being the highest level of anxiety. The following are some contextual conditions for you to suggest that clients consider when they report their anticipated level of anxiety: distance from home, ease of escaping, time of day, number of people, and accompanied or alone. The ratings for each feared situation will be used to develop the actual order of the hierarchy in step 5. The ratings will also serve the purpose of measuring progress by comparing pre- and post-scores during the exposure activities. A significant reduction in anxiety for a feared situation is typically a primary indictor to move on to the next feared situation.

4. Identify Unhelpful Coping Strategies

This can actually be done right before or after developing the hierarchy for exposure (next step), but the point here is to identify coping strategies that clients use that would impede the successful progress of the exposure activities. For example, some clients have superstitious objects, signals, and behaviors that they rely on to "get through" (i.e., reduces fear) particular anxiety-provoking situations. Such "safety behaviors" need to be identified in advance because they must be avoided (or at least eventually phased out) during the exposure activities (Blakey & Abramowitz, 2016).

If not, clients will not truly learn how to confront their fears independently and thus break the negatively reinforced behavior pattern. Clients will eventually need to learn that safety behaviors do not prevent danger because there is no true danger present in the first place. However, clients will come to realize this only when they engage in the exposure techniques without their safety behaviors. To help clients identify such safety behaviors, ask them what they never leave home without. You can also ask them what things or people make them feel less anxious when they are approaching or in a fearful situation.

5. Develop the Hierarchy for Exposure

Using the ratings from step 3, simply rank them from lowest to highest. Be sure that there is a full range of expected anxiety from very low (1–3) to very high (8–10). You want to avoid having steps in one range (i.e., only steps with low ratings or high ratings) in order to avoid making the exposure process "too easy" or "too difficult." Exposure activities that are too easy will not be strong enough physiologically to break the avoidance pattern. Activities that are too difficult will most likely not be successful, resulting in making the avoidance pattern even stronger, increasing distress and reducing motivation. If you find that many of the steps fall into one of the extremes, you will have to work with your clients to think of additional feared situations and/or consider breaking down existing steps into multiple steps. If necessary, you can integrate safety behaviors from the previous step. One option is to have clients face their feared situation with the safety behavior and then again without the safety behavior. The other option is to have clients face their feared situation without the safety behavior from the start. Table 9.5 can be used for developing a hierarchy for exposure. Note that there is space for rating anxiety before and after the exposure and for indicating any possible safety behaviors. As you develop a hierarchy of feared situations for graded exposure, remember that the effectiveness of your exposure is only as good as your hierarchy.

Imaginal Exposure

As the technique is named, imaginal exposure guides clients through a step in the hierarchy to immerse themselves in a particular event and imagine how they might react to their feared situation. In vivo exposure (discussed next) is generally ideal, but imaginal exposure can be used when in vivo exposure is not possible or practical, such as a particular traumatic experience that is not possible to reencounter or a specific phobia that is not readily accessible. (Note that with the advancement of technology, virtual reality therapy can sometimes be an option. See Chapter 10.) In other cases, imaginal exposure can be especially helpful when there is cognitive avoidance (i.e., thought exposure). There may also be times when your clients are not ready for in vivo exposure because it may be too intense too fast. Thus, the intervention of imaginal exposure itself can be used as a process to the eventual use of

Table 9.5. Hierarchy of Feared Situations for Graded Exposure

Feared Situation	Pre-Anxiety (0–10) and Ranking		Safety Behaviors to Avoid	Post-Anxiety (0–10) With Safety Behavior	Post-Anxiety (0–10) Without Safety Behavior

in vivo exposure. Finally, the more willing and able you are to do therapy "outside the office," the less you will need to rely on imaginal exposure.

Guiding clients through imaginal exposure uses a similar approach to guided imagery discussed in Chapter 7. Begin by providing your clients with an explanation as to why you will be beginning with imaginal exposure instead of in vivo exposure (e.g., not possible for this particular feared event or will eventually work toward in vivo exposure). You should begin with their lowest-feared situation for imaginal exposure (other situations may be used for in vivo) and then work your way up to higher-rated feared situations. Then tell your clients that you will verbally describe the feared event while also asking them questions to immerse them in the scenario. As a reminder, some questions to ask include these: Where are you? What do you see (hear, smell, or feel)? What are you doing (be detailed)? What are you feeling? What are you thinking? Who else is with you (describe)? Your goal is to give as many cues as possible to help the client mentally experience the scenario as vividly as possible. The more detailed the imagery, the better the chance for effectiveness. While guiding clients through this process, it is important to occasionally "check in" on their anxiety and physiological arousal by asking for ratings and any additional thoughts. This is also a good time to use Socratic techniques (e.g., decatastrophizing) to work through their thoughts. Additionally, if appropriate, psychoeducation and previously taught relaxation techniques and coping skills can be practiced. You may have to repeat imaginal exposure until their anxiety is sufficiently reduced. Whenever possible, it is best to move on to in vivo exposure unless the scenario is not appropriate. Even then, you can still attempt in vivo exposure for themes related to the original scenario. (You can also use some of the components of Sample Form 9.1, discussed next for in vivo exposure.)

In Vivo Exposure

In vivo exposure is a technique that has clients directly confront their feared stimulus. Whenever possible and therapeutically appropriate, in vivo exposure should be the primary choice for exposure. The most effective way to learn is through direct experience. As noted earlier, sometimes in vivo exposure is the next step following successful progress with imaginal exposure. Some types of in vivo exposure can be completed "inside the office" or surrounding area, but in many cases you will have to go "outside the office. The following are the key steps for implementing in vivo exposure.

1. Rationale for Using In Vivo Exposure

Again, like all previous techniques, begin by reminding your clients why they will be confronting some of their most feared situations. This information will mostly be a review because you have already completed developing a graded hierarchy of feared situations and you may have already done some imaginal exposure. Also, reassure them that when they begin the exposure, they may experience high levels of physiological arousal and associated catastrophic thoughts, which is normal and to be expected. The difference this time is that they now understand how their anxiety works, they have learned effective relaxation and coping skills, and they have been working on modifying their cognitive distortions. Also, at least to start, you will be there to provide emotional and therapeutic support. Your observations and feedback will be very important for your clients when you phase yourself out and they begin doing in vivo exposure between sessions as homework.

2. Implement In Vivo Exposure for the Next Situation on the Hierarchy

Sample Form 9.1 is a good resource for your clients to use once they are ready to begin exposure to their feared situations. You should start with your clients' lowest-rated feared situations and work your way up to higher-rated feared situations. If you have not done so already, remember to reword the feared situations as an exposure goal (i.e., specific, concrete, and measurable). Clients should identify with whom they completed the exposure (if anyone) and any specific safety behaviors that must be avoided. Also, it is important that clients assess their anxiety before and after the exposure. If you are present, you can also assess their anxiety in the moment. Clients should also share any thoughts they may have before and after the exposure (and in the moment if appropriate). You can also integrate any negative automatic thoughts as a behavioral experiment by asking clients to make a prediction about how threatening it will be, including ratings of expected anxiety. Thereafter, ask them to predict how well they will respond with the exposure considering their recently learned relaxation and coping skills. If necessary, clients can also identify any potential obstacles and coping skills in advance related to the specific feared situation.

SAMPLE FORM 9.1

Exposure Tracking Form

Feared Situation:

Hierarchy Ranking:

Exposure Goal:

Exposure Completed With (e.g., therapist, family, friend, alone):

Safety Behaviors to Avoid:

Pre-Anxiety (0–10):
Pre-Thoughts:

What is your prediction for the outcome of this exposure?

Potential Problems/Obstacles (e.g., safety behaviors, automatic thoughts, maladaptive behaviors, external factors)

1.

    Relaxation and coping skills:

2.

    Relaxation and coping skills:

3.

    Relaxation and coping skills:

Anxiety "in the moment" (0–10): _____
Thoughts "in the moment":

What was the outcome of this exposure? (e.g., effectiveness, role of others present, safety behaviors)

Post-Anxiety (0–10): _____
Post-Thoughts:

Thoughts and feelings to repeat exposure or move on to next feared situation on the hierarchy:

Depending on your clients' needs and type of feared situation, you can start off with being present for the exposure and then have them practice it alone. However, it is generally best for you to initially accompany the client during in vivo exposure for the following reasons: (a) to encourage and motivate clients to confront their fears (i.e., emotional support), (b) to provide psychoeducation, (c) to model and remind clients of their relaxation and coping techniques, (d) to assess physiological arousal and level of anxiety in the moment, (e) to identify and modify catastrophic thoughts, and (f) to provide feedback based on "live" observation. You will have to use your clinical judgment over time for when you will need to phase out your role and have clients do their exposure exercises on their own. Your presence will most likely make the feared situation feel safer, and this is okay to start. However, over time, if you are present too often, you may end up being a safety behavior just like their own family or friends and/or a superstitious object or behavior.

3. Assess Completed In Vivo Exposure

Before moving forward to the next step on the hierarchy, you must review the most recent step completed. This will be done by processing what you both observed/experienced and/or reviewing your clients' Exposure Tracking Form, especially if it was done between sessions alone as a homework assignment. (Note: clients' video recording of their own exposure experience can also provide much information without the concern of your being a safety behavior. See Chapter 10.) This review should include their prior predictions and the actual experience of the outcome. You should also assess their anxiety and thoughts after the exposure. Your ultimate goal is for your clients to significantly reduce their anxiety to at least 0–3 (depending on initial fear). The information gained from this review can provide insight into making necessary modifications if the experience did not go as planned and can reinforce the progress clients are making. You may or may not have to repeat the exposure, including consideration if others are still present and steps to remove or phase out safety behaviors. Sometimes, you will need to need to review relaxation and coping skills and/or modify any catastrophic thoughts. Other times, you may have to identify unanticipated obstacles and problem solve for future exposures. You will know that clients are truly making progress (i.e., low ratings of anxiety and no avoidance behaviors) when they are successfully completing multiple exposures outside of session unaccompanied and with no safety behaviors. Nevertheless, you will have to pace how fast you move through the hierarchy of feared situations based on the needs of your client, including diagnoses, initial baseline anxiety, responsiveness to exposure in general, strengths, and motivation. Overall, you want to make sure you "push" your clients enough so that they are challenged and achieve success but not pushed too much where challenges feel like frustration and failure.

The following is a vignette from Video Case Example PDA-11 demonstrating in vivo exposure. Following the vignette are discussion questions and an activity. (Note: See Video Vignette 4.6 (PDA-10) for another example of processing an in vivo exposure.)

VIDEO VIGNETTE 9.4

PDA-11: Behavioral Techniques—In Vivo Exposure

Therapist: Alright here we are! We are at the grocery store—one of the top items on your hierarchy but with the way things have been going, when we met in the office, it seems like you're ready to give it a shot.

Client: Yeah.

Therapist: I can tell you're a little bit anxious. I'll soon assess how you're feeling and then we're going to walk into the grocery store. Then, we will walk around in a few spots that are open initially, maybe like the produce section. I'll keep my distance a little bit, but one thing to remember is I will be there to coach you with your thoughts and remind you of your relaxation techniques. Then, depending on how things are going, we'll choose one of those aisles that can get a little bit busy and we'll walk through it and see how it goes from there. I'm not going to say too much more just other than I'll be there to help assess your anxiety, work on some of your thoughts, and remind you of some of the relaxation techniques. I think you're ready, but I want to see how you're feeling right now—how would you rate your anxiety from 0 to 10?

Client: Um. I would say I am feeling closer to a 6 or 7 right now.

Therapist: So 6 or 7?

Client: Yeah.

Therapist: What's going through your mind now?

Client: I am really scared about how many people are going to be in the grocery store around us and I'm scared of having a panic attack.

Therapist: Okay. I can tell it's a busy parking lot here so it might be busy today. Let's do a prediction then. How do you predict this will go?

Client: Well, I think I will be okay getting the cart. I think I will be okay. I am more nervous about what's going to happen when I go down an aisle with other people and how I'm going to feel in that moment. If there are too many people, I think I'm just going to have to get out and leave.

Therapist: Okay. So, you feel good walking in, making your way with a cart to the produce section, but if you go down an aisle that's maybe a little too busy—right now—your current prediction is "I might start feeling some of those panic symptoms and will have to get outta here."

Client: Yeah.

Therapist: Okay. I respect that. I'm not even going to work too much on modifying that thought. As you know, we've had similar exposure situations that have gone relatively well. I know this is a big one. What I want to do is, if you're ready to give it a shot, is walk to the grocery store and get a cart. I'll help you out if you need me and we'll see how things go from there. Does that sound good?

Client: Okay. Let's go.

Therapist: Let's do this.

Client: Okay.

_____

Therapist: Okay so you got a few things that you wanted, right?

Client: Yeah.

Therapist: I noticed a little bit of anxiety so I just wanted to quickly check in. We're still in the produce, doing okay, but I don't want to make any assumptions and see how you're doing.

Client: Um. I am feeling really anxious right now. And I think it's closer to an 8 right now.

Therapist: Okay. You say 8, but so far you seem to be keeping it together so . . .

Client: Yeah . . . there's a lot of people in here.

Therapist: Yeah. The was a rush of people just came in here. What would you say your thoughts are right now?

Client: Um. I'm starting to feel light-headed.

Therapist: Okay, so that's how you're feeling. What else are you feeling?

Client: Um. I'm feeling anxious. My hands are getting clammy right now.

Therapist: Have you noticed your heart rate change at all?

Client: Yeah, it's increasing . . . <nervous laughter>

Therapist: Because I noticed you're breathing faster and if you can—any quick thoughts that you have?

Client: I'm just scared of having a panic attack right here.

Therapist: What I want to do now is just remind you of what we talked about— some of the coping skills because you're doing a good job. I think this could be a point where maybe just taking the time to pause a little bit. If you can, just take some time to slow down those thoughts and breath- ing a little bit on your own.

Client: Okay. <deep breathing>

Therapist: That's good.

Client: Okay.

Therapist: And as you're doing that, I just want to remind you that this is normal for the fight-or-flight system. It's okay to have some of these feelings. They will pass and even though you might be having certain thoughts about having a panic attack, that doesn't mean it's going to happen, right?

Client: Right.

Therapist: And we did some other exposures like this and you did very well on those as well . . .

Client: Okay. <deep breathing>

Therapist: Okay?

Client: Yep.

Therapist: Do you want to take another breath or two? You're doing a really good job. That's excellent.

Client: Okay. <deep breathing>

Therapist: How would you rate your anxiety now? Zero to 10.

Client: I'm still kind of at the same pace but I don't feel like it's increasing.

Therapist: Okay. Let us then do another round of breathing here, okay? Remember it will pass. You've made it this far, right?

Client: You're right. <deep breathing>

Therapist:	One more shot, now what would you say?
Client:	Maybe closer to 7 or even a 6.
Therapist:	And that's okay. That means it's either stable or maybe it went down a little bit and that's perfectly fine. So if you're comfortable, let's continue with the produce. I'll check in with you there and then we can see how you do. Alright?
Client:	Okay.
Therapist:	Good job.
Client:	Let's do it.

Therapist:	Lindsey, I noticed it got pretty busy down the aisle over there and we just took a detour. You seem like you are feeling more anxious than before in the produce aisle so I just want to get an assessment of where would you say your anxiety is right now?
Client:	It's getting up there . . . <nervous laughter>
Therapist:	Yeah? Alright.
Client:	I'm feeling like maybe a 9. It's getting . . . I feel like I'm about to have a heart attack.
Therapist:	Okay, so I was going to ask what you're thinking and it sounds like you think you're having a heart attack?
Client:	Yeah.
Therapist:	I know you've been through some of these situations before. How many times have you had a heart attack before?
Client:	Never.
Therapist:	So, you've been through this before. You haven't had a heart attack before. I notice you're using some of your breathing techniques and that's working well.
Client:	Mhm . . . <deep breathing>
Therapist:	How are you doing?
Client:	I really want to leave right now. I just feel so light-headed.
Therapist:	And I completely respect that and you are, at any time you want, able to leave. Can you do one thing for me? Maybe, if you can, you've been experiencing these symptoms for 10 to 15 minutes, alright, so this will pass. Try a minute or two, if you can, before you leave—is that fair? I won't say anything unless you want me to. I'll let you relax a little bit.
Client:	This too shall pass. This too shall pass. This will pass. <deep breathing>
Therapist:	Okay. How would you rate your anxiety?
Client:	I think I'm going a little bit down—maybe a 7.
Therapist:	Okay. Do you still feel like you need to get out of here right away?
Client:	I don't particularly like being here right now . . .
Therapist:	You don't have to like being here.
Client:	This is very uncomfortable.

Therapist:	Do you still feel like you want to leave now? Do you still feel like giving it a shot?
Client:	I think I'm doing okay. I like having you here—for right now. <deep breathing>
Therapist:	Okay, for right now. Let's focus on that. That's good. Reminding you of how to relax and think through for a bit.
Client:	Yeah, it helps.
Therapist:	Any other thoughts?
Client:	I think reminding me that I've never had a heart attack in the past. So based on that evidence, I shouldn't have a heart attack now.
Therapist:	Right and you're not right now, are you? Because you know that it's partially a normal response in your body.
Client:	Right. It's all in my head. It's just in my head. <deep breathing>
Therapist:	Okay.
Client:	I think I'm okay.
Therapist:	Okay. One more time, just bear with me, how would you rate your anxiety now?
Client:	I feel like it's closer to a 6 or a 7 right now.
Therapist:	And that's fine too. When we leave here, it probably won't go down to a 0 or a 1. And that's okay. So I know there's a few more things you want to get while we are here for your dog.
Client:	Yeah.
Therapist:	We'll go from there. Do you just want to continue shopping?
Client:	Yeah. I'll be okay.

Therapist:	Alright, we made it! Here we are. You bought your groceries. We made it through everything. You're looking like you're feeling pretty good. How would you say you're feeling right now?
Client:	I can't believe I just did that. I'm feeling closer to like a 3.
Therapist:	That's great! Initially, you said 6 or 7 when we were out here, went up to a 7, 8, 9 while you're in there, and here you are now—didn't run out or anything like that. Do you recall what your initial prediction was when we were first standing by this car and how it was going to go?
Client:	I really thought I was going to have a panic attack.
Therapist:	Yep.
Client:	And, um, I didn't. I can't believe I got through that.
Therapist:	You thought not only that but that you were going to have a heart attack too. Did you have a heart attack?
Client:	No, I did not.
Therapist:	You thought you were going to end up running out of the store, right? Did that happen?
Client:	No, I really, really wanted to.

Therapist:	You wanted to, right? But that's actually the really cool thing about this exposure is that these feelings and sensations, considering all the past experiences you've had, is completely understandable and normal—and that's why we did the exposure. If you noticed, the big difference was that this time, you had those really strong anxious physiological symptoms, right? And then those anxious physiological symptoms triggered thoughts like having a heart attack.
Client:	Yep.
Therapist:	And then you wanted to get the heck out of there, but the difference was this time you didn't leave, right? You were cool enough to stay and say, "Alright, I'll give it a shot for a couple minutes," and then your anxiety went down. And even though you were a little bit anxious to stay and to buy the stuff, you seemed pretty cool, calm, and collected by the time we got out of there.
Client:	I just can't believe I did it.
Therapist:	Yeah.
Client:	I do feel pretty proud of myself right now.
Therapist:	You should. I am really impressed considering where we started and where we are now. We're almost there—maybe a few more sessions left but I think we're getting there. I'm really happy for you.
Client:	Yeah, I feel like I can finally start getting my life back.
Therapist:	Yeah, you're getting there. What I recommend is spend a little time later processing this. It was good that I was there and you said before that you were glad I was there . . .
Client:	Yeah.
Therapist:	That's okay to start. Eventually what you want to do is get yourself to start trying some of this stuff alone, just like you did with the restaurant and the menu a couple weeks ago. Maybe if it's just your husband parking the car initially and waiting outside, and then the next time, leaving, or just you coming by yourself.
Client:	Okay.
Therapist:	You've done a lot of work so that would be my homework assignment, if you choose to do so between now and next session, okay? I realize our time is up, but we will come back next week and process this a little bit more, see if you tried this on your own a little bit more, and we'll start talking about how we'll finish up for the last few sessions. You've made a lot of progress and I think you're almost there.
Client:	Okay, great!
Therapist:	Does that sound good?
Client:	Yes, yes.
Therapist:	I'm proud of you. That's good work.
Client:	Thank you.

Discussion Questions 9.4

- Why was it helpful to get a baseline of anxiety and a prediction before entering the grocery store?
- When the client was in the produce section, what was the most helpful technique to help her reduce her anxiety?
- When having a panic attack in the aisle, how was it therapeutically beneficial for the client to try and "wait it out" for a few minutes rather than immediately leaving the grocery store?
- What were some indicators after the in vivo exposure technique that it was effective for the client?

ACTIVITY 9.5: BEHAVIORAL TECHNIQUES— IMAGINAL AND IN VIVO EXPOSURE

Practice exposure to a feared situation with imaginal exposure and then in vivo exposure using the Exposure Tracking Form. Have one of you play the role of the "client" by picking a feared situation that is commonly avoided. While the other plays the "therapist," start with imaginal exposure by asking questions to immerse the client in the scenario. Be sure to check-in on the client's anxiety and physiological arousal by asking for ratings and additional thoughts. Afterwards, process the experience, especially with regard to the physiological experience and associated automatic thoughts. If practical, attempt in vivo exposure for the feared situation while using the Exposure Tracking Form. Be clear in identifying the exposure goal and possible safety behaviors to avoid. Identify pre-anxiety rating and pre-thoughts, including a prediction for the outcome of the exposure. Also review any potential obstacles and possible relaxation and coping skills. While doing the exposure, remember to provide encouragement and psychoeducation, model and remind client of relaxation and coping techniques, assess physiological arousal and level of anxiety, and identify and modify catastrophic thoughts. When the in vivo exposure is complete, process the outcome (e.g., effectiveness, safety behaviors), including post-anxiety rating and post-thoughts. Did the imaginal exposure elicit in any way some level of physiological arousal? If so, what were the specific sensations? In what ways could have imaginal exposure been more effective? While doing in vivo exposure, what therapist techniques were the most helpful? What techniques were not helpful? Were any of the following helpful in processing the in vivo experience: pre-post anxiety, pre-post thoughts, prediction and outcome? What was the most challenging aspect in guiding the client through imaginal exposure and in vivo exposure?

COMMON CHALLENGES FOR BEHAVIORAL EXPOSURE

Table 9.6 provides some common examples of challenges that can be experienced implementing behavioral exposure techniques. The two most common themes for challenges tend to be clients' hesitancy to initiate relaxation and in vivo exposure techniques.

Table 9.6.   Common Challenges for Behavioral Exposure

Challenge	Possible Considerations
Clients have difficulty assessing anxious and fearful patterns	Use clients' memories or images of a past or hypothetical event to trigger some anxiety.
	If clients have difficulty identifying their anxious thoughts, begin with their physiological arousal, which may be most prominent in their memory of the sequence of events.
	To help narrow your focus on anxious negative automatic thoughts, focus on the three most common cognitive distortions: catastrophizing, magnification (of risk), and minimization (of own skills to cope).
	Focus on clients' avoidance behavioral patterns in response to triggering events.
	Be sure to identity any "safety behaviors" to prevent, reduce, or escape/avoid perceived catastrophic events and associated distress.
	Determine the outcome of the clients' avoidance behaviors and their cognitive and emotion reaction.
Clients are hesitant to begin progressive muscle relaxation and/ or diaphragm breathing	Review rationale and method for these techniques. This can include emphasizing the importance of having effective coping skills to prevent or minimize anxious symptoms.
	Take the "give it a shot" or "what's the worst that could happen" approach. Sometimes, clients are put off by the technique because it looks silly or does not seem like it can work. After a few rounds of practice, the "silliness" often dissipates, and they may experience its benefits as they notice they have control in reducing their physiological arousal.
	Try visualization with a meditation component and then return to progressive muscle relaxation and/or diaphragm breathing.
Clients are hesitant to begin in vivo exposure techniques	Review rationale and method for these techniques. This can include reviewing their hierarchy of feared situations and the effective mechanisms of exposure.
	If clients show some motivation but are still hesitant for in vivo exposure, start with imagery and reassess their desire to move forward.

Challenge	Possible Considerations
	Start with a very small/simple step for in vivo exposure. This may include breaking the first step in the clients' hierarchy of feared situations into two smaller parts or developing a less threatening step before the first step.
	Remind clients of the progress they have made with learning relaxation skills and modifying their anxious thoughts. This conveys to them that they are more "equipped" to confront their feared situations than they were before therapy.

REFERENCES

Abramowitz, J. S., Deacon, B. J., & Whiteside, S. P. (2011). *Exposure therapy for anxiety: Principles and practice.* New York: Guilford Press.

Barlow, D. H. (2001). *Anxiety and its disorders* (2nd ed.). New York: Guilford Press.

Blakey, S. M., & Abramowitz, J. S. (2016). The effects of safety behaviors during exposure therapy for anxiety: Critical analysis from an inhibitory learning perspective. *Clinical Psychology Review, 49,* 1–15.

Craske, M. G., & Barlow, D. H. (2014). Panic disorder and agoraphobia. In D. H. Barlow (Ed.), *Clinical handbook of psychological disorders: A step-by-step treatment manual* (5th ed., pp. 1–61). New York: Guilford Press.

Craske, M. G., Liao, B., Brown, L., & Vervliet, B. (2012). Role of inhibition in exposure therapy. *Journal of Experimental Psychopathology, 3*(3), 322–345.

Craske, M. G., Treanor, M., Conway, C. C., Zbozinek, T., & Vervliet, B. (2014). Maximizing exposure therapy: An inhibitory learning approach. *Behaviour Research and Therapy, 58,* 10–23.

DiMauro, J. (2014). Exposure therapy for posttraumatic stress disorder: A meta-analysis. *Military Psychology, 26,* 120–130.

Fava, G. A., Rafanelli, C., Grandi, S., Conti, S., Ruini, C., Magelli, L., et al. (2001). Long-term outcome of panic disorder with agoraphobia treated by exposure. *Psychological Medicine, 31,* 891–898.

Gil, P. J. M., Carrillo, F. X. M., & Meca, J. S. (2001). Effectiveness of cognitive-behavioural treatment in social phobia: A meta-analytic review. *Psychology in Spain, 5,* 17–25.

Norton, P., & Price. E. (2007). A meta-analytic review of adult cognitive-behavioral treatment outcome across the anxiety disorders. *Journal of Nervous and Mental Disease, 195,* 521–531.

10

Homework

Therapy Between Sessions

Homework has been addressed throughout this text as the next step to practice outside of session what was learned in session. As explained in Chapter 4, homework is not a peripheral activity for CBT; it is a necessary specific factor. There are 168 hours in a week. In most cases, clients will only spend 50 to 60 minutes a week with you; that's at least 167 hours not in therapy. Clients will need to practice what they learn in session between sessions. In many ways, a good portion of therapy happens outside the office. Thus, not doing homework is not an option for a CBT therapist. Stated differently, a CBT therapist who does not do homework is not doing CBT. These statements are not hyperbole. Research consistently shows that CBT clients who are compliant with their homework assignments have better therapeutic outcomes than those who are not compliant (Kazantzis, Deane, & Ronan, 2000; Kazantzis, Whittington, & Dattilio, 2010; Rees, McEvoy, & Nathan, 2005). In summary, CBT without homework significantly reduces therapeutic effectiveness.

The focus of this chapter is not to discuss specific CBT techniques. Rather, the following content will address the general process of integrating homework as a key component of CBT, from assigning a task to maintaining client compliance.

ASSIGNING HOMEWORK

One of the key driving forces for assigning homework is your CBT conceptualization, treatment plan, and interventions. Of course, how and what homework is assigned varies based on the needs of each client. There are a variety of client specific factors that should be considered: (a) severity of psychological distress; (b) cognitive, emotional, and behavioral functioning; (c) motivation and readiness to change; (d) reading and writing skills; (e) CBT skills; (f) past therapy experience; and (g) personal constraints (e.g., living situation and available resources). However, there are some general considerations that apply across all clients. The expectation and necessity for homework assignments should be set by the first session. Assigning homework can begin as early as the first session and should really begin no later than the second session. Of course, you should take the initial lead in the process during the early phase of therapy. By the middle phase of therapy, clients should have an increasing collaborative role in homework assignments, and by the late phase, clients should have more of lead role with your support. Clients who initiate and develop their own homework assignments increase their level of self-efficacy and have a better chance of continuing this behavior pattern after therapy is over.

Always provide a rationale when assigning homework. In fact, most often, the task being assigned is an extension of what is being done in session. At the very least, the assignment should be reviewed in detail, including expectations for follow-up in the next session. Potential obstacles should be also be explored, including motivation and any relevant negative automatic thoughts. The following are some of the common types of homework assignments that are generally unique to CBT.

Bibliotherapy

Bibliotherapy is simply providing readings (e.g., handouts, books, or articles) for clients to review between sessions. Of course, bibliotherapy should never a substitute for providing your own psychoeducation. However, sometimes, important topics that are discussed in session can be supplemented with bibliotherapy to help refine understanding of key concepts or application of particular skills. Be sure to keep any reading assignments relatively brief (e.g., one chapter) with minimal jargon. Providing too much information at once and/or too complicated concepts can overwhelm many clients and possibly reduce motivation. It is usually most effective if clients are asked to take a few notes about what they got most out of the readings and any questions they may have. This information will allow you to assess their understanding of the material and make any necessary therapeutic adjustments when reviewed in the next session. Finally, always read and understand any material you assign for bibliotherapy. You must be familiar with anything you assign for bibliotherapy in order to provide appropriate feedback and support.

Activity Monitoring and Scheduling

For many clients, assessing their low energy and activity level is a vital technique in CBT. Like any assessment process, obtaining a baseline of daily activities and tasks can help you collaboratively determine what adjustments should be made. Thereafter, daily activity scheduling can be used for behavioral activation for target areas to help clients return to their daily routine with a sense of pleasure and accomplishment. This type of homework is especially important because it must take place between sessions; how much can be done in session is limited.

Automatic Thoughts and Core Beliefs: Monitoring, Evaluating, and Modifying

At the heart of any CBT approach, monitoring, evaluating, and modifying thoughts is a must for all clients experiencing distress. (This process can also include monitoring emotions and physiological sensations when appropriate.) Although these techniques begin and require much practice while in session, clients need to practice these skills between sessions. A common supplemental approach is for clients to test the validity of their thoughts by independently engaging in particular activities and assessing the outcome independently between sessions (e.g., behavioral experiments. Mastering these skills outside of session is vital for clients to eventually achieve autonomy and generalize cognitive and behavioral change well after therapy ends.

Exposure to Fearful Situations

Another common approach is to use exposure techniques to modify behavioral responses to anxiety-provoking and fearful situations. Before engaging in exposure techniques, clients typically learn relaxation exercises and modify their anxious automatic thoughts (e.g., catastrophizing). Although imaginal exposure can be an initial effective approach to practice new skills and reduce anxiety, the most effective approach is in vivo exposure, which almost always has to take place outside the office. There are occasions when you can accompany your clients outside the office, but they will have to eventually independently practice these exposure techniques. By the end of therapy, you want your clients to develop enough autonomy that they feel comfortable confronting their fears on their own.

Skills Training and Practice

Clients are always learning new skills in session, whether it is a new relaxation technique, coping skill, social skill, or problem solving (to name a few). Although psychoeducation, therapeutic worksheets, and role plays are helpful in session, clients will need to practice these new skills in their day-to-day lives. The more clients can apply their newly learned skills in "real life," the more their self-efficacy will increase.

Next Session Preparation

Just as how therapists are expected to prepare for the next session, so should clients, especially as they enter the middle and late phases of therapy. The Client Therapy Notes Worksheet, introduced in Chapter 4, has a section for clients to put down any thoughts they want to share in the next session. For example, clients can share their thoughts on treatment goal progress, new presenting problems or distress, technique effectiveness, or current and future homework assignments. Encouraging clients to prepare for their next session and provide feedback reinforces the important role of collaborative empiricism.

See Video Vignettes 4.4 (PDA-5), 4.5 (PDA-8), and 4.6 (PDA-10) demonstrating assigning homework during the late session stage across all three phases of therapy with the same client.

FOSTERING HOMEWORK COMPLIANCE

Some clients will have no problem completing homework assignments between sessions, while others may be inconsistent for a variety of reasons. Although there is no guarantee that all clients will complete all of their homework assignments, the following are some strategies that can be used to increase motivation and compliance.

Provide a Clear Rationale and Clear Instructions

Very early in therapy, clients should be provided a general rationale for the importance of homework for CBT treatment. As therapy progresses, you should be presenting a homework assignment at the end of nearly every session. The best way to provide a rationale is to link the homework assignment with what has just been covered in the current session and address how it will be related to the next session. Additionally, there should be a clear link between the homework assigned and the clients' case conceptualization and treatment goals. The more clients understand why they are doing something (i.e., it has relevance), the more likely they will comply. As therapy progresses, especially by the middle and late phases, you can begin asking clients to develop their own homework assignments and associated rationale.

What typically follows the rationale is the instructions on how to complete the assignment and what is expected to be addressed in the next session. Although providing clear instructions may seem obvious, it is easy to overlook basic information when you are very familiar with the assignment. Thus, it is important that you remind yourself to take the perspective of your client when giving instructions; do not make any assumptions. In most cases, you should be completing and reviewing a portion of the homework assignment before the session ends. Use this as an opportunity to review the specific steps and highlight what will be of primary focus during the next session. It also helps that clients use their Client Therapy Notes Worksheet to record all necessary steps on how to complete the assignment and include any other relevant information, such as where and when it should be completed, frequency, and if other people are included. Homework assignments that are vague are often not attempted because clients have forgotten how to complete them and/or they are avoided out of confusion about the purpose. Furthermore, when clients do attempt to complete a vague homework assignment, they often become frustrated and resentful of future homework. Thus, poorly assigned homework can cause more therapeutic damage than no assigned homework.

Initiate Homework in Session

At least some portion of a homework assignment should be initiated in session. Although homework is often assigned toward the late stage of a session, it is okay to begin earlier if you believe it is necessary to have enough time without rushing. It can help by planning ahead of time with your session agenda. In addition to providing a rationale and instructions, as previously noted, beginning homework in session is also a "live" opportunity to make sure that your clients understand how to do the assignment and that you can respond to any questions or feedback. Some clients may also share their negative automatic thoughts and emotions. This gives you the opportunity to troubleshoot for potential obstacles and develop a coping plan. Furthermore, depending on the homework assignment, it can be helpful to complete at least a portion of the homework together where you take the lead in order to model how to complete particular tasks. What is challenging for most clients is actually starting the task. You may find that completing a portion of a homework assignment can increase motivation, as it is much easier to continue a task that is already started than to initiate a task independently. This makes intuitive sense considering that many clients are experiencing distress that can inhibit initiation of a task, especially if it is new and/or may initially increase distress. As an added benefit, working on homework assignments together not only improves compliance but also can enhance the collaborative nature of the therapeutic alliance.

Individualize Homework Assignments

Although each homework assignment will have a specific set of instructions that must be addressed, this does not mean that you cannot tailor your approach to match your clients' needs. Some examples of client characteristics or factors to consider include disorder, level of distress, level of cognitive functioning, current motivation, attention span, life stressors, and external environmental factors. Beyond the type of homework assignment, how much is assigned can also be adjusted over time. This can include breaking down certain assignments into smaller, more manageable steps. You can even adjust expectations and goals to be completed between sessions. Some clients may find it helpful to use a personal journal to complete certain homework assignments. When reasonable, allow for creativity for alternative means to accomplish the same goals. For example, instead of using paper and pencil for thought records, some clients may benefit from typing them out on their computer or using a smartphone application (see Chapter 11). Similarly, the use of video and audio recordings for homework assignments can provide a lot of useful information to review during a session.

Develop and Initiate Homework Collaboratively

Like all aspects of CBT, there should be a collaborative process in developing, initiating, and reviewing homework assignments. Of course, how much of a "lead" you take will depend on the phase of therapy. Even during the early phase of therapy, where you are taking the lead in developing and initiating the assignment, it is still best to propose it in an inviting manner, including soliciting your clients' feedback. As you move toward the middle phase of therapy, you can offer some suggestions tentatively and explicitly encourage client input. Clients will think they have at least some control in solving their own problems and thus more to gain therapeutically. This will most likely decrease any homework-related anxiety, and they will be more likely to initiate and complete homework assignments if they contribute to its development. If clients are frequently active collaborative participants in developing their homework assignments, they may be ready by the last phase of therapy to develop and initiate their own. More often than not, as therapy evolves and clients continue to make therapeutic gains, they will have a better understanding of what would be an effective homework assignment. You can always provide guidance and suggestions for modification in response to their proposed homework assignment to ensure appropriateness and success. Overall, homework collaboration fosters clients' autonomy and will generalize to their day-to-day activities and continue after therapy is complete.

"Set Up" Your Clients for Success

You want to set up your clients for at least some level of success with their homework assignment, especially if they are doing something for the first time. If clients begin to view their homework attempts as "failures," this can cause much distress, including decreased self-efficacy and motivation. Anytime you assign homework, make sure you are confident that your client has both the capacity and the motivation to complete the assignment. You should emphasize to not focus on "success" or "failure" and/or "full completion" or "incomplete." Many times, what is important is the process of doing the homework assignment, not only the outcome. Even if clients do not fully complete their assignment, there is often still useful information available. If you can make it clear to clients to not focus only on the outcome (i.e., success vs. failure) this will often reduce anxiety and increase motivation. (This perspective can be generalized to life, especially for those with all-or-none tendencies. If something is not 100% completed or not 100% successful, this does not preclude the fact that much can be learned and integrated into future interactions or events.) You can also remind clients that it is okay for them to make "mistakes," have moments of confusion, and have additional questions. In fact, these types of responses are normal and one of the reasons that homework will be reviewed in the next session; it provides useful information to build off of. Ultimately, clients who have a sense of progress with their homework assignments are more likely to initiate and complete future homework assignments, including those that may be more challenging. There is also the potential of secondary gain of clients having increased confidence in your collaborative relationship and therapy in general.

Initially, it is always better to start off a little too easy than too hard. Especially with a new homework assignment, you want to ensure that your clients have at least some sense accomplishment. In some ways, you can look at this as a graded task approach; break large tasks into smaller parts and then increase the size and difficulty of tasks over time with each success. On the other hand, overly challenging assignments can create frustration and be a turnoff for future homework. With that said, you want to make sure that there is a balance between being challenging and too easy. As much as you do not want your clients to think that they have failed, assigned homework that is too easy will not provide much therapeutic benefit and may come off as patronizing.

Help Clients Remember to Do Homework

Ideally, clients should use their Client Therapy Notes Worksheet to write down their assignments at the end of each session. For some clients, this is enough for them to remember to do their homework. However, for other clients, once home, it is still possible for them to misplace their therapy notes or simply forget. Therefore, it is important to brainstorm strategies to help clients remember to complete assignments. Depending on your clients, you may have to think outside the box for strategies to improve their chances of remembering to do their homework. Some possible options to consider include using sticky notes on common items; using a smartphone app, computer, or appointment book for reminders; requesting reminders from a trusted friend/family member immediately after the session; associating another activity to cue when to review therapy notes; reviewing what they do to remember other tasks; and using automated e-mail, voice mail, or text messages from your office (if this is a reasonable option).

Anticipate Possible Problems

Reviewing with clients possible obstacles in homework increases the chances that the homework will actually be attempted and completed. In order to avoid potential ambiguity, Beck (2011) recommends directly asking clients if they have any potential concerns: "What are the chances of you attempting (completing) this homework assignment, 0% to 100%?" You will probably get the most accurate response after you explain and initiate/practice the homework assignment first. Initial impressions can change even after just a few minutes of engaging in a task. If clients are less than 90% to 100% confident, Beck recommends following up with clients by using previously learned CBT strategies to proactively troubleshoot. Before moving forward with a more intricate technique, you can simply ask, "Why?" Some clients may have a clear understanding of why they think they might not be able to initiate or appropriately complete the assignment (e.g., do not understand rationale or instructions, too complex, fear of failure, not sure will remember how to do it, or unmotivated). One commonly recommended technique is guided imagery, similar to what was described in Chapter 7. You can ask clients to think about doing the homework assignment while you verbally describe each of the steps from the beginning to completion. You can also ask them to talk aloud and describe their experience for each step. At the same time, you should be listening for any potential obstacles that are often associated with negative automatic thoughts and/or strong emotions. As a follow-up or a separate technique, you can ask clients to predict possible negative automatic thoughts while they attempt the homework assignment and if it does not go as planned. The information gained from these and other techniques can be used to clarify any concerns and proactively problem solve for any identified obstacles. If your clients still think they will not be able to initiate or complete their assignment at this point, it might be best to consider making a revision or an alternate assignment that will still meet their therapeutic goals.

Review Homework in the Next Session

Reviewing homework in the next session not only is therapeutically appropriate to achieve each clients' goals but also reinforces the importance of future homework assignments. Not following up on homework can communicate that it is not a worthwhile task. Clients put much effort into their homework, and so should you. Not giving homework appropriate attention can result in negative emotions and potentially damage the therapeutic relationship. Thus, clients will be less prone to complete future homework assignments if they do not receive the appropriate attention. As discussed in Chapter 4, you should review the homework assigned for the previous session during the pre-session stage and make it one of the first agenda items to be addressed. If planned appropriately in advance, reviewing homework can be a good bridge from the previous session to the current session.

When reviewing homework, it is best to start with a simple open-ended question that focuses on the process (e.g., "What was your experience working on last week's homework assignment?") instead of a closed-ended question that focuses on the outcome (e.g., "Did you complete last week's homework assignment?"). Although the outcome is still important, you want to set the stage that you are not looking for "success" or "failure." Rather, your emphasis should be on what was learned, what worked, and what did not work. Thus, you should initially focus on praising any attempts at completing the homework, on validating emotions, and on processing associated thoughts. In addition, do not blame or shame if the homework was not attempted or completed. If the homework assignment was not completed, have clients identify possible reasons, including exploring in detail their thought processes before, during, and after the attempt (e.g., Was it appropriately completed? If not, what prevented it from being appropriately completed? Did they make any modifications? Were there any unanticipated obstacles? What is their interpretation for not completing it?). Be sure to reinforce what was done right, provide supportive problem-solving suggestions for improvement, and make any necessary modifications. It is possible that the reason for not completing the homework assignment is related to their presenting problems and distress. Thus, you can turn missed homework assignments into a learning opportunity to continue working on CBT-related skills. Additionally, when practical, it is helpful to complete a portion of the homework in session and convey its relationship to what will be done in the current session. Also, consider assigning it again for the next session. This conveys the importance of completing homework while also demonstrating empathy and flexibility, which can decrease anxiety and increase motivation.

See Video Case Examples MDD-6 (Chapter 6) MDD-13 (Chapter 7), and MDD-16 (Chapter 8) demonstrating reviewing homework during the early session stage across all three phases of therapy with the same client.

Discussion Questions 10.1

- What are other possible reasons why clients might not initiate or complete their homework assignments? Is there anything you can do as a therapist in response to these reasons?
- What CBT technique(s) do you think would be the most challenging for clients to complete as a homework assignment for the first time? What makes this CBT technique(s) difficult for clients to complete independently between sessions? What can you do as a therapist to increase the chances of successful completion for this technique?
- What are some therapeutic options if clients have an especially difficult time understanding and/or completing a specific homework assignment?

ACTIVITY 10.1: RESPONDING TO CLIENTS NOT COMPLETING HOMEWORK

With another peer, pick a specific homework assignment (e.g., activity monitoring, negative automatic though record, or in vivo exposure) and take turns being a client while providing reasons for not initiating or completing the assignment. As the therapist, respond to the client in a manner that validates the client's experience while also trying to increase motivation and understating of the assignment. What was challenging about responding to different reasons for not initiating or completing the assignment? Was it challenging to provide validation while also noticing particular aspects of the homework assignment that were completed? What were some effective responses that might have increased motivation or understanding of the assignment? How can you "tell" if the client appears to be a little more motivated and/or understands the homework assignment?

COMMON CHALLENGES FOR HOMEWORK

Table 10.1 provides some common examples of challenges that can be experienced assigning and reviewing homework assignments. The two most common themes for challenges tend to be clients' difficulty initiating or completing homework and therapists' attitude and approach to assigning and reviewing homework.

Table 10.1. Common Challenges for Homework

Challenge	Possible Considerations
Client consistently struggles to initiate homework	Keep in mind that homework noncompliance is usually not deliberate or personal toward you.
	Be sure to not inadvertently reinforce homework noncompliance (e.g., "That's not a problem." "It's really not a big deal.").
	Consider if this behavior is part of your clients' presenting problems and distress (e.g., low energy level). Review your CBT formulation and determine if this is an external expression of their distress.
	Be sure clients fully understand the instructions and rationale.
	Assess possible reasons for not initiating homework. Reasons can range from fear of "failing" and being judged to simply not remembering it.
	While initiating homework in session, assess your clients' thought processes by asking them to "think out loud" and periodically check in on their thoughts and emotions.
	Review with clients specific steps to help them remember their homework assignment.
Client has difficulty fully completing homework or completes significant portions inaccurately	Praise clients for portions of homework completed and assess for any potential obstacles in completing other parts. If necessary, develop a coping and problem-solving plan to avoid and/or respond to each obstacle.
	Be sure clients fully understand the instructions and rationale.
	When initiating homework in session, spend more time working on it together than previous sessions.
	Assess if the homework assignment is too difficult. If necessary, adjust homework assignments so that there is a greater chance for "success."
Client explicitly states lack of desire to do homework	Try to understand your clients' position for not wanting to do homework (e.g., fear of failure, finds homework offensive, does not see value, or does not have time). You may need to approach the problem as you would other problems with CBT techniques (e.g., modifying negative automatic thoughts or imaginal exposure).

Challenge	Possible Considerations
	Review therapeutic expectations, including importance of a collaborative relationship and doing work between sessions.
	Be sure you provide a clear rationale for each homework assignment.
	Be sure to develop and initiate homework collaboratively. The more clients are involved in developing the homework, the more clients will be motivated to do it.
	Ask clients for suggestions on how to modify homework so that it is more appealing and/or practical.
	Reassess your therapeutic relationship to determine that there is enough mutual respect and trust.
Therapist difficulty following through with assigning and reviewing homework assignments	Remind yourself of the necessity to have clients learn and apply new skills between sessions.
	Assess your own thoughts for not consistently integrating homework into your therapy sessions (e.g., "I don't think it will help." "I tried earlier, but my clients didn't do it. What's the point now?" "I don't want to upset my clients by making them feel insulted or overburdened.").
	Consider that your clients' motivation to initiate and complete homework assignments is influenced by your own modeling in session. The more you sincerely believe in the effectiveness of homework, the more apt your clients are too.
	Consider supervision or consultation with an experienced CBT therapist to help you work through your own misgivings with homework.

REFERENCES

Beck, J. S. (2011). *Cognitive behavior therapy: Basics and beyond* (2nd ed.). New York: Guilford Press.

Kazantzis, N., Deane, F. P., & Ronan, K. R. (2000). Homework assignments in cognitive and behavioral therapy: A meta-analysis. *Clinical Psychology: Science and Practice, 7,* 189–202.

Kazantzis, N., Whittington, C., & Dattilio, F. (2010). Meta-analysis of homework effects in cognitive and behavioral therapy: A replication and extension. *Clinical Psychology: Science and Practice, 17,* 144–156.

Rees, C., McEvoy, P., & Nathan, P. (2005). Relationship between homework completion and outcome in cognitive behavior therapy. *Cognitive Behavior Therapy, 34,* 242–247.

11

CBT and Technology

It should come as no surprise that technology (e.g., computers, smartphones, and tablets) is an integral part of daily life for many Americans (Pew Research Center, 2017). Not only has technology become more readily available across populations, but it is also easier to use. Thus, it only seems natural that mental health professionals are more apt to use this available technology to assess and treat their clients. Furthermore, integrating technology into CBT appears to be a "good fit" due to its tracking and empirical nature (Aguilera & Muench, 2012; Luxton, McCann, Bush, Mishkind, & Reger, 2011). Using technology as a CBT treatment adjunct has shown to be effective for a variety of disorders by way of supplementing treatment techniques (e.g., Anderson & Price, 2013; Dettore, Pozza, & Andersson, 2015). Furthermore, research shows that clients are willing and able to integrate technology (e.g., smartphone apps) into their treatment (Aguilera & Muñoz, 2011; Proudfoot et al., 2010).

This chapter highlights a variety of modes of technology that are commonly used by CBT therapists for multiple therapeutic techniques. Examples of technology include smartphone and tablet applications, video and audio recordings, internet videos and pictures, and virtual reality. It is important to note here that these technologies are not meant to replace therapy; they are meant to supplement therapy. Additionally, the focus of this chapter is on using technology to enhance face-to-face therapy. Internet-based therapy is a separate topic and beyond the scope of this chapter.

TECHNOLOGY FOR CBT THERAPEUTIC TECHNIQUES

This section is divided into four parts for ease of explaining how technology can enhance particular CBT-related components: engagement and motivation, psychoeducation, self-monitoring and cognitive-behavior change, and relaxation.

Engagement and Motivation

Having clients engaged and motivated is important for developing the therapeutic relationship, participating in therapeutic techniques, and achieving treatment goals. Research is beginning to show that the general use of technology can have positive effects on the therapeutic alliance, including engagement and motivation (Chu et al., 2004; Richards, Simpson, Bastiampillai, Pietrabissa, & Castelnuovo, 2016). For example, the natural interactive nature of some forms of technology (e.g., computer programs and smartphone/tablet applications) can enhance engagement. More specifically, phone applications and automated text/e-mail can be used for homework and appointment reminders for clients who may need a boost in engaging in therapy-related activities between sessions. Simply watching a video and/or listening to music can prime communication and help clients feel more comfortable. Similarly, videos/music can create an opportunity for highly distressed clients to briefly "step away" from the treatment agenda as a way to hit the "reset button." Ideally, it is best if the videos or music are related to the clients' presenting distress and can be tied into the treatment goals.

Psychoeducation

There are many videos available through reputable mental health organizations that provide psychoeducation on a variety of topics, ranging from basic information about specific disorders to therapeutic techniques (many of which are available on YouTube). With your guidance, you can show clients appropriate websites and smartphone applications. Psychoeducation videos can offer a change of pace in treatment. These videos can make psychoeducation more appealing, relatable, and less intimidating to clients when they can be watched between sessions as part of a homework assignment (or independent task). Many of the psychoeducation smartphone applications also provide feedback and screening programs. There are also some applications specifically designed for therapists to assist with diagnostic information and medication interactions.

Self-Monitoring and Cognitive-Behavior Change

Self-monitoring of thoughts, emotions, and behaviors is one of the most used CBT techniques both in session and between sessions. Indeed, research continuously demonstrates that self-monitoring is attributed to a significant portion of cognitive and behavior change (e.g., Alsalamah, 2017; Craske & Tsao, 1999; Todd & Mullan, 2014). There are even formal technology-assisted self-monitoring programs that target specific disorders (e.g., Faurholt-Jepsen et al., 2015; Tregarthen, Lock, & Darcy, 2015). As a result of technological advances and increased accessibility, individuals are more easily able to record, store, and access notes, audio, and video files. Some clients may not be keen about writing out their self-monitoring homework between sessions. You may find it helpful to refer them to a particular smartphone application to digitally record their thoughts, emotions, and behaviors. Another great benefit for self-monitoring is to request that your clients use videos and audio recordings to track their thoughts, feelings, and behaviors in real time (e.g., audio diary or video thought record). When clients are experiencing a distressing event in the moment (or soon after), it is more of a "felt experience," and their memory tends to be more accurate than retroactively recalling past events. This approach can be more effective than self-report in session and written self-monitoring due to memory effects.

Clients can also audio or video record their exposure exercises (e.g., phobias) and practice specific skills (e.g., assertiveness). A key component of exposure activities is for clients to eventually engage in this behavior independently, which enhances clients' autonomy. One drawback is that therapists have to rely on client feedback, which can sometimes inhibit the quantity and quality of feedback. Similarly, although practicing specific skills in session has its merits, applying them in "real-world" settings provides the greatest opportunity for therapeutic gain. However, if clients are able to record their experiences independently, they can still obtain a true exposure/specific skill experience while also receiving the same quality of feedback as if the therapist is actually with them.

An option for some of these applications is to send reminders to clients via text message or e-mail to complete particular homework activities. Many of these applications also allow for displaying information graphically and can be sent to the therapist electronically (or a website) for easy review and feedback. Self-monitoring information presented this way can be especially effective in tracking treatment progress because it provides a concrete, objective perspective on specific domains of interest. A great resource for self-monitoring tools is the quantified-self website: http://www.quantifiedself.com/guide. The primary focus of this website is self-report and automatic tracking for self-monitoring.

Another popular technology used largely for exposure techniques is virtual reality. Virtual reality uses computer programs and artificially created environments with visual immersion to give clients a simulated but realistic experience. This allows clients to confront a digital version of a feared object or situation instead of using imagery or in vivo exposure. Virtual reality has been found to be especially effective in treating anxiety-related disorders, especially for phobias and some types of trauma (Maples-Keller, Bunnell, Kim, & Rothbaum, 2017). Typically, before a client uses virtual reality, the therapist prepares the client like one would for in vivo exposure (e.g., teach relaxation techniques, challenge cognitive distortions, and create a hierarchy of fears; see Chapter 9). Then, while the client is using virtual therapy, the therapist monitors the client and provides feedback. Virtual reality can be helpful for some clients before they are ready for in vivo exercises. In other cases, virtual reality may be the chosen intervention for comfort or safety reasons or for scenarios that are not easily accessible or practical for in vivo exposure (e.g., combat-related trauma). Due to improving technology and decreasing costs, this is becoming a more viable option for therapists. Using virtual reality as the primary mode of intervention is beyond the scope of this book (see Wiederhold & Bouchard, 2014).

Relaxation

There are many smartphone applications and internet audios/videos that can help facilitate clients' relaxation techniques (e.g., muscle relaxation, breathing exercises, visualization, meditation, and mindfulness). Although many of these techniques are initially taught and practiced in session, clients generally benefit the most when they can utilize these techniques independently between sessions. In fact, these techniques are generally more beneficial when done independently with there being more privacy and a more comfortable environment. Some of these programs provide good instructions on how to actually do specific techniques, whereas others provide soothing music and visuals while clients walk through each step.

CAUTIONS USING TECHNOLOGY IN THERAPY

Although using technology in therapy can have many enhancing effects for therapeutic outcomes, caution should be taken into consideration for selection and application. First, like choosing an assessment, you should put effort into selecting an appropriate mode of technology for your clients. For example, there are many smartphone applications and websites available touting their utility in helping people with a variety of disorders or problems. However, they are not all equal in quality of content and utility. Some may offer no benefit to clients, while others can potentially cause harm, especially without professional guidance. Table 11.1 provides a list of smartphone applications that are appropriate for supplementing a variety of CBT techniques.

Second, a common observed concern is overusing technology simply for the sake of using technology. Just because technology can be used does not mean it should be used. Not having a purposeful approach when using technology in therapy can result in a lack of direction, confusion, frustration, and possibly poor treatment outcomes. First consider what technique you want to use, then decide if the using a form a technology will have an enhancing effect (i.e., let the technique decide if technology is necessary, not the technology dictate the technique). Technology should be used only if it can truly supplement and enhance existing assessment and treatment goals.

Third, it is important that you are familiar with the technologies that you choose to use in therapy. In other words, the source of the technology and its purpose need to be considered. Furthermore, it is advisable that you become familiar with each chosen technology before using it with clients. The more you know about the technology, the more you will know about its strengths and limitations. In turn, you will be able to provide more constructive instructions on how to use each technology and relevant feedback.

Fourth, consider appropriateness based on your clients' idiosyncratic needs. This includes clients' demographic backgrounds (e.g., socioeconomic status), presenting problems, and specific symptoms. A technology that works for one client is not necessarily going to work for another client, even with the same disorder or presenting problems. In sum, if appropriate precautions are taken in selection and application, the use of technology in CBT can yield many therapeutic benefits.

Table 11.1. Smartphone Applications with CBT Utility

Name	Device(s)	Price	Uses	Features
Anxiety Coach	iOS (7.0 or later)	$4.99	Phobias, obsessive-compulsive disorder, generalized anxiety disorder (GAD), and panic disorder	"To-do" lists of fears (can add to an already comprehensive list). Customized for the individual; coaching before, during, and after exposure to fears; anxiety tracking over time during exposure.
Anxiety Resolver	iOS (6.0 or later)	$2.99	Anxiety and stress	Increases self-awareness of anxiety and provides educational advice and templates for altering unhealthy behaviors.
Belly Biofeedback	iOS (7.0 or later)	Free	Attention	Provides biofeedback for diaphragmatic breathing (place phone on abdomen and receive feedback on pace, etc.).
Breathe	iOS (9.0 or later)	Free (in-app purchases)	Stress and relaxation	Helps you stay calm and battle anxiety by sending you gentle deep-breathing reminders throughout the day. These notifications are customizable (frequency).
Breathe2Relax	iOS (7.0 or later) Android	Free	Wide variety	Guided breathing exercise over 16 cycles customized to user's breath speed; relaxing music/graphics; stress-level ratings; tips for relaxation.
CBT*ABC way	iOS (5.1 or later)	$6.99	Wide variety	Practice monitoring thoughts and feelings and modifying thoughts. Available in kid, teen, and adult versions as well as in Spanish.
CBT-i Coach	iOS (8.4 or later) Android	Free	Insomnia	Intended to augment therapy. Guides users through the process of sleep, developing positive sleep routines, and improving sleeping environments. Developed by the Veterans Administration (VA).
CBT Thought Diary Record	iOS (8.0 and later)	Free	Wide variety	Helps you evaluate, understand, and change your thoughts and feelings; identify emotions; analyze emotions; challenge negative beliefs; and change your thinking patterns for future situations.
Cognitive Diary	Android	Free	Wide variety	Dysfunctional thought record; write a thought, rate how much you believe it, identify and rate emotions, identify common cognitive distortions, write a more rational thought, and re-rate your belief.
eMoods	Android (Kindle and iOS [under development])	Free	Mood disorders	Track daily highs and lows, sleep, medications, and other symptoms related to mood disorders. Creates graphs; can e-mail monthly report to doctor to identify triggers/events.

(continued)

Table 11.1. *Continued*

Name	Device(s)	Price	Uses	Features
iCBT	iOS (8.0 or later)	$5.99	Wide variety	Inspired by the acclaimed "Feeling Good Handbook." Provides essential CBT self-help skills with sound structure and easy-to-follow steps. Connects through e-mail; no network required; secured access with password protection.
iCouchCBT	iOS (8.0 or later)	$2.99	Wide variety	Clear step-by-step process for easily keeping track of thoughts and modifying negative thinking patterns. Includes customizable emotions and distortions, e-mail exchange, and optional password protection.
iPromptU	iOS (7.1 or later) Android	Free	Homework	Can be used in conjunction with therapy as a 100% customizable tool for CBT homework.
Life Armor	iOS (6.0 or later) Android	Free	Wide variety	Provides a number of brief tips for coping with a specific stressor. User can select a specific target among a wide variety of stressors. Videos of military personnel talking about their struggles and how they cope.
Mindfulness Daily	iOS (7.1 or later)	Free (in-app purchases)	Daily living and stress	Quick and effective practices with daily reminders and records for tracking progress.
MindShift	iOS (6.0 or later) Android	Free	Anxiety, GAD, panic disorder, and worry	Targeted for adolescents and young adults. Provides active coping strategies tailored to the type of anxiety.
MoodKit	iOS (8.0 or later)	$4.99	Depression	Basic CBT tools, including positive activity scheduling, mood tracking, and thought evaluation/restructuring as well as mindfulness-based, values-based, and spirituality-based activities.
Moving Forward	iOS (4.3 or later)	Free	Posttraumatic stress disorder (PTSD) and adjustment	Designed by the VA for veterans and service members but useful for anyone with stressful problems. Take assessments, learn about effective stress management, and track stress over time.
Omvana—Meditation for Everyone	iOS (8.0 or later) Android	Free (in-app purchases)	Health and stress	Guided meditation for all aspects of life, with personalized background music and HealthKit integration that recognizes stress levels. Apple Watch features available.
Operation Reach Out	iOS (9.0 or later) Android	Free	Suicide	Geared toward military personnel. Addresses suicidality and other dangerous behaviors by providing a customizable list of helping resources.
Optimism	iOS (8.0 or later) Web based	Free	Wide variety	Mood recording app that generates customizable charts over time and helps you develop and monitor mental health strategies, learn the "triggers" of a decline in your mental health, and recognize the early warning signs of a decline.

Name	Platform	Price	Focus	Description
Pacifica—Anxiety, Stress, & Depression Relief	iOS (8.0 or later) Android	Free (in-app purchases)	Wide variety	Provides useful CBT tools for tracking mood and thoughts. Also incorporates mindfulness and relaxation techniques. Includes access to self-help work.
PE Coach	iOS (4.3 or later) Android	Free	PTSD	For use only in conjunction with structured and prolonged exposure therapy with a therapist. Can record sessions (requires a lot of free space on phone) and track homework assignments.
PTSD Coach	iOS (8.0 or later) Android	Free	PTSD	Developed by the VA, provides a self-assessment tool, tracking capabilities, and tools for coping through self-help.
Qi Gong Meditation Relaxation	Android	Free	Wide variety	Streams audio and video files from the internet, including mindful breathing exercise and other meditations.
Relax and Rest Guided Meditations	iOS (6.1 or later) Android	$1.99	Stress relaxation	Three meditations of varying lengths allow you to relax deeply (breathing awareness, deep rest, and whole-body relaxation).
Relax Me	Android	Free	Wide variety	Audio-guided progressive muscle relaxation with reminder features. Can select calming or energizing progressive muscle relaxation.
Simply Being	iOS (7.1 or later) Android	$1.99	Stress and relaxation	Choose between five meditation time lengths with the option to listen to guided meditation with or without music or nature sounds. You can also listen to the music or nature sounds alone. In addition, you can choose how long to listen to the music or nature sounds after the voice guidance finishes.
Stop, Breathe & Think	iOS (8.0 and later)	Free (in-app purchases)	Stress and relaxation	Check how you are thinking and feeling and select emotions that guide you to recommended meditations.
Stop Panic & Anxiety Self Help	Android	Free	Panic disorder and anxiety	Utilizes CBT approach to help individuals address destructive thought patterns. Has built-in audio relaxation.
Tactical Breather	iOS (6.1 or later) Android	Free	Wide variety	Similar to Breathe2Relax but uses a more structured, four-count breathing exercise. Breathing speed cannot be altered (unlike with Breathe2Relax).

(continued)

Table 11.1. Continued

Name	Device(s)	Price	Uses	Features
Thought Diary Pro	iOS (8.0 or later)	$4.99	Depression and anxiety disorders	Allows user to keep a thought record, facilitates understanding of cognitive errors/categories, prompts user to come up with more adaptive thoughts, and allows user to e-mail thought record to therapist.
T2 Mood Tracker	iOS (7.0 or later) Android	Free	Wide variety	Rating scales for various facets (anxiety, stress, depression, etc.); graph ratings over time, add customized scales on any topic, and e-mail results to a clinician.
Way of Life—The Ultimate Habit Maker & Breaker	iOS (9.0 or later) Android	Free	Wide variety	Helps implement behavior change through identifying goals, sending reminders, and tracking progress.
WebMD	iOS (7.0 or later) Android	Free	Reference information	Research conditions, check symptoms, access drug and treatment information, get first-aid essentials, and check local health listings on the go.
What's Up?	iOS (6.1 or later) Android	Free	Wide variety	Utilizes principles of CBT and acceptance and commitment therapy to address negative thinking patterns and track progress.
Worry Watch	iOS (7.1 or later)	$1.99	Anxiety, GAD, and worry	Provides self-monitoring tools and charts. Utilizes CBT theories to identify cognitive distortions that lead to worry.

Discussion Questions 11.1

- Can you think of any other ways technology can be appropriately integrated into CBT?
- Are there particular problems/disorders that are a "better fit" for technology than others?
- How do you think clients will respond to recommendations for integrating technology into therapy? Will responses vary by population (e.g., age, race/ethnicity, or socioeconomic status)?
- Can you think of any additional concerns or cautions when using technology with CBT?

ACTIVITY 11.1: PRACTICE USING CBT

Using Table 11.1, select one of the smartphone applications and download it to your smartphone. Spend some time learning about its features and how to use it. What problems/disorders is this application designed for? What features do you think would be the most helpful? Are there any features that might not be helpful or possibly harmful if not used appropriately? How would you integrate this application into therapy? Would you be able to show a client how to use this application effectively?

REFERENCES

Aguilera, A., & Muench, F. (2012). There's an app for that: Information technology applications for cognitive behavioral practitioners. *The Behavior Therapist, 35,* 65–73.

Aguilera, A., & Muñoz, R. F. (2011). Text messaging as an adjunct to CBT in low-income populations: A usability and feasibility pilot study. *Professional Psychology: Research and Practice, 42,* 472–478.

Alsalamah, A. (2017). Use of the self-monitoring strategy among students with attention deficit hyperactivity disorder: A systematic review. *Journal of Education and Practice, 8,* 118–125.

Anderson, P. L., & Price, M. (2013). Virtual reality exposure therapy for social anxiety disorder: A randomized controlled trial. *Journal of Consulting and Clinical Psychology, 81,* 751–760.

Chu, B. C., Choudhury, M. S., Shortt, A. L., Pincus, D. B., Creed, T. A., & Kendall, P. C. (2004). Alliance, technology and outcome in the treatment of anxious youth. *Cognitive and Behavioral Practice, 11,* 44–55.

Craske, M. G., & Tsao, J. C. I. (1999). Self-monitoring with panic and anxiety disorders. *Psychological Assessment, 11,* 466–479.

Dettore, D., Pozza, A., & Andersson, G. (2015). Efficacy of technology-delivered cognitive behavioural therapy for OCD versus control conditions, and in comparison with therapist-administered CBT: Meta-analysis of randomized controlled trials. *Cognitive Behaviour Therapy, 44,* 190–211.

Faurholt-Jepsen, M., Frost, M., Ritz, C., Christensen, E. M., Jacoby, A. S., Mikkelsen, R. L., et al. (2015). Daily electronic self-monitoring in bipolar disorder using smartphones—The MONARCA I trial: A randomized, placebo-controlled, single-blind, parallel group trial. *Psychological Medicine, 45,* 2691–2704.

Luxton, D. D., McCann, R. A., Bush, N. E., Mishkind, M. C., & Reger, G. M. (2011). mHealth for mental health: Integrating smartphone technology in behavioral healthcare. *Professional Psychology: Research and Practice, 42,* 505–512.

Maples-Keller, J. L., Bunnell, B. E., Kim, S.-J., & Rothbaum, B. O. (2017). The use of virtual reality technology in the treatment of anxiety and other psychiatric disorders. *Harvard Review of Psychiatry, 25,* 103–113.

Pew Research Center. (2017). *Mobile technology fact sheet.* Retrieved from: http://www.pew internet.org/fact-sheet/mobile

Proudfoot, J., Parker, G., Pavlovic, D. H., Manicavasagar, V., Adler, E., & Whitton, A. (2010). Community attitudes to the appropriation of mobile phones for monitoring and managing depression, anxiety, and stress. *Journal of Medical Internet Research, 12,* 111–122.

Richards, P., Simpson, S., Bastiampillai, T., Pietrabissa, G., & Castelnuovo, G. (2016). The impact of technology on therapeutic alliance and engagement in psychotherapy: The therapist's perspective. *Clinical Psychologist.* https://doi.org/10.1111/cp.12102.

Todd, J., & Mullan, B. (2014). The role of self-monitoring and response inhibition in improving sleep behaviors. *International Journal of Behavioral Medicine, 21,* 470–477.

Tregarthen, J. P., Lock, J., & Darcy, A. M. (2015). Development of a smartphone application for eating disorder self-monitoring. *International Journal of Eating Disorders, 48,* 972–982.

Wiederhold, B. K., & Bouchard, S. (2014). *Advances in virtual reality and anxiety disorders.* New York: Springer.

12

Common CBT Myths

Although CBT is the most well-established effective treatment approach for the most mental health problems (APA Presidential Task Force on Evidence-Based Practice, 2006; see http://www.div12.org/psychological-treatments/), there remain some common myths about its nature. It is especially important that those entering training in CBT are made aware of such myths in order to avoid any possible self-fulfilling prophecies and/or negatively biased influences. Keep in mind that the following are considered myths not because CBT theorists and therapists simply disagree or it evokes a negative emotional reaction but rather because they lack validity. Thus, the following myths are truly myths—that is, they are not true. (They are invalid negative automatic thoughts possibly stemming from core beliefs!)

CBT IS TOO RIGID/MECHANICAL/TECHNIQUE FOCUSED

This myth often comes from those with minimal to no training in CBT. Cognitive and behavioral therapies (now CBT) were the first theoretical therapeutic approaches to use manual-based treatment (Wilson, 2007) and may have resulted in precipitating this myth. Some therapists not familiar with CBT have a false belief that too scientific an approach means no flexibility, creativity, or innovation in therapy. For example, Gaston and Gagnon (1996) stated that manual-based treatments have the consequence of "stagnant, codified accepted treatments" (p. 17). This perspective has been shown to be patently wrong after many years of research. Ironically, CBT manual-based treatments have enhanced flexibility, creativity, and innovation for a variety of disorders across diverse client populations. With CBT, there is a balance between the science and the art of therapy. However, priority is not put on how creative therapists feel about themselves; priority is put on providing the best possible care for clients using evidenced-based practice. The art comes in when it is necessary to be flexible and innovative.

Models and protocols are important, but they are not the only driving force for effective therapy. Data gained in session (e.g., formal/informal assessment, monitoring behaviors, and thought records) help guide therapy with an ever-evolving CBT case formulation that is idiosyncratic to each client. Each client's presenting problems, distress, thoughts, emotions, and behaviors is unique to each. The art is knowing when to make modifications as therapy (and data) evolves. The focus of CBT is to fit the approach to the client (i.e., what, when, how, and sometimes where), not to fit the client to the approach.

Finally, agenda setting, which provides structure to individual sessions, also perpetuates the myth of CBT being too rigid. It is true that during the early phase of therapy, therapists direct many of the agenda items. However, collaborative empiricism allows for continuous feedback from clients. Furthermore, as therapy progresses to the middle and late phases of therapy, clients have increasing input over the agenda. Also, and most important, clients report feeling relieved and appreciative for having purposeful direction, as it helps ensure that important issues are addressed and there is improvement in overall well-being.

CBT FOCUSES ONLY ON THOUGHTS AND EXCLUDES EMOTIONS

As can be seen in this book, thoughts obviously receive a lot of attention in CBT. The development of this myth may also be an emotional response in and of itself: emotions must receive attention in therapy! Again, research shows that emotions are definitely relevant; in fact, therapy often begins with emotions before transitioning to thoughts. A primary therapeutic approach to CBT is to modify maladaptive thoughts. However, this is done as a means to an end, not as an end in itself. As demonstrated throughout this book, emotions and behaviors receive much attention as well. For example, a key way to identify automatic thoughts and core beliefs is by eliciting strong emotions. Thereafter, clients learn that modifying thoughts will moderate the intensity of their emotions. If CBT therapists are not able to integrate clients' emotions in their therapeutic approach, they will be ineffective. In other words, it is impossible to ignore emotions in CBT.

CBT THERAPIST–CLIENT RELATIONSHIPS ARE OF LITTLE VALUE

As discussed extensively in Chapter 2, CBT acknowledges that the relationship is important, including such key Rogerian conditions as empathy, genuineness, and unconditional positive regard. However, these common factors are necessary but not sufficient for long-term change for most clients experiencing distress. The specific factors of CBT are necessary for true change, but they are of little value if there is a poor-quality therapist–client relationship. A vital component of the therapeutic relationship in CBT is collaborative empiricism, which requires clients to trust both the therapist and the techniques that are implemented (e.g., exposure to clients' worst fears, making decisions together through guided discovery, and giving and receiving feedback). Collaborative empiricism is the driving force for behavioral experiments and developing new thoughts and core beliefs. Research shows that collaborative empiricism is most effective when there is a strong therapeutic relationship that is valued by clients (i.e., clients are able to autonomously solve their problems; Dattilio & Hanna, 2012; Wright & Davis, 1994). Thus, not only is the therapist–client relationship of great value for CBT, but it is necessary for efficient and effective therapy.

CBT TREATS ONLY SURFACE SYMPTOMS, NOT THE SOURCE

This is an "old-school," unsupported view that initially developed when behaviorism began to establish itself in response to psychoanalysis (i.e., science vs. nonscience). Historically, psychoanalysis has focused on the id, ego, superego, and repression (to name a few), which conceptually helped one understand how clients developed their neuroses deep within themselves (e.g., unconscious and conflict). However, these are essentially made-up constructs to explain internal distress (i.e., neuroses) that actually do not exist and have no empirical support (there is some support for an unconscious but not in the Freudian sense). Behaviorism took the opposite approach by focusing only on what is observable and measurable, which naturally fits within the scientific method, allowing for experiments. The rise of behaviorism resulted in complaints (i.e., myths) that it treated only the symptoms, not the source ("symptom substitution"). These complaints have been shown to be unfounded, as behaviorism has continuously demonstrated its effectiveness to treat many problems, especially anxiety-related distress (Montgomery & Crowder, 1972).

Today, as many behavioral approaches evolved into cognitive-behavioral approaches, research strongly supports that CBT treats well beyond symptoms relative to other therapeutic approaches (APA Presidential Task Force on Evidence-Based Practice, 2006). In fact, many times, treating what would initially be considered "only the symptoms" is actually treating the source. CBT does this by focusing largely on present problems and maintaining factors by targeting the source— thoughts. Providing clients insight into why they are feeling distressed and behaving maladaptively is important, but it is insufficient for change if they do not know what to do with such insight. The premise of the CBT theoretical model is that distress comes largely from how one appraises and responds to one's environment. Changing thoughts and how one behaviorally interacts with the environment does produce long-term change. Thus, by definition, CBT treats the whole person. Correspondingly, CBT has some of the best therapeutic outcomes for the generalization and maintenance of change, especially for anxiety and depressive disorders (e.g., Cuijpers et al., 2013; Hofmann, Asnaani, Vonk, Sawyer, & Fang, 2012; Tolin, 2010). The long-term, post-therapy success of CBT is due largely to the fact that CBT actually gets very deep and addresses underlying problems (i.e., core beliefs), promoting client autonomy (i.e., clients become their own therapists and do not need to rely on therapists and be in therapy for many years), protection from relapse, and overall improved quality of life.

CBT DOES NOT CONSIDER THE PAST IMPORTANT

CBT does focus largely on the present and future change over time but also acknowledges the importance of the past and, when necessary, will explore specific relevant events. Our past experiences definitely influence and shape who we are in the present. Compared to other theoretical approaches, CBT is different in how the past is perceived and how information about the past is used in conceptualizing clients' distress and problems. For example, other approaches (e.g., psychoanalysis) focus heavily on the past and believe that what happens as a child largely determines who we are as adults and that we are continually working on our conflicts. CBT recognizes that the past does play a role in shaping us, but it is a continuous process (and not an end in itself). For example, core beliefs, often formed due to significant past events, are an important part of CBT in understanding how clients perceive themselves, the world, and their future. However, CBT does not get so caught up in the past that the focus on the present is skewed or missed (i.e., does not miss the forest for the trees). While the past can be helpful in conceptualizing what may be contributing to clients' problems and distress, the maintaining factors in the present may be different than what contributed to its initial development. Thus, while past events can inform conceptualization, the present is used to solve current problems, modify relevant cognitions, and apply new behaviors while also planning for the future (e.g., troubleshooting and generalizing change).

CBT IS SIMPLY A FANCY APPROACH
TO POSITIVE THINKING

As stated a few times in this book, CBT is not positive thinking. This myth appears to be due largely to the lack of knowledge of the actual mechanisms of change for CBT. Generally, positive thinking is making a negative thought positive simply by changing the words. For example, instead of thinking, "I'm a bad person," think, "I'm a good person." This is far from how CBT works. The example focuses only on the surface outcome and ignores the internal process of change. CBT focuses on "realistic thinking" by having clients modify their invalid negative automatic thoughts so that they are more accurate with adaptive behaviors and consequences.

This process helps clients think differently about themselves, the world, and the future. However, notice that the focus is on valid thoughts, not to be more "positive." If modification results in a positive thought, it was the natural outcome of the actual process of change by examining the nature and validity (or lack thereof) of the initial thought. In other cases, some negative automatic thoughts are valid because the situation is not positive (e.g., may cause actual physical and/or psychological harm). Thus, trying to think positive for valid negative automatic thoughts can actually cause more harm than good. If clients are experiencing valid negative automatic thoughts, the focus should be not on making them positive but rather on learning ways was to cope and acceptance. Overall, simply thinking positive rarely provides any short-term reduction in distress and does not provide any long-term reduction in distress. In fact, false positive thinking can actually result in clients feeling frustrated and reduce their motivation and hope for change. On the other hand, modifying invalid negative automatic thoughts and learning how to cope and accept valid negative automatic thoughts can significantly reduce stress and maintain its benefits over time.

CBT IS ONLY FOR INTELLIGENT/ PSYCHOLOGICALLY MINDED/MOTIVATED PEOPLE

This myth may have developed due to the logical nature of CBT and the importance of clients being active participants in their own therapy. There is no doubt that individuals who are more intelligent, self-aware, and motivated, are in a better position to more readily engage and "pick-up" on certain CBT concepts. However, this is no different than any other theoretical orientation. With that said, CBT is malleable enough to adapt to a wide range of levels of intelligence, cognitive functioning, self-awareness, mental health distress, and motivation. A client's capacity to be psychologically minded and desire to change can be developed over time with CBT. There is extensive research demonstrating the effectiveness of CBT with a variety of populations: young and older people, individuals with learning disabilities, psychosis, personality disorders, and substance abuse (Beck, Davis, & Freeman, 2015; Friedberg & McClure, 2015; James, 2010; Kroese, Dagnan, & Loumidis, 1997; Najavits, 2001; Rector & Beck, 2001).

CBT IS ADVERSARIAL

The perception by those who do not have a sophisticated understanding of CBT is that therapists argue with their clients and tell them that their thoughts are wrong. This also comes from a lack of understanding of the collaborative nature of CBT, where feedback is continuously provided and elicited (or maybe watching too many old videos of Albert Ellis, who had a more direct and confrontational approach!).

Hopefully, this book has shown that challenging thoughts and the collaborative nature of CBT does not involve arguing with clients. Rather, CBT is a continuous process of guided discovery that focuses on identifying specific cognitive and behavioral patterns, modifying those patterns that are most distressing to the client, and validating and reinforcing such changes. More specifically, CBT therapists may notice that clients have clear maladaptive thoughts (i.e., cognitive distortions) but do not state to their clients that their thinking is wrong. This is not an effective way to produce change. It also lacks empathy and perspective taking—both important qualities for CBT therapists. CBT therapists validate clients' feelings and try to understand the development and maintaining factors of related thoughts. Thereafter, therapists and clients collaboratively work on understanding the relationship between thoughts, emotions, and behaviors and guide clients in making the necessary changes (i.e., clients ultimately have control). If therapists find themselves arguing with their clients, they are not appropriately implementing CBT techniques.

CBT IS QUICK TO LEARN AND EASY TO PRACTICE

Again, this comes from individuals with little to no training in CBT. This view may stem from an earlier-stated myth that CBT is rigid/mechanical/technique focused (assumes that there is a prescribed mechanistic approach). Not only is CBT a flexible therapeutic approach, but it takes much skill to balance the science–art relationship. Having solid common factor skills, the primary focus of some therapeutic approaches, is one thing. However, CBT goes well beyond these basic skills with its own specific factors and techniques requiring extensive training, practice, and supervision to master. This book and other CBT resources show that much effort and skill goes into being a quality therapist. This can be initially intimidating to some, but over time with practice, the effectiveness and improved quality of life that CBT provides for clients can be both personally and professionally satisfying.

WHY CARE ABOUT THESE MYTHS?

Worrying about what myths are perpetuated by other therapists not trained in CBT should not consume your own practice. However, well-trained CBT therapists represent how other mental health professionals (and clients) perceive CBT. When reasonable, you should address these stated myths to reduce ignorance and increase quality care for clients. You will be working for agencies with other mental health providers, some of whom may be using therapeutic approaches that are not evidence-based practices. You will want to make sure that the decisions made in your agency are based on science and facts, not on anecdotes and false assumptions.

Overall, the therapy provided for our clients should be based on therapeutic approaches supported by science. Doing otherwise, knowing that evidence-based practices are available, is unethical. You can have a role in refuting such myths and making sure that clients receive quality care by educating other therapists through your interactions and participating in training. You can also demonstrate the effectiveness of CBT by having others observe your therapy sessions ("showing" can be more effective than "telling"). Just like negative automatic thoughts and core beliefs, you can help make modifications to these invalid myths.

Discussion Questions 12.1

- Why do you think some of these myths continue to exist?
- Can you think of any other CBT myths? How do you think these myths originated?
- What negative effects can such myths have on the mental health field and quality of care provided to clients?
- What can you do to help dispel some of these myths?

ACTIVITY 12.1: REFUTING CBT MYTHS

With another peer, practice debunking these myths while role-playing. Have one peer pick a myth to "believe" and another peer explain in a professional manner why that particular myth is not true. Then switch roles using a different myth. What was challenging about refuting the myths? What are different ways people can respond when you refute a myth? What CBT techniques can you use in response to those believing such myths? How did it feel playing the role of someone believing the myths?

REFERENCES

APA Presidential Task Force on Evidence-Based Practice. (2006). Evidence-based practice in psychology. *American Psychologist, 61,* 271–285.

Beck, A. T., Davis, D. D., & Freeman, A. (Eds.). (2015). *Cognitive therapy of personality disorders* (3rd ed.). New York: Guilford Press.

Cuijpers, P., Hollon, S. D., van Straten, A., Bockting, C., Berking, M., & Andersson, G. (2013). Does cognitive behavior therapy have an enduring effect that is superior to keeping patients on continuation pharmacotherapy? A meta-analysis. *British Medical Journal Open, 3,* 1–8.

Dattilio, F. M., & Hanna, M. A. (2012). Collaboration in cognitive-behavioral therapy. *Journal of Clinical Psychology, 68,* 146–158.

Friedberg, R. D., & McClure, J. M. (2015). *Clinical practice of cognitive therapy with children and adolescents: The nuts and bolts* (2nd ed.). New York: Guilford Press.

Gaston, L., & Gagnon, R. (1996). The role of process research in manual development. *Clinical Psychology: Science and Practice, 3,* 13–24.

Hofmann, S. G., Asnaani, A., Vonk, I. J. J., Sawyer, A. T., & Fang, A. (2012). The efficacy of cognitive behavioral therapy: A review of meta-analyses. *Cognitive Therapy and Research, 36,* 427–440.

James, I. A. (2010). *Cognitive behavioral therapy with older people: Interventions for those with and without dementia.* London: Jessica Kingsley.

Kroese, B. S., Dagnan, D., & Loumidis, K. (Eds.). (1997). *Cognitive-behaviour therapy for people with learning disabilities.* London: Routledge.

Montgomery, G. T., & Crowder, J. E. (1972). The symptom substitution hypothesis and the evidence. *Psychotherapy: Theory, Research and Practice, 9,* 98–102.

Najavits, L. M. (2001). *Seeking safety: A treatment manual for PTSD and substance abuse.* New York: Guilford Press.

Rector, N. A., & Beck, A. T. (2001). Cognitive behavioral therapy for schizophrenia: An empirical review. *Journal of Nervous and Mental Disease, 189,* 278–287.

Tolin, D. F. (2010). Is cognitive-behavioral therapy more effective than other therapies? A meta-analytic review. *Clinical Psychology Review, 30,* 710–720.

Wilson, G. T. (2007). Manual-based treatment: Evolution and evaluation. In T. A. Treat, R. R., Bootzin, & Baker, T. (Eds.). *Psychological Clinical Science: Papers in Honor of Richard M. McFall.* New York: Psychology Press.

Wright, J. H., & Davis, D. (1994). The therapeutic relationship in cognitive-behavioral therapy: Patient perceptions and therapist responses. *Cognitive and Behavioral Practice, 1,* 25–45.

13

Being a Competent CBT Therapist

CBT and its techniques is an evidence-based practice—its effectiveness is supported by many years of research. However, that effectiveness is determined by each therapist's level of competence, which includes both knowledge and skills to provide therapy at a level that produces its desired effects (Fairburn & Cooper, 2011). Not all therapists' skills are equal both within CBT-trained therapists and between CBT-trained therapists and therapists trained in other theoretical orientations. No therapist can be an expert in every area of therapy. However, competence in the populations and problems you are working with is a must. All therapists have the responsibility to provide the best possible therapy to all clients. Research shows that the number of years in practice and level of education (i.e., master's vs. PhD) does not determine therapeutic effectiveness (Seligman, 1995). Rather, it is theoretical orientation based on evidence-based practice (e.g., CBT) and quality of training (Lilienfeld, 2007, 2014). However, although training begins in graduate school, it does not end there. Training should continue indefinitely after graduation as long as one is in practice. You do not want to become stagnant in your knowledge and skills after you receive your graduate degree. This chapter addresses key domains to consider, both professionally and personally, while progressing as a competent CBT therapist throughout your career.

PRACTICE WHAT YOU PREACH

Part of being a competent therapist is not only fine-tuning one's in-session skills but also practicing many of these skills on yourself, especially when distressed. It is not pragmatic to practice every CBT technique on yourself, but there are many techniques that can be naturally integrated into your own daily life. Having experience of what it is like to be on the receiving end of some CBT techniques provides therapists with greater self-awareness and insight that can translate into greater skill competency and empathy when working with clients. Examples of CBT techniques you can practice on yourself include monitoring daily activities and behavior activation, monitoring and modifying negative automatic thoughts (and emotions), identifying and modifying core beliefs, and using exposure techniques for many anxieties. There are also books specifically developed to help therapists with self-awareness CBT techniques. For example, Bennett-Levy, Thwaites, Haarhoff, and Perry's (2015) book *Experiencing CBT from the Inside Out: A Self-Practice/Self-Reflection Workbook for Therapists* is specifically designed for CBT therapists to practice a variety of CBT techniques, including step-by-step instructions and opportunities for self-reflection. In fact, research has shown that even experienced CBT therapists who engage in self-practice/self-reflection are able to enhance both technical cognitive therapy skills and interpersonal empathic skills (Davis, Thwaites, Freeston, & Bennett-Levy, 2015). Of course, no matter how good a therapist you may be, you can never be your own therapist. If you notice that you are experiencing significant distress, it always best to seek therapy from another trained CBT therapist.

If you find yourself having a strong aversion to practicing even some of the simpler CBT techniques, this could be a possible area of concern. If you do not see the benefit of using these empirically supported techniques on yourself (e.g., "this is stupid" or "this won't work on me"), this will most likely be noticed by your clients, resulting in your coming off as disingenuous and, in turn, reducing their hope and motivation for change and having poor treatment outcomes.

CONSIDER THERAPY WITH A CBT THERAPIST

If possible, consider being in the client's chair to be on the receiving end of therapy with a CBT therapist. Of course, consider this option only if you are experiencing enough distress where you think you could benefit from some therapeutic assistance. (If you are a graduate student, you are probably experiencing at least some type of distress!) It is helpful to know the experience of what it is like to be in the other chair. By being a client, you can learn what you find helpful and what you do not find helpful, ranging from basic therapeutic alliance skills to specific CBT skills. You may consider modifying your therapeutic approach after having more awareness of particular experiences from your clients' perspective. Also, receiving CBT from a competent therapist can help you manage your own personal distress. This is good for your own personal growth and the well-being of your clients.

ACTUALLY DO CBT WITH YOUR CLIENTS

CBT requires significant training and a strong skill set in order to be effective. It is easy to "stray" from adherence to the CBT model if you are feeling insecure about your CBT skills and overwhelmed with many clients or a lot of paperwork. Nevertheless, it is important to continue developing you CBT skills, especially early in training. Like learning any new skill, you will learn the most through continuous practice and application. Just like with your clients, if there is some initial anxiety (which is completely normal!), "confront" your apprehension by gradually integrating new behaviors/skills into your daily practice. With time and support (i.e., supervision), you will find that your anxiety will decrease while your self-efficacy as a CBT therapist increases. A helpful aid to ensure that your sessions are appropriately following the CBT model is the Cognitive Therapy Rating Scale (CTRS; Young & Beck, 1980). The CTRS provides feedback across 11 domains: agenda, feedback, understanding, interpersonal effectiveness, collaboration, pacing and efficient use of time, guided discovery, focusing on key cognitions or behaviors, strategy for change, application of cognitive-behavioral techniques, and homework. The rating system allows for detailed feedback on strengths and areas in need of improvement. The CTRS can also be used as part of your supervision.

RECEIVE CBT SUPERVISION

It is vital that you receive CBT supervision as part of your training and post-graduate practice. The more experienced your supervisor is in CBT, the greater potential for you to learn and master CBT skills (Moldovan & David, 2013). (If you truly want a CBT supervision experience, be wary of potential supervisors who say that they are "familiar" with CBT or insist that their theoretical orientation is not important.) No therapist in training can truly develop and master their CBT skills only by reading books. Reading appropriate materials and practicing skills in class and internships is a good start. But in order to truly develop CBT skills, you will need to be supervised by a skilled licensed therapist who specializes in CBT. Of course, supervision is important at any point in your career, but it is especially important early in your career (or early in your transition to starting CBT) to get the best start possible. A good supervisor will help ensure your adherence to CBT theory and skills and overall treatment fidelity. Ideally, it is best to have your supervisor observe your sessions live (e.g., one-way mirror, video feed, or earbud). If this is not possible, then video or audio recorded sessions are also appropriate. Essentially, any type of live/recorded session is better than a verbal report because it can provide more contextual information. Often, verbal reports can result in forgetting important information, misinterpreting information, and the desire to present oneself in a positive light. Additionally, live/recorded sessions allow for continuous assessment of therapeutic skills and self-reflection. Overall, research consistently shows that live/recorded session supervision is better than verbal reports (Bartle-Haring, Silverthorn, Meyer, & Toviessi, 2009; Champe & Kleist, 2003). A highly recommend resource for CBT supervision is the Cognitive-Behavior Therapy Supervision Checklist (CBTSC; Sudak, Wright, Bienenfeld, & Beck, 2001). The purpose of this checklist is to monitor and evaluate

CBT competencies. It is divided into two parts: (a) competencies demonstrated for each session and (b) competencies demonstrated throughout the process of therapy (i.e., early, middle, and late phases). The CBTSC and the CRTRS (noted earlier) allow supervisors to formally assess and provide feedback to their supervisees session by session and throughout the course of therapy.

Another great option is group CBT supervision, which can both help you develop your technical skills and assist your conceptualization and treatment plan skills. Group supervision may also provide the added option of watching other therapists at varying skill levels do CBT (see the next section). If necessary, you can also develop your own peer supervision group with other colleagues within your community. Such CBT supervision groups allow for discussing challenging cases, exchanging knowledge about specific skills, and emergency consultation. As much as supervision is important while in training and pursing licensure, it should not end there. Supervision should always be an integral part of your practice regardless of skill level and years of experience.

OBSERVE OTHER THERAPISTS CONDUCT SESSIONS

Observing other CBT therapists conduct sessions, either live or recorded, is a great way to learn and refine your therapeutic skills. Ideally, the best way to promote the opportunity to observe CBT in action is to work with other therapists who actively practice CBT. Although it is helpful to watch well-trained and experienced professionals, especially for refining skills, it is also important to observe other therapists who are at a similar level of experience as you. It can sometimes be intimidating if you watch only experts successfully complete a skill. Sometimes, learning is most effective when the individuals performing the task are similar to the observer.

CONTINUE BUILDING CONCEPTUALIZATION SKILLS

Most suggestions for building and refining competence focus on building in-session therapeutic skills. This is necessary, but just as important is continuing to refine your conceptualization skills through a CBT lens. Remember that the effectiveness of your CBT skills is only as strong as your CBT case formulation and treatment plan. In other words, expert CBT skills have little value if clients' problems and associated distress are not appropriately assessed. A good resource to monitor your CBT conceptualization skills is the Cognitive Formulation Rating Scale (CFRS) developed by the Academy of Cognitive Therapy (http://www.academyofct.org). The CFRS focuses on three domains: case history, formulation, and treatment plan and course of therapy. Receiving feedback from your supervisors and other experienced CBT therapists on your CBT case formulation is a great way to enhance your CBT conceptualization skills.

CONTINUE TRAINING AFTER GRADUATION

Your training in CBT skills should not end after graduation, nor does it have to be confined to your CBT supervision. There are many options to continue professional training in CBT well after graduation and licensure. Be sure to continuously read peer-reviewed articles, books, and treatment manuals. There are also quality professional newsletters and blogs that cover modern CBT-related topics. The Beck Institute provides a high-quality active blog across multiple CBT-related topics (http://www.beckinstitute.org/blog). Additionally, attend CBT-related talks and workshops for additional live, up-to-date training. You will most likely find that your local colleges/universities and mental health agencies host CBT training. Finally, attending professional conferences is a great way to keep up to date with both the most recent research in the field and therapeutic skills being used in practice. For example, the Association for Behavioral and Cognitive Therapies (http://www.abct.org) is a great organization to maintain a professional affiliation with as a practicing CBT therapist, including their active listservs, newsletter, and opportunities to network. Also, as referenced throughout this book, the Academy of Cognitive Therapy (http://www.academyofct.org) provides a wealth of information related to training and research in CBT. Overall, a competent CBT therapist is able to stay up to date with evidence-based practices. Like all theoretical approaches, CBT evolves over time. You do not want to be using all of the same techniques 15 years from now that you are using today. Although some techniques may not change and others may be only slightly modified, there may be a few significant shifts in the field that you will need to keep up with.

Discussion Questions 13.1

- Are there any particular CBT techniques that you think would be challenging to try on yourself? How can it be a problem if a CBT therapist has a strong aversion to practicing CBT techniques?
- What are your thoughts about considering being a client with a CBT therapist? What do you hope you could get out of this experience?
- What CBT technique(s) are you the most anxious to try with your clients? What are ways for you to confront and overcome this anxiety?
- What are some possible indicators to determine if you are receiving quality CBT supervision? What type of feedback from your supervisor do you think would be most beneficial to your professional development? What are your anxieties about recording your sessions for review during supervision?
- How would observing other therapists providing CBT be most beneficial to your development as CBT therapist?
- What CBT conceptualization skills do you think is the most challenging for you?
- Can you think of any other ways to maintain your competence as a CBT therapist?
- What are some possible negative outcomes if you do not stay up to date with CBT knowledge and skills?

ACTIVITY 13.1: PRACTICE FOR CBT COMPETENCE

If possible, video or audio record one of your CBT sessions (preferably middle phase) with one of your clients (be sure to receive informed consent!). If this is not possible, you can role-play a session with one of your peers. After the session, complete a Cognitive Therapy Rating Scale. You can also ask your supervisor and/or a more experienced colleague to rate the session. Compare your ratings with those of your supervisor and/or colleague. What is similar? What is different? Review your current strengths and consider options to reinforce them. Review you current areas in need of improvement and develop a corrective plan of action with goals that are objective and measurable. In the future, record future sessions and compare your scores to track improvement in your CBT skills.

REFERENCES

Bartle-Haring, S., Silverthorn, B. C., Meyer, K., & Toviessi, P. (2009). Does live supervision make a difference? A multilevel analysis. *Journal of Marital and Family Therapy, 35*, 406–414.

Bennett-Levy, J. Thwaites, R., Haarhoff, B., & Perry H. (2015). *Experiencing CBT from the inside out: A self-practice/self-reflection workbook for therapists.* New York: Guilford Press.

Champe, J., & Kleist, D. M. (2003). Live supervision: A review of the research. *The Family Journal: Counseling and Therapy for Couples and Families, 11*, 268–275.

Davis, M. L., Thwaites, R., Freeston, M. H., & Bennett-Levy. J. (2015). A measureable impact of a self-practice/self-reflection programme on the therapeutic skills of experienced cognitive-behavioural therapists. *Clinical Psychology and Psychotherapy, 22*, 176–184.

Fairburn, C. G., & Cooper, Z. (2011). Therapist competence, therapy quality, and therapist training. *Behaviour Research and Therapy, 49*, 373–378.

Lilienfeld, S. O. (2007). Psychological treatments that cause harm. *Perspectives on Psychological Science, 2*, 53–70.

Lilienfeld, S. O. (2014). The dodo bird verdict: Status 2014. *The Behavior Therapist, 37*, 91–95.

Moldovan, R., & David, D. (2013). The impact of supervisor characteristics on trainee outcome in clinical supervision: A brief report. *Journal of Cognitive and Behavioral Psychotherapies, 13*, 517–527.

Seligman, M. E. P. (1995). The effectiveness of psychotherapy: The *Consumer Reports* study. *American Psychologist, 50*, 965–974.

Sudak, D. M., Wright, J. H., Bienenfeld, D., & Beck, J. S. (2001). *Cognitive Therapy Supervision Checklist.* Unpublished. Available from Donna M. Sudak (donna.sudak&drexelmed.edu).

Young, J., & Beck, A. T. (1980). *Cognitive Therapy Scale Rating manual.* Philadelphia: Center for Cognitive Therapy.

Index

Academy of Cognitive Therapy: case formulation guidelines of, 57; conceptualization skills rating scale from, 332; training and research resources from, 333

acceptance: of diagnosis, *119–20*; for events and outcomes, 206

accomplishments: in activity monitoring and scheduling, 133, 136, 143, *143*, 150; core belief work and, *228*, 230; with homework as focus, 304–5, 306

activity monitoring and scheduling, 121; assessments with, 125, *126–27*, 128, 132–33, 137–39; behavior baseline assessed with, 128, 132–33; case examples of, 128–31, 137–41, 150–53; challenges and obstacles with, 136, 148, 154, *154–55*; ease/difficulty of task in, 148–49, *149*; homework assignment on, 300; interpersonal relationships and, 143, 144–46; motivation and responsibility with, 143, 148, 154, *154*; overwhelm addressed in, 148, 151, *154*; pleasure and accomplishment assessment for, 133, 136, 143, *143*, 150; practice exercises for, 131, 142, 147; psychoeducation on, 124–25, *125*, *126–27*, 128–31; review/evaluation process of, 131–33, *132*, 137–39, 142–47, *143*; stages of, 124. *See also* Daily Activity Schedule; graded task assignments; Weekly Activity Monitoring Log

adaptive functioning and thinking, 199; empathy validating, 14; interpersonal relationship examples of, 4, *5*, 6; new core beliefs leading to, 245, *246*; practice exercise for developing examples of, 6–7; quantitative difference between maladaptive and, 7; reciprocal model with, 4, *5*, 6–7, 269; Socratic techniques and encouragement of, 236. *See also* maladaptive functioning and thinking

adversarial approach, 325–26

agenda: check-in informing session, 79, 84; collaborative empiricism in, *73*, 76, 78, *102–3*, 322; in early session stage, *73*, 81–82, 84; flexibility, 81; homework review informing, 84–85; in-session shift of, 84; middle session stage summary of, 91; middle to late phase therapy shift in setting, 82, 322; prioritizing, *102*; problem review and, 90; psychoeducation on setting, 81; timing of, *103*

agoraphobia: behavioral exposure for, 278; formal symptom measures for, 94;

335

presenting symptoms assessment of, 44, 45; psychoeducation case example on, 114–16

anger: events associated with, *171*; presenting symptoms and challenges of, 22; treatment goal example for, *64*

anticipating obstacles. *See* obstacles

anxiety/anxiety disorders: assessment of patterns with, 42–45, 262–64, *265*, 266–69; avoidance behaviors with, 259–60, *261*, 281–82; behavioral exposure for, 2, 259, 277–81, 283, *283*; breathing with and for, 272–76; case example of in vivo exposure for, 99–101, 290–94; CBT effectiveness with, 3; client awareness of patterns with, *296*; coping and safety behavior with, 263, *264*, *265*, 278, 283–84, *285*; events associated with, *171*; fear differentiation from, 259; formal symptom assessment for, 54–55; intervention specificity for, *65*; motivation for change assessment with, 50–51; negative automatic thoughts with, 2, 259, 262–63, *265*, 277–81, 283, *283*; physiological response with, 263, *265*, 277, 282; PMR for, 269–72, *271*; presenting problems assessment case example for, 42–45; psychoeducation case example on, 114–16; relaxation training/techniques for, 269–77, *271*; smartphone applications for, *315–18*; sympathetic nervous system with, 263, *265*, 277, 282; as therapeutic alliance obstacle, 66; thought modification with, 2, 277–81, 283, *283*; treatment goal examples for, 63, *64*. *See also* catastrophizing; fearful behavior patterns; panic attacks

Anxious Patterns Record, *265*

articles. *See* books/articles

assessments: with activity monitoring, 125, *126–27*, 128, 132–33, 137–39; of anxiety behavior patterns, 42–45, 262–64, *265*, 266–69; automatic thoughts, 41–42; case examples of, 42–48; CBT compatibility, *36*, 36–38, *60*, *68*; CBT-specific, 35–36, *36*, 38–49, *41*;

challenges to, 67, *68*; during check-in, 79–80; client self-report, 42, 78, 80–81, 91, 95, 99–100, 125, 128, 312–13; DSM diagnosis and, 35, 59; of event–thought–emotion–behavior patterns, 40–42, *41*, 46–48, 79–80; formal, for core beliefs, 225, *256*; formal symptom, *36*, 53–57, 94; of goal and problem-solving ability, 38; of hope/optimism, 49, 50, 52, 53; mood and symptom, in early session stage, *73*, 79–81; of motivation and responsibility for change, *36*, 49–53; of presenting problems and symptoms, 35–36, *36*, 38–49, *41*, *73*, 79–81; pre-session formal, 72, *73*, 78, 80; therapeutic alliance, 37; on Therapy Session Worksheet, *75*; treatment plan based on, 63. *See also* intake session

assets. *See* strengths/assets

Association for Behavioral and Cognitive Therapies, 333

attractiveness, therapist, 18

attributional biases, 151–52; identifying and shifting, *180*, 185–88, *186*, *187*, 192; types of, 185–86, *194*; worksheets on, *186*, *187*

automatic thoughts/negative automatic thoughts: alternative explanations for events creating, *180*, 182, 184, *184*, 205–6; with anxiety, 2, 259, 262–63, *265*, 277–81, 283, *283*; assessments, 41–42; attributional biases behind, *180*, 185–88, *186*, *187*, *192*; in avoidance/escape patterns, 260, *261*; behavioral activation impact on, 122, *125*; behavioral experiments for testing, 204–5; behavioral exposure evaluation of, 287, *288*; case example of modifying, 188–91; case example of recording, with NATR, 200–202; in case formulation, 57, 58, 173; catastrophizing and, *180*, 181–82, *183*, *194*, 277–78; challenges/considerations for working with, 165–66, *166*, 206, *206*; client ability for identifying, 37–38, 40–42, 165–66, *166*, 206, *207*; client-specific emotions associated with, 160, *170*, 170–71; cognitive distortions relationship to, 179, *181*, 192–93, *194*, 195; cognitive rehearsal for, 203–4, *204*; coping methods for, 159, *160*, 205, 206, 322; core beliefs identified through, 209, 210, 211, *213*, 217–20, *221*, *234*, *256*; defining, 158; of depressed clients, 1; distress levels with, 38; early phase assessment of, 41–42; elements of, 158–59, *159*; eliciting/identifying techniques for, 163–73, *166*, *170*, *171*, *172*; emotions relationship to, 158, *159*, 160, 165, *170*, 170–71; evaluation and modification techniques for, 2, 179–205, *180*, *181*, *183*, *184*, *186*, *187*, *194*, *196–97*, *204*, 277–81, 283, *283*, 287, *288*; evaluation process for, 173–78; events perception and, 157, 161; follow-up questions with discovery of, 165, *166*; homework on, 97–98, 172, *172*, 301; hypothesizing technique for, 166; images and imagery relationship with, 158, *159*, 161–62, 164, 168; impact of believing, *180*, 184–85; intake focus on, *36*, 40; in maladaptive functioning, 6, 7, 157, 209; modification of anxious, 2, 277–81, 283, *283*; mood shifts in discovery of, 164, *166*; overview for working with, 157; past experience basis for, 159, *159*, 161; practice exercise for modifying, 192; psychoeducation on, *108*, 111, 159, 160–63; recording with NATR, 195, *196–97*, 198–200, 202–3; role play for eliciting, 168–69; self-monitoring and modification of, 7–8; self-perpetuation of, 158, *159*, 161; self separation from, *180*, 185; "shorthand" form of, 158, *159*, 161–62, 164; Socratic techniques for evaluation of, 179–88, *180*, *181*, *183*, *184*, *186*, *187*, 198; timing of distress with, 164–65, *166*; tracking of, 97–98, 172, *172*, 301; treatment goal examples for, *64*; utility measure for, 159, *160*; validity assumption with, 158, *159*; validity

evaluation for, 159, *160*, 179–81, *180*, *181*, 204–6. *See also* event–thought– emotion–behavior patterns
Automatic Thoughts Questionnaire, 225
avoidance/escape behaviors: with anxiety, 259–60, *261*, 281–82; as maintaining factor, 40; reinforcement of, 260, *261*

Bandura, Albert, 2, 3
Beck, Aaron T.: on behavioral activation, 121; on cognitive distortions, 193; cognitive therapy origins with, 1–3; on core beliefs, 210; on psychoanalysis, 1–2
Beck, J. S.: on automatic thoughts, 159, 164, 166, 179; on core beliefs, 210, 212; on homework concerns, 305
Beck Depression Inventory, 63, *64*
Beck Institute, 333
behavior: activity monitoring log for baseline, 128, 132–33; anxiety/fear coping, 263, *264*, *265*, 278, 283–84, *285*; assessment questions on, *41*; in case formulation, 58; homework considerations with, 300; inactivity and distress cycle of, *123*, *125*; self-monitoring and modification of, 7–8; therapist expertness in, 17; thoughts and emotions reciprocal relationship with, 2, 3, *4*, *5*, 6–7, 40–42, *41*, 269
behavioral activation: behavioral exposure compared with, 122; case examples of, 128–31, 137–41, 144–46; challenges/ considerations for, 154, *154–55*; collaborative relationship and, 123, *154*; in depression treatment, 121–22; forms of, 123–24; implementation timing and factors for, 122–23; intervention specificity for, *65*; for maladaptive functioning, 122, *125*, 131; on negative automatic thoughts, 122, *125*; principles of, 121, 122, *125*; psychoeducation influence on, 124–25. *See also* activity monitoring and scheduling; Daily Activity Schedule; graded task assignments; Weekly Activity Monitoring Log

behavioral experiments: for activity planning, 136, 143, *143*; for automatic thought "testing," 204–5; for client autonomy, *27*; for core belief modification and creation, *237*, 244, 245, 249–51, *251–52*, 253–55; practice exercise on core belief, 255

behavioral exposure: anxious thought modification and, 2, 277–81, 283, *283*; automatic thoughts evaluation in, 287, *288*; for avoidance/escape patterns, 260, 281–82; behavioral activation compared to, 122; case examples/vignettes of, 99–101, 274–76, 290–94; caution with, 281–82, 289; challenges/considerations with, *288*, 289, 296, *296–97*; client autonomy goal with, 301; goals/desired outcomes for, 283, *283*, 301; hierarchy of feared situations for graded, 282–84, *283*, *285*; as homework, 99–101, 301; imaginal, 284, 286, 301, 313; practice exercises for, 269; relaxation techniques for, 269–77, *271*; safety behaviors with, 263, 287, *288*; Socratic techniques during, 286; therapy phases for introducing, 259; tracking form for, *288–89*; virtual reality, 313. *See also* in vivo exposure

behaviorists/behavioral therapy: cognitive components integrated with, 2–3; on depression, 121; history of, 2

beliefs. *See* core beliefs

Bennett-Levy, J., 330

biases: in core beliefs, 211, *211*; in maladaptive compared to adaptive functioning, 7; self-awareness of, 25–26, *27*. *See also* attributional biases

bibliotherapy, 118, 300

biological vulnerability, 210, *211*, 212

bipolar (mania), *22*

books/articles: for homework, 300; for psychoeducation, 118, 300

borderline personality disorder, *22*

brain injury, 34

breathing: for and with anxiety, 272–76; diaphragm, 273–76, *296*; meditation, 274; in PMR, 272

case examples/vignettes: of activity monitoring and scheduling, 128–31, 137–41, 150–53; of automatic thought recording with NATR, 200–202; on automatic thoughts modification, 188–91; of behavioral activation, 128–31, 137–41, 144–46; of behavioral exposure, 99–101, 274–76, 290–94; on diaphragm breathing, 274–76; of expectations discussion, 111–12; of formal symptom measures, 54–57, 94, 95, 99; on homework assignments, 95–96, 97–98, 99–101; of presenting problems assessment, 42–48; of psychoeducation, 110–12, 114–16, 128–31, 161–62, 215–16; of session structure, 85–89, 93–101; of in vivo exposure, 99–101, 290–94

case formulation: assessment/intake as base for, 35, 57, 59, *60*; automatic thought discovery shaped by, 57, 58, 173; challenges to, 67, *68*; collaborative empiricism in, 26, *27*, *68*; DSM diagnosis in, 59, *61*; form for, *60–61*; homework relationship with, 302; practice exercise for creating, 67; process and timing for, 57; psychoeducation on, *108*, 113–14; review on Therapy Session Worksheet, *76*; review with clients, 106–7, 114; sections of, 58–59; treatment plan success based on, 35, 59, 63

catastrophizing: Decatastrophizing Worksheet for addressing, *183*, 281; modification of, 278; negative automatic thoughts evaluation and, *180*, 181–82, *183*, *194*, 277–78

CBT. *See* cognitive-behavioral therapy

CBTSC. *See* Cognitive-Behavior Therapy Supervision Checklist

check-ins, session: agenda informed by, 79, 84; assessments during, 79–80; client distress and increase of, 103; early stage, *73*, 78–79

childhood: core beliefs development in, 210–11, *211*, 212; intake interview on, 32–33, *33*

classical conditioning, 2

client: activity across phases of therapy, 19–21, *20*; automatic thought/ emotions identification ability of, 37–38, 40–42, 165–66, *166*, 206, *207*; CBT compatibility assessment of, *36*, 36–38, *60*, *68*; cognitive model understanding of, 113, *119*; labeling of, 22–23; motivation challenges for, *27*, 154, *154*, *308–9*; personality traits response from therapist, 21–22, *22*; problem identification challenge for, 36; problem-solving ability of, 38, 40; progress internalization by, 142–43, 144; self-report assessments of, 42, 78, 80–81, 91, 95, 99–100, 125, 128, 312–13; therapeutic alliance impacting commitment of, 11–12; vulnerability, 71. *See also* note taking, client; therapeutic alliance; therapist–client relationship; *specific topics*

client autonomy: with behavioral exposure, 301; challenges with, *27*; encouragement of, 7–8, *27*, 301, 324; homework collaboration and, 304; psychoeducation aiding, 105; psychoeducation on, *108*; within session structure, 71, 72

client information: demographic and background, 32, *33*, *60*; intake session gathering of, 31–35, *33*; omission of, 53; pre-session review of, 72, *73*, 77–78

client-specific factors: anticipated obstacles based on, 66; CBT focus on, 321–22; homework considerations with, 300–301; interventions based on, 64; in session structure challenges, *103*; in technology use, 314; in therapeutic alliance, 21–26, *22*, 35, 66

Client Therapy Notes Worksheet, *83*, 91, 93, 302. *See also* note taking, client

cognitions: in case formulation, 58; hot, in automatic thought discovery, 164

cognitive-behavioral hypothesis. *See* case formulation

cognitive-behavioral therapy (CBT): competency tips for therapists practicing, 329–34; history of, 1–3; model overview, 3, *4*; myths about, debunked,

8, 321–27. *See also* psychoeducation; *specific topics*

Cognitive-Behavior Therapy Supervision Checklist (CBTSC), 331–32

cognitive distortions, 217; with anxiety/ anxiety disorders, 277–78; in core belief tracking, *234*; identifying, 192–93, *194*, 195; as maintaining factor, 40; negative automatic thoughts relationship with, 179, *181*, 192–93, *194*, 195; types and examples of, *194*

cognitive model: case example of discussing, 111–12; client understanding of, 113, *119*; formal assessments in review of, 80; psychoeducation on, 106, *108*, 109–12

cognitive rehearsal, 203–4, *204*

cognitive restructuring specificity, 64–65, *65*

Cognitive Therapy of Depression (Beck, A., Rush, Shaw, and Emery), 2

Cognitive Therapy Rating Scale (CTRS), 331, 332, 334

collaborative empiricism/relationship, 11; in agenda setting, *73*, *76*, *78*, *102–3*, 322; arguing impact on, 326; behavioral activation and, 123, *154*; in case formulation and treatment plan, 26, *27*, *68*; client-specific factors in, 21–26, *22*, 35, 66; for conceptualization, 26, *27*, 57; focus of, 19, 37, 322–23; with homework assignments, 303–4; intake session as start of, *26*, 31, 57; interpersonal skills in, 17–18; motivation impacted by, 57; in negative thought modification, 179–80; with problem-solving, *73*, 90, 94; psychoeducation and, 105–6, *108*, 110; in session structure, 71; therapist–client activity level in, 19–21, *20*; in therapy expectations, *108*. *See also* therapeutic alliance

compatibility, CBT, *36*, 36–38, *60*, *68*, 325

competency, therapist: CBT dedication and, 330–31; colleague observations for, 332; with continuing education after licensure, 333; practice exercise for, 334; rating and feedback systems for, 331, 332, 334; self-practice of CBT skills and, 329–30; supervision impact on, 331–32; training quality and duration relation to, 329

conceptualization: client understanding of case, 170; collaborative empiricism for, 26, *27*, 57; core beliefs integrated in, 215; evolution of, 113; homework relationship with, 302; in middle session stage, 90; past experiences informing, 324; of problem/distress, 8; psychoeducation on, 113; skills building and refinement, 332; skills rating scale, 332

conditioning, 2

confidentiality, 18

consistency: across case formulation and treatment plan, 63; in session structure, 71

continuing education, 333

coping skills and behavior: anxiety/fear, 263, *264*, *265*, 278, 283–84, *285*; for core belief work, *227*, 229, 249, *251*; emotion-focused, *64*, 159, *160*, 205, 206, 322; identifying, *227*, 229, 283–84; problem-focused, *64*, 159, *160*, 205, 206; for worst-case scenarios, 181–82, 279, 280

Core Belief Flowchart, *226*, *227–28*

core beliefs: advantages/disadvantages list for, 238–39, *239*, 243–44; automatic thoughts origin with, 209, 210, 211, *213*, 217–20, *221*, *234*, *256*; behavioral experiments for, *237*, 244, 245, 249–51, *251–52*, 253–55; benefits of treating negative, 212, 214; categories, elements, and lens of, *210*, 210–12, *211*, *227*, 228, *234*, 235, *256*; challenges/ considerations for working with, 256, *256–57*; client awareness of, 218, 220, 234, *256*; client note taking on, *238*, 238–39, *239*; continuum view for, 240–41, *241*; coping skills for working with, *227*, 229, 249, *251*; development of, 210–11, *211*, 212, *213*, 225–26, *226*, *227–28*, 228–33; downward-arrow technique for identifying, 218–20, *221*, 222–24; emotions reinforcing, 211, 217; evaluation and modification of,

205, 209, 211, *211*, 220, 234–36, *237*, *238*, 238–50, *239*, *241*, *246*, *251–52*, 253–55, *257*; events activating, 211, 212, *227*, 229; formal assessments of, 225, *256*; history and domain of, 225–26, *226*, *227–28*, 228–33; homework on, 234, *234*, *251–52*, 301; identifying, 217–20, *221*, 222–26, *226*, *227–28*, 229–34, *234*, *256*; intermediate beliefs impact on, 214; interpersonal relationships behind, 212, *213*, 225–26, *226*, *227*, 228; modification of old/ creation of new, 245–49, *246*, *257*; new, evidence and enforcement, 236, 238, *238*, 245–50, *246*, *251–52*, 253–55, *257*; old compared to new, 245, *246*, *251–52*, *257*; positive, reinforcement, 211, *211*, 212, 234; practice exercises for identifying, 224, 233; practice exercises for modifying, 248–49; practice exercises for review of, 255; process overview for working with, 209; psychoeducation on, 214–16; self-perpetuation of negative, 211, *211*, 215; self separated from, 239–40; sociocultural factors in, *228*, 229–30; Socratic techniques for working with, 211, 217, 236, *237*, *238*, 238–41, *239*, *241*, *256–57*; tracking, 234, *234*; validity/evidence of, 235, 236, *237*, 238, *238*, 241–43, 244, *256*

cross-sectional view, 58, *61*

CTRS. *See* Cognitive Therapy Rating Scale

Daily Activity Schedule: case example of creating, 139–41; challenges with, *154–55*; features of, 133; form for, *134–35*; GTAs supplementing, 148; practice exercise in creating, 142; practice exercise in reviewing, 147; review/evaluation process with, 142–47, *143*; Weekly Activity Monitoring Log informing, 133

Decatastrophizing Worksheet, *183*, 281

demographic and background information, 32, *33*, *60*

depression: behavioral activation treatment for, 121–22; CBT history and effectiveness with, 2–3; development of, 2; events associated with, *171*; formal symptom measures for, 55–56; internalization of environmental stressors in, 24; intervention specificity for, 64, *65*; motivation for change with, 51–52; negative automatic thoughts with, 1; presenting problems assessment case example for, 45–48; presenting symptoms and challenges of, *22*; psychoeducation on activity monitoring case example for, 128–31; smartphone applications for, *316*, *318*; treatment goal example for, 63, *64*

desensitization, systematic, 2

development and life history: in case formation, *60*; in intake interview, 32–33, *33*

diagnosis: case example of discussing, 114–16; client acceptance of, *119–20*; DSM, 35, 59, *61*; psychoeducation on, *108*, 113–16; technology aids for, 312

Diagnostic and Statistical Manual of Mental Disorders (DSM) diagnosis: assessment limited by, 35, 59; case formulation including, 59, *61*

diaphragm breathing: case example of teaching, 274–76; challenges/considerations with, *296*; for panic attacks, 272; practice exercise for, 276; steps and guidance for, 273–76

dichotomous thinking, *194*

diplomas, display of, 17

distress: check-in priority with, *103*; conceptualization of, 8; inactivity and, *123*, *125*; levels with automatic thoughts, 38; problem-focused coping during, 206; timing with automatic thoughts, 164–65, *166*

domain, core belief, 225–26, *226*, *227–28*, 228–33

downward-arrow technique, 218–20, *221*, 222–24

DSM diagnosis. *See Diagnostic and Statistical Manual of Mental Disorders* diagnosis

Dysfunctional Attitude Scale, 225

Early Phase Psychoeducation Worksheet, *108*

early phase therapy: activity level in, 20, *20*; activity monitoring and review case example in, 137–39; behavioral activation techniques in, 122; for behavioral exposure introduction, 259; client note taking introduced in, 82; early session stage case example in, 85–86; homework beginning in, 300; late session stage case example in, 93–96; psychoeducation in, 106–7, *108*, 109–16

early session stage: activity monitoring and review case example in, 137–39; agenda setting and modification in, *73*, 81–82, 84; check-in at, *73*, 78–79; core belief behavioral experiment in, 253–55; early phase therapy case example of, 85–86; homework in, *73*, 84–85; late phase therapy case example of, 88–89; medications review in, 81; middle phase therapy case example of, 86–88; mood and symptom check in, *73*, 79–81; role play activity for, 89; structure overview of, *73*

Ellis, Albert, 2, 3, 325

Emery, G., 2, 121

emotion-focused coping: for automatic thoughts, 159, *160*, 205, 206, 322; as therapy goal/strategy, 64, *160*

emotions: assessment questions for, *41*; automatic thoughts elicited/identified with, 163–68, *166*; automatic thoughts experienced as, 158, *159*, 160, 165, *170*, 170–71; in case formulation, 58; client ability to identify, 37–38; in core belief discovery, 220; core beliefs reinforced by, 211, 217; empathy in validation of, 13, 14, 326; events associated with negative, 171, *171*; thoughts and behavior reciprocal relationship with, 2, 3, *4*, *5*, 6–7, 40–42, *41*, 269; thoughts differentiated from, 169–71, *207*; thoughts modification over, 169, 322

empathy: defining, 12–13; difficulty finding, 23, *27*; in emotions validation,

13, 14, 326; expressions of, 13–14; for financial stressors, 15; sample scenarios involving, 14–16; in therapist–client relationship, 12–16, 23, *27*, 326; vigilant, 23

environmental stressors. *See* external/ environmental stressors

escape. *See* avoidance/escape behaviors

events/situations: alternative explanations for negatively perceived, *180*, 182, 184, *184*, 205–6; core beliefs activated by, 211, 212, *227*, 229; memory creation from, 33; negative emotions associated with, 171, *171*; outcomes from threatening, 264, *265*, 278; perception of, impact on thoughts, 157, 161; problem-focused coping for negative, 206; triggering types of, 262, 264, *265*. *See also* hierarchy of feared situations

event–thought–emotion–behavior patterns: assessment of, 40–42, *41*, 46–48, 79–80; check-in assessment of, 79–80; cognitive rehearsal for, 203–4, *204*; focus priority on, 157; guide imagery and, 168; late session stage work on, 98–99; NATR for identifying/modifying, 195, *196–97*, 198–200; psychoeducation on, 114–16, 171; responsibility pie worksheet for evaluating, 186–88, *187*; tracking of, 172, *172*

evidence. *See* science-based approach; validity/evidence

examples, real-life: psychoeducation use of, 117; therapy use of, 41–42

expectations, therapy: case example of discussing, 111–12; motivation relationship with, 49, 107; psychoeducation outlining, 107, *108*, 109–12

Experiencing CBT from the Inside Out: A Self-Practice/Self-Reflection Workbook for Therapists (Bennett-Levy, Thwaites, Haarhoff, and Perry), 330

expertness, therapist: agenda setting and, 82; session structure and, 71; therapeutic alliance enhanced by, 17, 71

external/environmental stressors: consideration in therapeutic alliance, 23–25; empathy for, 15; intake interview on, 34; internalization and externalization of, 24–25; as obstacles to treatment, 66–67; in reciprocal model cycle, 3, *4*, *5*, *7*. *See also* sociocultural factors

family relationships. *See* childhood; interpersonal relationships

family therapy, 14–16

fearful behavior patterns, 2; anxiety contrasted with, 259; assessment of, 42–45, 262–64, *265*, 266–69; behavior exposure goals for, 283, *283*; client awareness of, *296*; coping and safety behavior with, 263, *264*, *265*, 278, 283–84, *285*; intervention specificity for, 65; outcomes and probability evaluation with, 182, 278–79; physiological response with, 263, *265*, 277, 282; relaxation training for, 269–77, *271*; smartphone applications for, *315–18*; sympathetic system and, 282. *See also* hierarchy of feared situations

feedback and questions, 165, *166*; assessment continuum with, 53; client challenges with providing, *27*; on formal symptom measures, 53, *68*, 78; in late session stage, 93, 96, 98–99; in middle session stage, 91; for therapist competency, 331, *332*, 334

Ferster, C. B., 121

financial stressors: empathy for, 15; as obstacle to treatment, 66–67

flexibility: in agenda, 81; in session structure, 72, 81–82, *102*; in treatment approach, 8, 18, 35, 68, 321–22

formal symptom measures: administration and applicability of, *36*, 53–54, 57; case examples of, 54–57, 94, 95, 99; in case formation, *60*; feedback on, 53, *68*, 78; pre-session, 72, *73*, 78, 80

friendships. *See* interpersonal relationships

future, 2

generalized anxiety disorder (GAD). *See* anxiety/anxiety disorders

genuineness, 12–13, 16

goals/desired outcomes: for behavioral exposure, 283, *283*, 301; client ability to work toward, 38, 40; of client autonomy, 7–8, *27*, 301; emotion-focused coping in, *64*, *160*; external stressors impacting, 66–67; foundation for, 63; intake interview informing, 35; interventions linked to, 64, 67, *68*, 77–78; problem-focused coping as, *64*, 159; process objectives aiding, 77–78; psychoeducation on, *108*, 110; sociocultural factors informing, 35; on Therapy Session Worksheet, *75*; treatment plan outlining, *62*, 63–64, *64*; wording of, *63*, 63–64

graded task assignments (GTAs): Daily Activity Schedule supplemented with, 148; introducing, 148–49, *149*, 150–53; motivation issues addressed with, 148–49, 150; pleasure/accomplishment assessment for, 150; practice exercise in creating, 154; visual aid for explaining, *149*

Haarhoff, B., 330

Haigh, E. A. P., 7

Harper, R. A., 2

health history. *See* medical and mental health history

helplessness, 210, *210*, 227

hierarchy of feared situations: for behavioral exposure, 282–84, *283*, *285*; in vivo exposure use of, 286–87; intervention specificity for, *65*; timing with exposure to, 289

history: CBT, 1–3; client, 32–33, *33*, 34, 60; of core beliefs, 225–26, *226*, *227*–28, 228–33

homework: on activity monitoring and scheduling, 300; agenda informed with review of, 84–85; Anxious Patterns Record, *265*; assignment factors, 300–301; on automatic thoughts tracking/evaluating, 97–98, 172, *172*, 301; behavioral exposure as, 99–101, 301; books/articles for, 300; case examples of assigning, 95–96, 97–98, 100–101; CBT skill practice as, 301; challenges/considerations with, 300, 305–8, *308–9*; clarity in assigning, 302; collaborative development of, 303–4; completion obstacles/considerations, 307; compliance strategies, 302–4, *308–9*; core belief, 234, *234*, *251–52*, 301; on diaphragm breathing, 274; in early session stage, *73*, 84–85; on events and negative emotions connection, 171, *171*; focus on success/accomplishment with, 304–5, 306; individualization of, 303; in-session initiation of, 303; late session stage assignment of, 92, 94, 95–96, 97–98, 99–101; motivation considerations with, 84–85, 300, 302–4, *308–9*; notebook provided for, 117–18; obstacle foresight with, 305–6; PMR for, 272; practice exercise for non-compliance of, 307; psychoeducation on, *108*, 110–11; on relaxation techniques, 301; reminders, 305; reviewing, 86, 87–88, 230–33, 306–7; session preparation as, 301; smartphone application for, *316*; on Therapy Session Worksheet, *76*; therapy success with compliance with, 299; time allocated for, 299; timing for introduction of, 300; visualization meditation for, 277. *See also* activity monitoring and scheduling; graded task assignments

hope/optimism, 96; assessment of therapy, 49, 50, 52, 53; negative automatic thoughts impact on, 122; psychoeducation aiding, 106

humanistic approach, 12–13

hyperventilation, 272–73

hypothesis, working, 58–59, *61*, 166

imagery: automatic thoughts appearing as, 158, *159*, 161–62, 164, 168; automatic thoughts elicited with guided, 168;

behavioral exposure through, 284, 286, 301, 313; meditation using, 277; in PMR, 272

imaginal exposure, 284, 286, 301, 313

insomnia, *315*

intake session: automatic thought patterns identified in, *36*, 40; case formulation from, 35, 57, 59, *60*; collaborative empiricism beginning at, *26*, 31, 57; formal symptom assessment at, 53–54; information gathered at, 31–35, *33*; information left-out at, 53

intelligence: CBT compatibility and, 36–37, 325; psychoeducation and, 118

interpersonal relationships: activity scheduling and, 143, 144–46; adaptive compared to maladaptive functioning in, 4, *5*, 6; anxiety coping behaviors with, 263, *264*; in case formation, *60*; core belief developments with, 212, *213*, 225–26, *226*, *227*, 228; depression and, 46, 47–48; intake interview on, 32–33, *33*, 34; panic attacks and, 44, 45; presenting problems impacting, 34

interpersonal skills, 17–18

interventions: Daily Activity Schedule review informing, 142; goals linked to, 64, 67, *68*, 77–78; sociocultural factors informing, 35; on Therapy Session Worksheet, *75*; in treatment plan, *62*, 64–65, *65*; wording specificity of, 64, 64–65

in vivo exposure: case examples of, 99–101, 290–94; challenges/considerations with, *296–97*; as homework, 301; imaginal compared with, 284, 301; review of, 289; steps for, 286–87, 289–94; tracking form for, *288–89*; virtual reality therapy for, 313

labeling, 22–23

late phase therapy: activity level in, 20, *20*; agenda setting shift in, 82, 322; core belief behavioral experiment in, 253–55; early session stage case example in, 88–89; homework in, 99–101, 302; late

session stage case example in, 99–101; mentor–protégé relationship in, 21, 82; psychoeducation in, 117

late session stage: client note taking in, 93; early phase therapy case example in, 93–96; feedback and questions in, 93, 96, 98–99; homework assignment in, 92, 94, 95–96, 97–98, 99–101; late phase therapy case example of, 99–101; middle phase therapy case example of, 97–99; role play activity for, 101; structure overview for, *73*, 91–92; summaries in, 92, 93–94, 97, 100

learning theory, 259

Lewinsohn, P. M., 121

longitudinal view, 58, *61*

lovability/unlovability, 210, *210*, *227*

magnification/minimization, *194*, 277

maintaining factors. *See* precipitating and maintaining factors

maladaptive functioning and thinking: adaptive thinking quantitative difference with, 7; automatic thoughts in, 6, 7, 157, 209; behavioral activation for, 122, *125*, 131; in case formulation, 58; core beliefs reinforced by, 211, 217; developing examples of, 6–7; empathy and reinforcement of, 13; identification and "testing" of, 19, 25, 26; interpersonal relationship examples of, 4, *5*, 6; treatment goal examples for, *64*

mania. *See* bipolar

medical and mental health history: in case formation, *60*; in intake interview, *33*, 34

medications: in-session review of, 81; intake interview on, 34; technology assisting in, 312

meditation: breathing, 274; visualization, 277

Meichenbaum, Donald, 2, 3

memory: assessment from client, 42; automatic thoughts discovery through, 164; events creating "permanent," 33. *See also* past experience

mental status exam, 34–35

mentor–protégé relationship, 21, 82

middle phase therapy: activity level in, 20, *20*; agenda setting shift in, 82, 322; for behavioral exposure introduction, 259; early session stage case example in, 86–88; homework in, 302; late session stage case example in, 97–99; psychoeducation in, 117; summaries in, 91

middle session stage: feedback in, 91; problem review in, 90; structure overview for, *73*, 89–90

mind reading, 167, *194*

mood and symptom check: in early session stage, *73*, 79–81; formal ranking approach to, 79

mood disorder tracker, *315*

mood shifts, 164, *166*

motivation/responsibility for change: with activity monitoring and scheduling, 143, 148, 154, *154*; in activity scheduling, 143, 148; assessment of, *36*, 49–53; with behavioral exposure, *296–97*; in case formation, *60*; client challenges with, *27*, 154, *154*, *308–9*; collaboration impacting, 57; expectations impacting, 49, 107; GTAs and, 148–49, 150; homework and, 84–85, 300, 302–4, *308–9*; internal and external compared in, 49, 53; negative automatic thoughts impact on, 122; psychoeducation aiding, 106; technology aiding, 312; validation improving, *27*

multicultural therapy, 26

muscle tension. *See* progressive muscle relaxation

myths, CBT, 8, 321–27

Negative Automatic Thought Record (NATR), 195, *196–97*; case example of, 200–202; practice exercises for, 202–3

negative automatic thoughts. *See* automatic thoughts/negative automatic thoughts

notebook, therapy: negative automatic thought list in, *170*, 170–71; for psychoeducation, 117–18; review process of, 118

note taking, client, 77; attributional worksheet in, *186*, *187*; automatic thoughts evaluation in, 181; cognitive rehearsal and, 204; core belief work in, *238*, 238–39, *239*; introduction of, 82; late session stage review of, 93; in middle session stage, 91; notebook provided for, 117; psychoeducation on, *108*; session preparation in, 302; worksheet, *83*

note taking, therapist: after-session, 93; in-session, 77

obsessive-compulsive disorder, *315*

obstacles: anticipated, outlined in treatment plan, *62*, 65–67; therapeutic alliance, 26, *27*, 65–66

online resources. *See* technology

operant conditioning, 2

outcomes: acceptance for, 206; behavioral exposure, *288–89*; coping plan for negative, 181–82, 279, 280; perception of negative, *180*, 264, *265*; probability assessment for feared event, 182, 278–79; from triggering event, 264, *265*, 278

outcomes, desired. *See* goals/desired outcomes

overgeneralization, *194*

pacing. *See* timing and pacing

panic attacks: assessment of presenting problems for, 42–45; behavioral exposure for, 278; diaphragm breathing for, 272; formal symptom measures for, 54–55, 94; intervention specificity for, 65; psychoeducation case example on, 114–16; smartphone applications for, *315–18*; treatment goal examples for, *64*

past experience: automatic thoughts based on, 159, *159*, 161; conceptualization informed by, 324; core beliefs development from, 210, 225–26, *226*, *227–28*, 228–33; homework considerations with, 300; intake interview on, 32–34, *33*; present focus over, 324; psychoanalysis focus on, 1; with therapy impacting therapeutic alliance, *27*

Pavlov, 2

perception: alternative explanations for event, *180*, 182, 184, *184*, 205–6; automatic thoughts origins with, 157, 161; of negative outcomes, *180*, 264, *265*

perfectionism, 66

permanent stable/unstable attribution, 185–86

Perry, H., 330

personal internal/external attribution, 185–86, *194*

Personality Belief Questionnaire, 225

personality disorders, *22*, 325

personality traits, 21–22, *22*

pervasive general/specific attribution, 185–86

phases, therapy: behavioral activation techniques across, 122; for behavioral exposure introduction, 259; session structure case examples across, 85–89, 93–101; session structure shifting across, 72, 101; therapist–client activity levels in, 19–21, *20*. *See also* early phase therapy; late phase therapy; middle phase therapy

phrase, 158, *159*, 161–62

physical appearance. *See* attractiveness; presentation, physical

physiological response: with anxiety/fear, 263, *265*, 277, 282; automatic thought discovery and, 168; questions for assessment of, *41*; tracking automatic thoughts and, 172, *172*. *See also* event–thought–emotion–behavior patterns

pity, 13

pleasures assessment, 133, 136, 143, *143*, 150

PMR. *See* progressive muscle relaxation

positive thinking: alternative conclusions compared to, 205–6; false, impact, 325; myth about CBT and, 8, 324–25; realistic and rational thinking focus over, 8, 324–25

posttraumatic stress disorder (PTSD), *264*, *316–17*

precipitating and maintaining factors: assessment of, 39–40, 45–46; in case formulation, 58, *61*; for depression, 121

presentation, physical, 18; in case formation, *60*; intake interview and, *33*, *34*–35

presenting problems and symptoms: assessment case examples, 42–48; assessment in early session stage, *73*, 79–81; in case formulation, 58, *60*; CBT-specific assessment of, 35–36, *36*, 38–49, *41*; challenges/considerations in understanding, *22*, 68; client ability for identifying, 36; client sharing primary concern of, 32, *60*; daily life impact of, 39, 44, 45–46, 48; focus on, over diagnosis, *120*; formal measures of, 53–57, 94; frequency/duration and intensity of, 39, 40, 42–44, 45; homework considerations with, 300; medical history significance to, 34; multiple and intertwined, 39, 59; past experiences impact on, 324; precipitating and maintaining factors of, 39–40, 45–46; psychoeducation on, *108*, 113–16; response to, 21–22, *22*; role play activity for assessment of, 48–49; treatment focus on source of, 323–24

pre-session stage: challenge in following through with, *102*; client information review in, 72, *73*, 77–78; formal assessment in, 72, *73*, 78, 80; task overview for, *73*; Therapy Session Worksheet review in, 77–78

problem-focused coping: emotion-focused combined with, 206; as therapy goal/strategy, *64*, 159; with valid automatic thoughts, 159, *160*, 205, 206

problems. *See* presenting problems and symptoms

problems list: middle session stage review of, 90; purpose of, 63; in treatment plan, *62*, 63, 67

problem-solving techniques: client ability for, 38, 40; collaborative empiricism with, *73*, 90, 94; empowerment in distressing events with, 206; in middle session stage, 90–91; psychoeducation on, 90, 94

process objectives: goal achievement with, 77–78; middle session stage consideration of, 90; in session structure, 75, 77–78

professional affiliations, 57, 332, 333

progress: assessments, *36*, 53; client internalizing, 142–43, 144; goals wording for monitoring, *63–64, 64*

progressive muscle relaxation (PMR): applicability and steps for, 269–72, *271*; challenges/considerations with, *296*; practice exercise for, 272; template for, *271*

psychoanalysis, 1–2

psychoeducation: activity monitoring and, 124–25, *125, 126–27*, 128–31; on agenda setting, 81; on automatic thought patterns, *108*, 111, 159, 160–63; behavioral activation influenced by, 124–25; books/articles for, 118, 300; case examples of, 110–12, 114–16, 128–31, 161–62, 215–16; on case formulation, *108*, 113–14; of CBT skills, 117–18, *119–20*; challenges with, 119, *119–20*; client autonomy and, 105, *108*; on cognitive model, 106, *108*, 109–12; collaborative empiricism/relationship and, 105–6, *108*, 110; confidence with, 107; on core beliefs, 214–16; delivery methods and tips for, 109, 113, 117, 119; on diagnosis and presenting symptoms, *108*, 113–16; early phase, 106–7, *108*, 109–16; Early Phase Psychoeducation Worksheet for, *108*; on event–thought–emotion–behavior patterns, 114–16, 171; expectations for therapy outlined in, 107, *108*, 109–12; on homework, *108*, 110–11; intervention specificity for, *65*; middle and late phase therapy, 117; notebook provided for, 117–18; practicing for, 116; of problem-solving techniques, 90, 94; smartphone

application for, *318*; technology aiding, 118, 312, *318*; therapeutic alliance fostered with, 105–6, 109; therapist reluctance for, 105

PTSD. *See* Posttraumatic stress disorder

questions, session. *See* feedback and questions

racial discrimination, 67

reading and writing skills, 300

reciprocal determinism, 2

reciprocal inhibition, 2, 269

reciprocal model: breaking negative patterns of, 6, 7; of thoughts, emotions, and behaviors, 2, 3, *4, 5*, 6–7, 40–42, *41*, 269

relaxation training/techniques, 2; for anxious distress, 269–77, *271*; challenges/considerations with, *296*; diaphragm breathing in, 273–76; as homework, 301; with PMR, 269–72, *271, 296*; technology-assisted, 314, *315, 317*; visualization in, 277

responsibility attribution, 186–88, *187*, 192

rigidity, 321–22

Rogerian qualities, 12–17, 322

Rogers, Carl, 12–13

role play: automatic thoughts elicited with, 168–69; early session stage, 89; late session stage, 101; presenting problems and symptoms assessment, 48–49

Rush, A. J., 2, 121

sadness. *See* depression

safety behaviors: with anxiety/fear, 263, *264, 265*, 278, 283–84, *285*; behavioral exposure impacted by, 263, 287, *288*; therapist role in, 289

scaffolding, information, 20, 117, 172

schemas. *See* core beliefs

science-based approach, 322, 326–27

selective abstraction, *194*

self: core beliefs separate from, 239–40; core belief through lens of, *227*; depression development in relation to, 2; negative automatic thoughts separation from, *180*, 185

self-awareness, client: of anxiety patterns, *296*; CBT success and, 325, 329–30; of core beliefs, 218, 220, 234, *256*; with PMR, 270; visualization aiding, 277

self-awareness, therapist, 16; of biases and stereotypes, 25–26, *27*; in empathy challenges, 23; in presenting symptoms response, 21–22

self-disclosure, therapist, 18

self-monitoring and modification: for anxious behavior patterns, 264, *265*; of negative thoughts/behaviors, 7–8; technology and online resources for, 312–13, *318*

self-perpetuation: of automatic thoughts, 158, *159*, 161; of negative core beliefs, 211, *211*, 215

self-practice, therapist, 329–30

session structure: activity level in, 19–20, *20*; case examples of, across phases of therapy, 85–89, 93–101; challenges/considerations for, 102, *102–3*; client autonomy within, 71, 72; consistency significance in, 71; expertness in, 17; flexibility in, 72, 81–82, *102*; overview of stages of, *73*; pacing in, *102*, 117; preparation importance in, 72, *73*, 74; process objectives in, *75*, 77–78; psychoeducation on, *108*; purpose and benefits of, 71–72; shifts through phases of therapy, 72, 101; Therapy Session Worksheet aid for, *75–76, 77–78*, 91, 93. *See also* early session stage; late session stage; middle session stage; pre-session stage

Shaw, B. E., 2, 121

"shoulds and musts," *194*

sincerity, 16; in empathy expression, 13; in therapeutic alliance, *27*

Skinner, 2

smartphone applications, 313–14, *315–18*, 319

social cognitive theory, 2

social phobia: as therapeutic alliance obstacle, 66; treatment plan challenge and, *68*

sociocultural factors: in case formation, *60*; in core beliefs, *228*, 229–30; examples of, 25; goals informed by, 35; intake interview on negative, *33*, 35; as obstacle to treatment, 67; in therapeutic alliance, 25–26

Socratic techniques: adaptive thinking encouragement with, 236; during behavioral exposure, 286; challenges in applying, 206, *207*; in cognitive rehearsal, 203–4; for core beliefs work, 211, 217, 236, *237*, *238*, 238–41, *239*, *241*, *256–57*; for negative automatic thought evaluation, 179–88, *180*, *181*, *183*, *184*, *186*, *187*, 198; reference table for, *180*

stereotypes, 25–26, *27*

strengths/assets: in case formation, *60*; in core beliefs, *228*; for goal-setting and problem-solving, 38; intake interview on, *33*, 35

stress-diathesis hypothesis, 212

stressors: biases triggered with, 7; core beliefs and contributing, *227*, 229; in presenting problems and symptoms, 39; psychoeducation on, *108*; structured approach to, 71. *See also* external/environmental stressors

substance abuse: externalization of environmental stressors with, 24–25; presenting symptoms and challenges of, *22*

suicide resources, *316*

summaries, session: late, 92, 93–94, 97, 100; middle, 91

sympathetic nervous system, 263, *265*, 277, 282

symptoms. *See* formal symptom measures; presenting problems and symptoms

systematic desensitization, 2

tasks. *See* activity monitoring and scheduling; graded task assignments; homework

technology: cautions in using, 314; practice exercise using, 319; in psychoeducation, 118, 312, *318*; relaxation training/

techniques with, 314, *315*, *317*; self-monitoring assistance with, 312–13, *318*; with therapeutic utility, 311–14, *315–18*, 319

therapeutic alliance: assessment of ability for, 37; client commitment impacted by, 11–12; client-specific factors in, 21–26, *22*, 35, 66; for conceptualization and treatment, 26, *27*, 57; defining, 11; disorder-specific symptoms and challenge to, *22*; expertness enhancing, 17, 71; interpersonal skills in, 17–18; labeling of client impact on, 22–23; obstacles in creating, 26, *27*, 65–66; across phases of therapy, 19–21, *20*; pre-session information review and, 77; psychoeducation fostering, 105–6, 109; repair of, 26, 28; Rogerian qualities in, 12–17, 322; sociocultural factors in, 25–26; treatment plan agreement in, *68*; trust in, 17–18, *22*, 26, *27*, 71, 323

therapist: attractiveness, 18; client labeling by, 22–23; empathy challenges for, 23, *27*; expertness, 17, 71, 82; genuineness, 12–13, 16; note taking for, 77, 93; safety behaviors role of, 289; self-awareness, 16, 21–22, 23, 25–26, *27*; self-disclosure from, 18; self-practice of, 329–30; therapy received by, 330; vulnerability, 105. *See also* competency, therapist; *specific topics*

therapist–client relationship: activity levels across therapy phases in, 19–21, *20*; empathy in, 12–16, 23, *27*, 326; homework challenges and, *309*; to mentor–protégé relationship in late phase, 21, 82; self-awareness key to, 16; similarity of experience/interest in, 18; treatment success impacted by quality of, 11–12, 18, 66, 323; unconditional positive regard in, 12–13, 16, 18, *27*, 322. *See also* therapeutic alliance

Therapy Session Worksheet, 91; pre-session review of, 77–78; after session notes in, 93; template, *75–76*

thoughts: behavior and emotions reciprocal relationship with, 2, 3, *4*, *5*, 6–7, 40–42, *41*, 269; emotions differentiated from, 169–71, *207*; modification of, over emotions, 169, 322; questions for assessment of, *41*; validation of emotions over, 13. *See also* automatic thoughts/negative automatic thoughts

Thwaites, R., 330

timing and pacing, 117; of agenda points, *103*; of behavioral activation introduction, 122; for diaphragm breathing, 274; in empathy expression, 13, 14; with hierarchy of feared situations exposure, 289; for homework, 299, 300; of negative automatic thought distress, 164–65, *166*; session structure, *102*, *103*

training, CBT: after graduation and licensure, 333; quality and duration of, 329; supervision significance in, 331–32

transdiagnostic treatment approaches, 59

treatment plan: agenda informed by, 81; anticipated obstacles in, *62*, 65–67; bibliotherapy and technology in, 118; case formulation and success of, 35, 59, 63; challenges/considerations with, 67, *68*; collaborative empiricism for, 26, *27*, *68*; form for, *62*; goals outlined in, *62*, 63–64, *64*; interventions in, *62*, 64–65, *65*; practice exercise for creating, 67; problems list outlined in, *62*, 63, 67; psychoeducation on, *108*; review on Therapy Session Worksheet, *76*; review with client, 106–7

trust, 17–18, *22*, 26, *27*, 71, 323

unconditional positive regard: attractiveness with, 18; in therapist–client relationship, 12–13, 16, 18, *27*, 322

utility, automatic thought, 159, *160*

validation: of emotions with empathy, 13, 14, 326; increasing motivation with, *27*

validity/evidence: automatic thoughts and assumed, 158, *159*; of core beliefs, 235, 236, *237*, 238, *238*, 241–43, 244, *256*; negative automatic thoughts evaluated for, 159, *160*, 179–81, *181*, 204–6 video recording: self-monitoring with, 312–13; therapist competency and session, 331, 334

virtual reality therapy, 313

visualization, 277

vulnerability: biological, 210, *211*, 212; session structure impact on client, 71; therapist, 105

Weekly Activity Monitoring Log: challenges with, *154–55*; Daily Activity Schedule informed by, 133; form for, *126–27*; practice exercise in creating, 142; psychoeducation and, 125, 128;

review/evaluation of, 131–33, *132*, 137–39

world: core belief through lens of, *227*; depression development in relation to, 2

worry. *See* anxiety/anxiety disorders; fearful behavior patterns

worst-case scenarios: coping plan for, 181–82, 279, 280; probability assessment for, *180*, 182, 278–79. *See also* catastrophizing

worthlessness, 210, *210*, 227

writing skills. *See* reading and writing skills

Young Schema Questionnaire, 225

About the Author

Adam M. Volungis, PhD, is a counseling psychologist and licensed mental health counselor. He has worked with a variety of populations in multiple settings using cognitive-behavioral therapy (CBT) for the past 15-plus years. He is an assistant professor and the CBT concentration coordinator in the Clinical Counseling Psychology Program (CCPP) at Assumption College (Worcester, Massachusetts), where he teaches multiple CBT graduate courses. The CCPP is home to the Aaron T. Beck Institute for Cognitive Studies and is one of the few master's-level programs in the country with a primary concentration in cognitive-behavioral studies. He is also a member of the Association for Behavioral and Cognitive Therapies and the American Psychological Association.